Polly Galalbance

# ICD-10-PCS
# Coder Training Manual
# 2016

D0904684

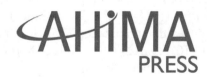

AHIMA
PRESS

Copyright ©2016 by the American Health Information Management Association. All rights reserved. No part of this publication may be reproduced, stored in a retrieval system, or transmitted, in any form or by any means, electronic, photocopying, recording, or otherwise, without the prior written permission of the publisher.

AHIMA Product No.: AC207816
ISBN: 978-1-58426-446-0

AHIMA Staff:
Katherine Greenock, MS, Production Development Editor
Jason O. Malley, Director, Creative Content and Development
Maria Ward, MEd, RHIT, CCS-P, Technical Review
Caitlin Wilson, Assistant Editor
Pamela Woolf, Director of Publications

The American Health Information Management Association (AHIMA) makes no representation or guarantee with respect to the contents herein and specifically disclaims any implied guarantee of suitability for any specific purpose. AHIMA has no liability or responsibility to any person or entity with respect to any loss or damage caused by the use of this publication, including but not limited to any loss of revenue, interruption of service, loss of business, or indirect damages resulting from the use of this workbook.

CPT® is a registered trademark of the American Medical Association. All other copyrights and trademarks mentioned in this book are the possession of their respective owners. AHIMA makes no claim of ownership by mentioning products that contain such marks.

The websites listed in this book were current and valid as of the date of publication. However, webpage addresses and the information on them may change or disappear at any time and for any number of reasons. The user is encouraged to perform his or her own general web searches to locate any URLs listed here that are no longer valid.

For the sake of brevity and to limit the amount of time required to review the record, some cases have been condensed. Reviewing the History and Physical and Discharge Summary as well as the entire medical record is required for accurate diagnosis reporting.

The Centers for Medicare and Medicaid Services (CMS) and the National Center for Health Statistics (NCHS), two departments within the US Federal Government's Department of Health and Human Services (HHS) provide the *International Classification of Diseases, Tenth Revision, Clinical Modification* (ICD-10-CM) for coding and reporting. ICD-10-CM is the US modification to the World Health Organization's (WHO) International Classification of Diseases, Tenth Revision (ICD-10). *Coding Clinic for ICD-10-CM and ICD-10-PCS* is a publication of the American Hospital Association (AHA).

American Health Information Management Association
233 North Michigan Avenue, 21st Floor
Chicago, Illinois 60601-5809
www.ahima.org

# Contents

**Part I: ICD-10-PCS Coding**

**ICD-10-PCS Training—Day 1 .........................................................................86**

## Part II: ICD-10-PCS Coding

# Acknowledgments

The exercises in this book were created using several AHIMA resources as a base. All of the adapted materials underwent a vigorous review to bring them into alignment with the latest versions of the ICD-10-PCS code sets and guidelines which were available at the time of publication.

The author team utilized or adapted many of the exercises and case studies from the AHIMA publication, *ICD-10-PCS: An Applied Approach*. This publication was co-authored by Lynn Kuehn, MS, RHIA, CCS-P, FAHIMA and Therese Jorwic, MPH, RHIA, CCS, CCS-P, FAHIMA. The author team also adapted many of the application exercises in this book from case scenarios originally created by Anita Hazelwood, MLS, RHIA, FAHIMA and Carol Venable, MPH, RHIA, FAHIMA. The authors also would like to thank Sue Bowman, MJ, RHIA, CCS, FAHIMA for her contribution to the content and review of this publication. In addition, the authors would like to thank June Bronnert, RHIA, CCA, CCS-P; Ann Zeisset, RHIT, CCS, CCS-P; Anita Majerowicz, MS, RHIA; Kathryn DeVault, RHIA, CCS, CCS-P; Ann Barta, MSA, RHIA, CDIP; Patricia E. Buttner, RHIA, CDIP, CCS, Angie Comfort, RHIA, CDIP, CCS; Melanie Endicott, MBA/HCM, RHIA, CDIP, CCS, CCS-P, FAHIMA; and Tina L. Cressman, CCS, CCS-P, CPC CPC-H CPC-P CEMC for their contributions.

# Preface to the Training Manual

On January 16, 2009, the US Department of Health and Human Services (HHS) published a Final Rule for the adoption of ICD-10-CM and ICD-10-PCS code sets to replace the 30-year-old ICD-9-CM code sets under rules 45 CFR Parts 160 and 162 of the Health Insurance Portability and Accountability Act of 1996 (HIPAA). The initial compliance date for the two classification sets was established as October 1, 2013 and that was subsequently revised to a compliance date of October 1, 2014. On April 1, 2014, the Protecting Access to Medicare Act of 2014 (PAMA) (Pub. L. No. 113-93) was enacted, which stated the Secretary may not adopt ICD-10 prior to October 1, 2015. Accordingly, the U.S. Department of Health and Human Services released a final rule on July 31, 2014 that included a new compliance date that would require the use of ICD-10 beginning October 1, 2015. The rule will also require HIPAA covered entities to continue to use ICD-9-CM through September 30, 2015.

To read the final rules published in the *Federal Register*, please go to the following websites:

- Modifications to the Health Insurance Portability and Accountability Act (HIPAA) Electronic Transaction Standards (http://edocket.access.gpo.gov/2009/pdf/E9-740.pdf)
- HIPAA Administrative Simplification: Modifications to Medical Data Code Set Standards to Adopt ICD–10–CM and ICD–10–PCS (http://edocket.access.gpo.gov/2009/pdf/E9-743.pdf)
- ICD-10-CM/PCS final compliance date: http://www.gpo.gov/fdsys/pkg/FR-2009-01-16/pdf/E9-743.pdf

The adoption of ICD-10-CM (diagnoses) will affect all components of the healthcare industry. However, the adoption of ICD-10-PCS will affect only those components of the healthcare industry that currently utilize ICD-9-CM Volume 3—inpatient procedures. Therefore, CPT® and HCPCS Level II will continue to be used for reporting physician and other professional services in addition to procedures performed in hospital outpatient departments and other outpatient facilities.

The three key issues HHS believes necessitate the need to update from ICD-9-CM to ICD-10-CM and ICD-10-PCS are

- ICD-9-CM is out of date and running out of space for new codes.
- ICD-10 is the international standard to report and monitor diseases and mortality, making it important for the United States to adopt ICD-10-based classifications for reporting and surveillance.
- ICD codes are core elements of many health information technology (HIT) systems, making the conversion to ICD-10-CM/PCS necessary to fully realize benefits of HIT adoption.

The use of ICD-10-CM will offer greater detail and granularity and will greatly enhance HHS's capability to measure quality outcomes, such as the quality performance outcome measures used in the hospital pay-for-reporting program. The greater detail and granularity of ICD-10-CM/PCS will also provide more precision for claims-based, value-based purchase initiatives such as the hospital-acquired condition (HAC) payment policy.

In addition, the transition to ICD-10-CM/PCS will ultimately facilitate realizing the benefits of using interoperability standards specified by the Healthcare Information Technology Standards Panel (HITSP), including SNOMED CT®. The benefits of using SNOMED CT increase if such use is linked to classification systems such as ICD-10-CM and ICD-10-PCS. Mapping would be used to link SNOMED CT to these new code sets, and plans are underway to develop these maps.

# How to Use This Manual

The AHIMA Academy for ICD-10-PCS Trainers is primarily designed to prepare individuals to train others in ICD-10-PCS through course content that focuses on instruction in the code set. The *ICD-10-PCS Coder Training Manual 2016* is designed to be used by students who are trained by AHIMA Academy ICD-10-PCS trainers to build upon their basic knowledge of ICD-10-PCS fundamentals. It is necessary that individuals responsible for training are fully knowledgeable of the code sets in order to prepare students and the workforce for the transition. Transitioning curriculum from ICD-9-CM to ICD-10-CM/PCS will present unique challenges for academicians. Educating the workforce will also require that the healthcare industry begin planning and preparing for the new code sets.

The content of the *ICD-10-PCS Coder Training Manual 2016* is based on the June 2015 release of the *International Classification of Diseases, Tenth Revision, Procedure Coding System (ICD-10-PCS)*, which can be downloaded from the following website: http://www.cms.gov/ICD10/.

The *ICD-10-PCS Coder Training Manual 2016* contains many references to and explanations of ICD-10-PCS coding guidelines and conventions. It includes ICD-10-PCS coding exercises at the basic, intermediate, and advanced level. These coding exercises emphasize all aspects of the coding classification system so students can apply their knowledge of coding principles and definitions. Answers to the coding exercises are provided.

Students should recognize that additional, self-directed study will be required to master the guidelines and principles of ICD-10-PCS coding beyond the materials provided in this manual. In addition, many students will require additional coursework to increase their level of knowledge in anatomy, physiology, pathophysiology, pharmacology, and medical terminology. Because ICD-10-PCS requires a stronger background in the biomedical sciences, instructors should develop plans for assessing their students' strengths/weaknesses in these areas. Identifying students' learning needs and levels of knowledge is crucial to preparing a solid educational transition plan.

# Introduction: ICD-10-PCS Overview

# Section 1 – ICD-10-PCS History, Structure, and Organization

## History of ICD-10-PCS and General Structure

### Introduction to ICD-10-PCS

The reporting of procedures for hospital inpatients has been done using Volume 3 of the *International Classification of Diseases, Ninth Revision, Clinical Modification* (ICD-9-CM) since 1979. This system is highly outdated and incapable of further expansion to identify specific levels of detail to classify procedure codes. In 1992, the Centers for Medicare and Medicaid Services (CMS) funded the project to develop the *International Classification of Diseases, Tenth Revision, Procedure Coding System* (ICD-10-PCS) with 3M Health Information Systems. ICD-10-PCS will be implemented in the United States on October 1, 2015, to capture hospital inpatient procedure codes. ICD-10-PCS has a multiaxial seven-character alphanumeric code structure providing unique codes for procedures. ICD-10-PCS currently undergoes annual updates.

There were four key attributes that were considered during the development of ICD-10-PCS. The following table defines these characteristics:

**Key Attributes of ICD-10-PCS**

| Attribute | Definition |
|---|---|
| Completeness | A unique code for each substantially different procedure |
| Expandability | Structure should allow easy expansion |
| Multiaxial | Should contain independent characters and an individual axis that maintains its meaning across ranges of codes |
| Standardized Terminology | Definitions are well defined, with no multiple meanings, and each term is assigned a specific meaning |

**Note:** Meeting these objectives should allow coders to construct accurate codes with minimal effort.

In the development of ICD-10-PCS, several general principles were followed:

- Diagnostic Information is Not Included in Procedure Description – When procedures are performed for specific diseases or disorders, the disease or disorder is not contained in the procedure code. There are no codes for procedures exclusive to aneurysms, cleft lip, strictures, neoplasms, hernias, etc. The diagnosis codes, not the procedure codes, specify the disease or disorder.
- Not Otherwise Specified (NOS) Options are Restricted – ICD-9-CM often provides a Not Otherwise Specified code option. Certain NOS options made available in ICD-10-PCS are restricted to the uses laid out in the ICD-10-PCS guidelines. A minimal level of specificity is required for each component of the procedure.

• Limited Use of Not Elsewhere Classified (NEC) Option – ICD-9-CM often provides a Not Elsewhere Classified code option. Because all significant components of a procedure are specified in ICD-10-PCS, there is generally no need for an NEC code option. However, limited NEC options are incorporated into the classification system where necessary. For example, new devices are frequently developed, and therefore it is necessary to provide an Other Device option for use until the new device can be explicitly added to the coding system.

- Level of Specificity – All procedures currently performed can be specified in ICD-10-PCS. The frequency with which a procedure is performed was not a consideration in the development of the system. Rather, a unique code is available for variations of a procedure that can be performed.

Source: CMS 2016a

## ICD-10-PCS Code Structure

One of the reasons ICD-10-PCS was created was because there were structural problems with ICD-9-CM. In addition, specific objectives, essential characteristics, and general guidelines were established for the development of a procedural coding system in order to meet today's coded data requirements. Therefore, one would expect the structure of ICD-10-PCS to be quite different than ICD-9-CM Volume 3.

From the 2016 *ICD-10-PCS Reference Manual (CMS 2016b)*:

> With the ICD-10 implementation, the US clinical modification of the ICD will not include a procedure classification based on the same principles of organization as the diagnosis classification. Instead, a separate procedure coding system has been developed to meet the rigorous and varied demands that are made of coded data in the healthcare industry. This represents a significant step toward building a health information infrastructure that functions optimally in the electronic age.

The following table provides a comparison between the structure of ICD-9-CM and ICD-10-PCS.

| ICD-9-CM Volume 3 | ICD-10-PCS |
|---|---|
| Follows ICD structure (designed for diagnosis coding) | Designed and developed to meet healthcare needs for a procedure coding system |
| Codes available as fixed/finite set in list form | Codes constructed from flexible code components (values) using Tables |
| Codes are 3 to 4 digits long with a decimal point placed after the second digit | Codes are seven characters long |
| Codes are numeric | Codes are alphanumeric |

Source: CMS 2016b

The following is a table from the CMS 2016 Development of the ICD-10 Procedure Coding System (ICD-10-PCS), which provides a comparison of ICD-9-CM and ICD-10-PCS using the NCVHS (National Committee on Vital and Health Statistics) characteristics.

| NCVHS Characteristics | ICD-9-CM | ICD-10-PCS |
|---|---|---|
| **Hierarchical Structure:** Ability to aggregate data from individual codes into larger categories. | **Hierarchical Structure:** The ability to aggregate by body system is provided but there is no ability to aggregate by other components of a procedure. | **Hierarchical Structure:** The ability to aggregate across all essential components of a procedure is provided. |
| Each code has a unique definition forever—not reused. | Some codes do not have a unique definition because the codes have been reused. | All codes have a unique definition. |
| **Expandability:** Flexibility to new procedures and technologies ("empty" code numbers). | **Expandability:** Minimal flexibility. New procedures and technologies are difficult to incorporate. Virtually no empty code numbers. | **Expandability:** Extensive flexibility. New procedures and technologies are easily incorporated. Unlimited empty code values available. |
| Mechanism for periodic updating. | Updated annually through Coordination and Maintenance Committee. | Updated annually, upon implementation, through Coordination and Maintenance Committee. |
| Code expansion must not disrupt systematic code structure. | Code expansions are difficult to incorporate without disrupting systematic code structure. | Code expansions do not disrupt systematic structure. |

| | | |
|---|---|---|
| **Comprehensive:** Provides NOS and NEC categories so that all possible procedures can be classified somewhere. | **Comprehensive:** Extensive use of NOS and NEC categories. All procedures can be categorized somewhere. Broad NOS and NEC categories result in procedure codes which are ambiguously defined. | **Comprehensive:** Limited use of NOS and NEC categories. NEC and NOS categories are specific to each axis of code. All procedures can be categorized somewhere. Procedure codes are precisely defined even when NOS and NEC options are used. |
| Includes all types of procedures. | All types of procedures are included although there is minimal detail for many types of procedures. | All types of procedures are included except evaluation and management procedures. Complete detail is provided for all types of procedures. |
| Applicability to all settings and types of providers. | All settings and types of providers are covered, although there is minimal detail for many settings and types of providers. | All settings and types of providers are covered except physician office services for evaluation and management. Complete detail is provided for all settings and types of providers. |
| **Non-Overlapping:** Each procedure (or component of a procedure) is assigned to only one code. | **Non-Overlapping:** The same procedure when performed for different diagnoses is sometimes assigned to multiple codes. | **Non-Overlapping:** Each procedure is assigned to only one code. |
| **Ease of Use:** Standardization of definitions and terminology. | **Ease of Use:** No standard definitions provided. Terminology is inconsistent across codes. | **Ease of Use:** All terminology is precisely defined. All terminology is used consistently across all codes. |
| Adequate indexing and annotation for all users. | Full Index but specificity of Index varies across codes. | Full Index is computer-generated so specificity of Index is consistent across codes. |

| Setting and Provider Neutrality: Same code regardless of who or where procedure is performed. | Setting and Provider Neutrality: Codes are independent of who or where procedure is performed. | Setting and Provider Neutrality: Codes are independent of who or where procedure is performed. |
|---|---|---|
| **Multiaxial:** Body system(s) affected. | **Multiaxial:** Body system affected can be determined from code number. | **Multiaxial:** A specific character in the code specifies the body system affected. |
| Technology used. | Limited and inconsistent specification of technology used. | Technology used is specified in the approach character of the code. |
| Techniques/approaches used. | Limited and inconsistent specification of techniques/approaches used. | Techniques/approaches used are specific in the approach character of the code. |
| Physiological effect or pharmacological properties. | Limited and inconsistent specification of physiological effect and pharmacological properties. | Physiological effect and pharmacological properties are specified when relevant to the procedure. |
| Characteristics/composition of implant. | Limited and inconsistent specification of characteristics/ composition of implant. | Characteristics/ composition of implants are specified in the device character of the code. |
| **Limited to Classification of Procedures:** Should not include diagnostic information | **Limited to Classification of Procedures:** Diagnostic information is included in some codes | **Limited to Classification of Procedures:** No diagnostic information is included in the code |
| Other data elements (such as age) should be elsewhere in the records | No other data elements included in code | No other data elements included in code |

Source: CMS 2016a

The process of constructing codes in ICD-10-PCS is logical and consistent: individual letters and numbers, referred to as *values*, are selected in sequence to occupy the seven spaces of the code, referred to as *characters*.

**Characters**

All codes in ICD-10-PCS are seven characters in length and each of the seven characters represent an aspect of the procedure. The following diagram illustrates the seven characters of a code from the main section of ICD-10-PCS, the Medical and Surgical section.

| Character 1 | Character 2 | Character 3 | Character 4 | Character 5 | Character 6 | Character 7 |
|---|---|---|---|---|---|---|
| Section | Body System | Root Operation | Body Part | Approach | Device | Qualifier |

An ICD-10-PCS code is best understood as the result of a process rather than as an isolated, fixed quantity. The process consists of assigning values from among the valid choices for that part of the system, according to the rules governing the construction of codes.

**Values**
One of 34 values can be assigned to each character in an ICD-10-PCS code; the numbers 0 through 9 and the alphabet (except [the letters] I and O) are utilized. I and O are not used to eliminate the possible confusion with the numbers 1 and 0. An example of an ICD-10-PCS code is 0T9B70Z. This code was constructed by choosing a specific value for each of the seven characters. Based on details about the procedure performed, values for each character specifying the section, body system, root operation, body part, approach, device and qualifier are assigned.

Due to the fact that the definition of each character of the code is a function of its physical position in the code, the same value placed in a different position in the code has a different meaning. For example, the value 0 in the first character means something different than the value 0 in the second character.

**Code Structure: Medical and Surgical Section**
Next, the code 0LB50ZZ, "Excision of right lower arm and wrist tendon, open" will be utilized to illustrate the meanings of each of the seven characters of a code from the Medical and Surgical section of ICD-10-PCS.

**Character 1: Section**
The first character of a code determines the broad procedure category, or section, where the code is located. In this example, the section is the Medical and Surgical with "0" representing Medical and Surgical section in the first character.

**Character 2: Body System**
The second character defines the body system which is the general physiological system or anatomical region involved. Examples of body systems include Central Nervous System, Upper Arteries, Respiratory System, Tendons, Muscles, and Upper Joints. In this example, the body system is Tendons, represented by the value of L for the second character.

### Character 3: Root Operation

The third character defines the root operation, or the objective of the procedure being performed. Examples of root operations are Excision, Bypass, Division and Fragmentation. For this example the root operation is Excision, which has the character value of B.

### Character 4: Body Part

The fourth character defines the body part or specific anatomical site where the procedure was performed. The body system, second character, provides only a general indication of the procedure site and the body part, fourth character, indicates the precise body part. When the second character is L, the value 5 as the fourth character represents the Right Lower Arm and Wrist Tendon.

### Character 5: Approach

The fifth character defines the approach, or the technique used to reach the operative site. Seven different approach values are used in the Medical and Surgical section of ICD-10-PCS. In this example, the approach is Open and is represented by the value 0.

### Character 6: Device

The sixth character defines the device and depending on the procedure performed, there may or may not be a device left in place at the end of the procedure. Device values fall into four basic categories:

- Grafts and Prostheses
- Implants
- Simple or Mechanical Appliances
- Electronic Appliances

In this example, there is no device left at the operative site, therefore, the value Z is used to represent No Device.

### Character 7: Qualifier

The seventh character defines a qualifier for a particular code. A qualifier specifies an additional attribute of the procedure, if applicable. In this example, there is no specific qualifier applicable to the procedure, so the value is Z, No Qualifier.

| Character 1 Section | Character 2 Body System | Character 3 Root Operation | Character 4 Body Part | Character 5 Approach | Character 6 Device | Character 7 Qualifier |
|---|---|---|---|---|---|---|
| Medical and Surgical | Tendons | Excision | Lower Arm and Wrist, Right | Open | No Device | No Qualifier |
| 0 | L | B | 5 | 0 | Z | Z |

Source: CMS 2016b

# Overall Organization

*General Organization*

ICD-10-PCS is composed of 16 sections, represented by the numbers 0 through 9 and the letters B through D and F through H. The broad procedure categories contained in these sections range from surgical procedures to substance abuse treatment. The 16 sections are subdivided into three main sections: Medical and Surgical section, Medical and Surgical-related sections and Ancillary sections.

The first section, Medical and Surgical section, contains the majority of procedures typically reported in an inpatient setting. As mentioned, all procedure codes in this section begin with the section value of 0. The following diagram illustrates the seven characters of a code from the Medical and Surgical section.

| Character 1 | Character 2 | Character 3 | Character 4 | Character 5 | Character 6 | Character 7 |
|---|---|---|---|---|---|---|
| Section | Body System | Root Operation | Body Part | Approach | Device | Qualifier |

Sections 1 through 9 of ICD-10-PCS comprise the Medical and Surgical-related sections. These sections include the following:

| Section Value | Description |
|---|---|
| 1 | Obstetrics |
| 2 | Placement |
| 3 | Administration |
| 4 | Measurement and Monitoring |
| 5 | Extracorporeal Assistance and Performance |
| 6 | Extracorporeal Therapies |
| 7 | Osteopathic |
| 8 | Other Procedures |
| 9 | Chiropractic |

In sections 1 and 2, all seven characters have the same definition or meaning as the procedures in the Medical and Surgical section.

Codes in sections 3 through 9 are structured for the most part like their counterparts in the Medical and Surgical section, with a few exceptions. For example, in sections 5 and 6, the fifth character is defined as the duration instead of approach.

Additional differences include these uses of the sixth character:
- Section 3 defines the sixth character as substance
- Sections 4 and 5 define the sixth character as function
- Sections 7 through 9 define the sixth character as method

Sections B through D and F through H comprise the Ancillary sections of ICD-10-PCS which includes the following sections:

| Section Value | Description |
|---|---|
| B | Imaging |
| C | Nuclear Medicine |
| D | Radiation Therapy |
| F | Physical Rehabilitation and Diagnostic Audiology |
| G | Mental Health |
| H | Substance Abuse Treatment |

The definitions of some characters in the Ancillary sections also differ from those seen in the previous sections. For example, in the Imaging section, the third character is defined as the root type, and the fifth and sixth characters define contrast and contrast/qualifier respectively.

Additional differences include:
- Section C defines the fifth character as radionuclide
- Section D defines the fifth character as modality qualifier and the sixth character as isotope
- Section F defines the fifth character as type qualifier and the sixth character as equipment
- Section G and H define the third character as a type qualifier

Source: CMS 2016b

*Components of ICD-10-PCS and Table Organization*

So far you have learned that the overall organization of the codes within ICD-10-PCS is by section. The next step is to understand how the codes are incorporated into ICD-10-PCS.

There are several components to ICD-10-PCS, including: the Tables, the Index, the Body Part Key, and the Device Key. The ICD-10-PCS Index can be used to access the Root Operation Tables and consists of alphabetized main terms that represent either a root operation value or a common procedure term. The Root Operation Tables provide the valid choices of values available to construct a code. The Tables consist of four columns and a varying number of rows with each row specifying the valid choices for the characters 4 through 7.

**Coding Tip:** The values for characters 1 through 3 are located at the top of each table. The Index often only provides the first three to four characters of the code with the first three characters indicating the correct Table to reference.

**Note:** Contrary to ICD-9-CM, after a coding professional is acquainted with the Table structure, it is no longer necessary to first consult the Index when coding in ICD-10-PCS.

**Tables** – The tables are organized in a series, beginning with section 0, Medical and Surgical, and body system 0, Central Nervous, and proceeding in numerical order. Sections 0 through 9 are followed by sections B through D and F through H. The same convention is followed within each table for the second through the seventh character, numeric values in order first, followed by alphabetical values in order.

The Root Operation Tables consist of four columns and a varying number of rows. Following is an example of the Table for the root operation Bypass, in the Central Nervous body system.

| 0: Medical and Surgical (Section) | | | |
|---|---|---|---|
| 0: Central Nervous (Body System) | | | |
| 1: Bypass: Altering the route of passage of the contents of a tubular body part (Root Operation) | | | |
| Body Part<br>Character 4 | Approach<br>Character 5 | Device<br>Character 6 | Qualifier<br>Character 7 |
| 6 Cerebral<br>  Ventricle | 0 Open<br>3 Percutaneous | 7 Autologous<br>  Tissue Substitute<br>J Synthetic<br>  Substitute<br>K Nonautologous<br>  Tissue Substitute | 0 Nasopharynx<br>1 Mastoid Sinus<br>2 Atrium<br>3 Blood Vessel<br>4 Pleural Cavity<br>5 Intestine<br>6 Peritoneal Cavity<br>7 Urinary Tract<br>8 Bone Marrow<br>B Cerebral Cisterns |
| U Spinal Canal | 0 Open<br>3 Percutaneous | 7 Autologous<br>  Tissue<br>  Substitute<br>J Synthetic<br>  Substitute<br>K Nonautologous<br>  Tissue Substitute | 4 Pleural Cavity<br>6 Peritoneal Cavity<br>7 Urinary Tract<br>9 Fallopian Tube |

The values of characters 1 through 3 are provided at the top of each table. Four columns contain the applicable values for characters 4 through 7.

A Table may be separated into rows to specify the valid choices of values for characters 4 through 7. In order to build a valid ICD-10-PCS code, the values for characters 4 through 7 must come from the same row. An ICD-10-PCS code built with values from more than one row is considered to be an invalid code.

**Index** – The ICD-10-PCS Index can be used to access the Tables. The Index mirrors the structure of the Tables, so it follows a consistent pattern of organization and use of hierarchies. The Index is organized as an alphabetic lookup with two types of main terms:

- Based on the value of the third character (root operation)
- Common procedure terms

For the Medical and Surgical-related sections, the root operation values are used as main terms in the Index. In other sections, the values representing the general type of procedure performed, such as nuclear medicine or imaging type, are listed as main terms.

For the Medical and Surgical-related sections, values such as Bypass, Division, Excision and Transplantation are included as main terms. The applicable body systems or body parts are listed beneath the main term, and refer to a specific Table. For the Ancillary sections, values such as Fluoroscopy and Positron Emission Tomography are listed as main terms.

The second type of main terms in the Index are common procedure terms such as Appendectomy, Colonoscopy, or Hysterectomy. These entries are listed as main terms and generally refer to a Table or Tables from which a valid code can be constructed. For example, the following appears under the main term Cholecystectomy in the Index:

**Cholecystectomy**
- see Excision, Gallbladder 0FB4
- see Resection, Gallbladder 0FT4

Source: CMS 2016b

---

*Index and Table Conventions*

ICD-10-PCS utilizes a number of Index and Table conventions. Following is a summary of selected conventions:
- All codes are seven characters long.
- The definition of each character is a function of its physical position in the code.
- The Tables are organized beginning with the numeric values in order first, followed by the alphabetic values in order. For the second through the seventh character value, this same convention is followed within each Table.
- Root Operation Tables contain values for characters 1 through 3 and four columns providing the valid combinations of values for characters 4 through 7 required for code creation.
- Each column in the Table may have a varying number of rows. However, a combination of characters not in a single row of a Table is not a valid code.
- Main terms are based on the second- and third-character value.
- The root operation values, character 3, are included as main terms for the Medical and Surgical-related sections. For other sections, the general type of procedure performed is listed as a main term.
- Common procedure terms such as Appendectomy are also listed as main terms in the Index.

**Activity 1: Matching Procedures with Sections**

Match the following procedures with the section of ICD-10-PCS where it is found:
(Hint: The first character identifies the section.)

1. 0B110F4, Tracheostomy

2. 8E0H30Z, Acupuncture

3. F07L0ZZ, Manual physical therapy for range of motion and mobility, patient right hip, no special equipment

4. 3E1M39Z, Peritoneal dialysis via indwelling catheter

5. 4A02XM4, Cardiac stress test, single measurement

6. BW03ZZZ, Chest x-ray, AP/PA and lateral views

# Section 1 Review Questions

1.  Which of the following codes is located in the Medical and Surgical-related sections of ICD-10-PCS?
    a.  B342ZZZ
    b.  C23GQZZ
    c.  HZ94ZZZ
    d.  5A2204Z

2.  True or false? ICD-10-PCS Medical and Surgical codes can be looked up in the Index by common procedure names, such as "Appendectomy."
    a.  True
    b.  False

3.  Complete the following sentence. The third character for codes located in the Medical and Surgical section defines the _____.
    a.  Root Operation
    b.  Section
    c.  Body System
    d.  Body Part

4.  Which government agency was responsible for funding the development of ICD-10-PCS?
    a.  CDC
    b.  NCHS
    c.  CMS
    d.  NCVHS

5.  ICD-10-PCS will be implemented in the US on what date?
    a.  January 1, 2014
    b.  October 1, 2014
    c.  January 1, 2015
    d.  October 1, 2015

6.  All ICD-10-PCS codes have _____ characters.
    a.  3 to 5
    b.  3 to 7
    c.  5 to 7
    d.  7

7.  True or False? The Index must always be referenced first before proceeding to the Tables in ICD-10-PCS to locate a code.
    a.  True
    b.  False

8.  Each character of ICD-10-PCS has _____ possible values.
    a.  31
    b.  32
    c.  34
    d.  36

9.    All of the following are key attributes of ICD-10-PCS, *except:*
        a.    Completeness
        b.    Expandability
        c.    Standardized Terminology
        d.    Uniaxial

10.   Codes from the Radiation Therapy section of ICD-10-PCS begin with what value?
        a.    B
        b.    C
        c.    D
        d.    F

# Section 2 – ICD-10-PCS Structural Attributes, Characteristics, and Definitions

## *Structural Attributes of ICD-10-PCS*

Based on the information covered in Section 1, you now know that ICD-10-PCS is quite different in structure and organization than ICD-9-CM Volume 3. In Section 2, further explanation is provided on the structural attributes of ICD-10-PCS. The three structural attributes described—multiaxial structure, completeness, and expandability—were among those that the National Committee on Vital and Health Statistics recommended for a new procedural coding system.

---

**Multiaxial Structure** – The key attribute that provides the framework for all other structural attributes is multiaxial code structure. This attribute makes it possible for the ICD-10-PCS to be complete, expandable and to provide a high degree of flexibility and functionality.

ICD-10-PCS codes are composed of seven characters with each character representing a category of information that can be specific about the procedure performed. A *character* defines both the category of information and its physical position in the code.

A character's position can be understood as a semi-independent axis of classification that allows different specific values to be inserted into the space, and whose physical position remains stable. Within a defined code range, a character retains the general meaning that it confers on any value in that position. For example, the fifth character retains the general meaning "approach" in sections 0 through 4 and 7 through 9.

Each group of values for a character contains all the valid choices in relation to the other characters of the code, giving the system completeness. Additionally, each group of values for a character can be added to as needed, giving the system expandability. Finally, each group of values is confined to its own character, giving ICD-10-PCS a stable, predictable readability across a wide range of codes. ICD-10-PCS' multiaxial structure houses its capacity for completeness, expandability and flexibility, giving it a high degree of functionality for multiple uses.

**Completeness** – Completeness is considered a key structural attribute for a new procedural coding system. The specific recommendations for completeness include the following characteristics:
- A unique code is available for each significantly different procedure
- Each code retains its unique definition; codes are not reused

In ICD-10-PCS, a unique code can be constructed for every significantly different procedure. Within each section of ICD-10-PCS, a character defines a consistent component of a code, and contains all applicable values for that character. The values define individual expressions (i.e., open, percutaneous) of the character's general meaning (approach) that are then used to construct unique procedure codes. Therefore, all approaches by which a procedure is performed are assigned a separate approach value in the system resulting in every procedure which uses a different approach having its own unique code.

This is true of the other characters of ICD-10-PCS as well. For example, the same procedure performed on a different body part has its own unique code and the same procedure performed using a different device also has its own unique code.

Because ICD-10-PCS codes are constructed of individual values, the unique, stable definition of a code in the system is retained. New values may be added to ICD-10-PCS to represent a specific new approach, device or qualifier, but whole codes by design cannot be given new meaning and reused.

**Expandability** – Expandability is another key structural attribute of ICD-10-PCS. The specific recommendation for expandability includes the following characteristics:
- Accommodate new procedures and technologies
- Add new codes without disrupting the existing structure

ICD-10-PCS has been designed to be easily updated as new codes are required for new procedures and techniques. All changes to this classification system can be made within the existing structure, because whole codes are not added. Instead, one of the two possible changes is made:
- A new value for a character is added as needed to the classification system
- An existing value for a character is added to a table(s) in the classification system

Source: CMS 2016b

## *Design Characteristics of ICD-10-PCS*

Besides the three structural attributes implemented into ICD-10-PCS, there were several additional design characteristics recommended by the National Committee on Vital and Health Statistics and others. As you familiarize yourself with these characteristics, keep in mind how many of the problems identified with ICD-9-CM Volume 3 have been addressed in ICD-10-PCS.

ICD-10-PCS also possesses several additional characteristics in response to government and industry recommendations as follows:
- Standardized terminology within the coding system
- Standardized level of specificity
- No diagnostic information

- No explicit Not Otherwise Specified (NOS) code options
- Limited use of Not Elsewhere Classified (NEC) code options

**Standardized Terminology** – Words commonly used in clinical vocabularies may have multiple meanings resulting in confusion and inaccurate data. ICD-10-PCS is standardized and self-contained with characters and values used in the system having specific definitions.

For example, the word *excision* is used to describe a wide variety of surgical procedures. In ICD-10-PCS, *Excision* describes a single, precise surgical objective, defined as "cutting out or off, without replacement, a portion of a body part."

The terminology used in ICD-10-PCS is standardized to provide precise and stable definitions for all ICD-10-PCS code descriptions. As a result, ICD-10-PCS code descriptions do not include eponyms or common procedure names. This is not the case with ICD-9-CM. For example, ICD-9-CM code descriptor for 22.61 is "Excision of lesion of maxillary sinus with Caldwell-Luc approach" and the code descriptor for 51.10 is "Endoscopic retrograde cholangiopancreatography." In these two examples, the code descriptor refers to either a physician's name or common terms. In ICD-10-PCS physician's names, common terms, and acronyms are not included in a code description. Instead, such procedures are coded to the root operation that accurately identifies the objective of the procedure.

With rare exception, ICD-10-PCS does not define multiple procedures with one code which allows preserving standardized terminology and consistency across the classification system. Therefore, a procedure that meets the reporting criteria for a separate procedure is coded separately in ICD-10-PCS allowing the system to respond to changes in technology and medical practice with the maximum degree of stability and flexibility. This is not the case with ICD-9-CM where we often see procedures that are typically performed together coded with a combination code such as 28.3, Tonsillectomy with adenoidectomy.

**Standard Level of Specificity** – In ICD-9-CM one procedure code with its description and includes notes often encompasses multiple procedure variations while another code defines a single specific procedure. In contrast, ICD-10-PCS provides a standardized level of specificity for each code, with each code representing a single procedure variation.

In ICD-9-CM code 39.31, Suture of an artery, does not specify the artery, whereas the code range 38.40–38.49, Resection of artery with replacement, specifies the artery by anatomical region at the fourth-digit level of the code. In ICD-10-PCS, the codes identifying all artery suture and artery replacement procedures have the same degree of specificity.

In general, ICD-10-PCS code descriptions are more specific than their ICD-9-CM counterparts, but occasionally an ICD-10-PCS code description is actually less specific. In most instances this is because the ICD-9-CM code contains diagnostic information. ICD-10-PCS uses a standardized level of code specificity which cannot always take into account the fluctuations in the ICD-9-CM level of specificity. Instead, ICD-10-PCS provides a standardized level of specificity that can be predicted across the system.

**Diagnosis Information Excluded** – Another key feature of ICD-10-PCS is that information regarding a diagnosis is excluded from the code description. This is not true of ICD-9-CM which often contains diagnosis information in its procedures codes. Including diagnosis information within a procedure code limits the flexibility and functionality of a procedural coding system. It has the effect of placing a code "off limits" if the diagnosis in the medical record does not match the diagnosis in the procedure code description.

Diagnosis information is not contained in any ICD-10-PCS codes. The actual diagnoses codes, not the procedure codes, will specify the reason for the procedure.

**NOS Code Options Restricted** – ICD-9-CM often designates codes as Unspecified or Not Otherwise Specified (NOS). In contrast, the standardized level of specificity of ICD-10-PCS restricts the use of broadly applicable NOS or unspecified code options. ICD-10-PCS requires a minimal level of specificity in order to construct a code.

Each character in ICD-10-PCS defines information about the procedure with all seven characters containing a specific value obtained from a single row of a table to build a valid code. Even values such as the sixth character value Z, No Device, and the seventh character value Z, No Qualifier, provide important information regarding the procedure performed.

**Limited NEC Code Options** – ICD-9-CM often designates codes as Not Elsewhere Classified (NEC) or Other Specified throughout the classification system. NEC options are provided in ICD-10-PCS, but only for specific, limited use.

In the Medical and Surgical section of ICD-10-PCS, two significant Not Elsewhere Classified options are the root operation value Q, Repair and the device value Y, Other Device.

The root operation Repair is a true NEC value and is only used when the procedure performed is not one of the other 30 root operations in the Medical and Surgical section.

Other Devices is intended to be used to temporarily define new devices that do not have a specific value assigned, until one can be added to the system. No categories of medical or surgical devices are permanently classified to Other Devices.

Source: CMS 2016b

---

**Activity 2: Identifying Problems with ICD-9-CM Procedure Codes**
Review and identify the problem with ICD-9-CM procedure codes for the following questions, and then select the characteristic in ICD-10-PCS that addresses the problem.

1. 28.11, Biopsy of tonsils and adenoids
   a.    NOS code option excluded
   b.    Diagnosis information excluded
   c.    Standardized terminology
   d.    Standardized level of specificity

2. 51.22, Cholecystectomy
   a.    NOS code option excluded
   b.    Diagnosis information excluded
   c.    Standardized terminology
   d.    Standardized level of specificity

3. 38.91–38.99, Puncture of vessels, does not specify site whereas 38.00–38.09, Incision of vessel, provides fourth digit subclassification for specifying the vessel
   a.    NOS code options excluded
   b.    Diagnosis information excluded
   c.    Standardized terminology
   d.    Standardized level of specificity

4. 23.01, Extraction of deciduous tooth
   a.    NOS code options excluded
   b.    Diagnosis information excluded
   c.    Standardized terminology
   d.    Standardized level of specificity

5. 42.40, Esophagectomy, not otherwise specified
   a.    NOS code options excluded
   b.    Diagnosis information excluded
   c.    Standardized terminology
   d.    Standardized level of specificity

**Activity 3: ICD-10-PCS Key Attribute – Completeness**
Compare the following pairs of codes for drainage and identify the differences and similarities in the codes.

1. 0C9P00Z vs. 0B9100Z

2. 0B9300Z vs. 0B933ZX

3. 0H90X0Z vs. 0H90XZZ

# *Definitions Used in ICD-10-PCS*

As previously mentioned, ICD-10-PCS has standardized, specific definitions for *values and characters*. Review the following definitions:

**Character** – One of the seven components that comprise an ICD-10-PCS procedure code

**Value** – Individual units defined for each character and represented by a number or letter

**Procedure** – The complete specification of the seven characters

**Section (1st character)** – Defines the general type of procedure

**Body System (2nd character)** – Defines the general physiological system on which the procedure is performed or anatomical region where the procedure is performed

**Root Operation/Type (3rd character)** – Defines the objective of the procedure

**Body Part or Region (4th character)** – Defines the specific anatomical site where the procedure is performed

**Approach (5th character)** – Defines the technique used to reach the site of the procedure

**Device (6th character, sections 0-2)** – Defines the material or appliance used to accomplish the objective of the procedure that remains in or on the procedure site at the end of the procedure.

**Qualifier (7th character)** – Defines the additional attribute of the procedure performed, if applicable

Source: CMS 2016b

Having standard and strict definitions of terms in ICD-10-PCS provides clarity and makes the system easier to use. Let's take an example of the term *resection* and see how having an exact definition to work from leads to consistent use and coding accuracy.

Sample definitions of the term *resection*:

| Definition | Source |
|---|---|
| Cutting out or off, without replacement, all of a body part | *ICD-10-PCS Reference Manual* (CMS 2016) |
| The surgical removal of part of an organ or structure | *Merriam-Webster's Medical Dictionary* (Merriam-Webster 2010) |
| 1. A procedure performed for the specific purpose of removal, as in removal of articular ends of one or both bones forming a joint.<br>2. To remove a part.<br>3. Syn: excision | *Stedman's Medical Dictionary* (Stedman's 2006) |
| Removal of a portion or all of an organ or other structure. Called also excision and ectomy. | *Dorland's Illustrated Medical Dictionary* (Dorland 2007) |

As you can see, each of the medical dictionaries has a slightly different definition for resection. However, ICD-10-PCS has only one definition. Therefore, you would need to closely review the documentation in the medical record to ensure that the type of procedure being coded to the root operation Resection meets the definition. If it does not, even though the physician may have called the procedure a resection, when classifying it in ICD-10-PCS, it will be coded to a different root operation.

> *Example:* Some examples of procedures classified to the root operation Resection are
> - Right hemicolectomy
> - Total mastectomy
> - Total lobectomy of lung
> - Laparoscopic-assisted total vaginal hysterectomy

The resection definition is just one of many found in the Medical and Surgical section of ICD-10-PCS. It is important to become familiar with the definitions for all the root operations and approaches in order to correctly translate the procedures documented in the medical records into ICD-10-PCS codes.

To build upon the knowledge already gained regarding standardized terminology, refer to Appendix B, Root Operations, and Appendix C, Approaches, located in this training manual, and read through the definitions.

> **Note:** Becoming familiar with these definitions is critical to success in ICD-10-PCS coding. Building codes correctly relies on the correct interpretation and understanding of these definitions.

# Section 2 Review Questions

1.  Which of the following key attributes is the one that provides the framework for all other structural attributes?
    a.  Multiaxial structure
    b.  Completeness
    c.  Expandability
    d.  Standardized terminology

2.  True or false? Every procedure that uses a different approach will have its own unique code.
    a.  True
    b.  False

3.  Which of the following would you find in ICD-10-PCS?
    a.  Combination codes
    b.  Eponyms
    c.  Information pertaining to a diagnosis in a code description
    d.  Limited NEC code options

4.  The root operation _____ is a true NEC value in ICD-10-PCS.
    a.  Bypass
    b.  Change
    c.  Insertion
    d.  Repair

5.  True or false? ICD-10-PCS includes a code for every significantly different procedure.
    a.  True
    b.  False

6.  True or False? Eponyms are found in ICD-10-PCS.
    a.  True
    b.  False

7.  All of the following procedures would be classified to the root operation Resection, except:
    a.  Left hemicolectomy
    b.  Total mastectomy
    c.  Partial lobectomy of lung
    d.  Total abdominal hysterectomy

8.  Which character of an ICD-10-PCS Medical and Surgical section code describes the Body Part?
    a.  Character 1
    b.  Character 2
    c.  Character 3
    d.  Character 4

9.	True or false? A colonoscopy procedure would utilize a Percutaneous Endoscopic approach value for the sixth character.
	a.	True
	b.	False

10.	True or false? Each ICD-10-PCS code has a unique definition and will not be reused.
	a.	True
	b.	False

# Section 3 – Review of Medical and Surgical Section – Section Value 0

## *Overview of the Medical and Surgical Section*

In this section an overview of the Medical and Surgical section of ICD-10-PCS is provided. Additionally, this section briefly reviews the 31 ICD-10-PCS body system values and illustrates root operations that share similar attributes.

### General Overview of the Medical and Surgical Section

The Medical and Surgical codes have a first character value of 0. Characters 2 through 7 represent body system, root operation, body part, approach, device, and qualifier. The following diagram summarizes the organizational structure of the Medical and Surgical section.

| Character 1 | Character 2 | Character 3 | Character 4 | Character 5 | Character 6 | Character 7 |
|---|---|---|---|---|---|---|
| Section | Body System | Root Operation | Body Part | Approach | Device | Qualifier |

The Medical and Surgical section is by far the largest of the 16 sections of ICD-10-PCS.

Some of the procedures found in this section are:
- Thrombectomy
- Lithotripsy
- Inguinal hernia repair
- Gastrostomy tube change
- Cardiac mapping
- Insertion of central venous catheter

### Body Systems

The meaning of the second character in the Medical and Surgical section is general body system. This character may be represented by one of 31 values, 0 through 9, B through D, F through H, J through N, and P through Y. However, the way in which ICD-10-PCS defines a "body system" is a bit different than the usual meaning of the term. A review of the following list shows how some customary body systems are given multiple body system values. For example, note the circulatory system does not have a single value.

| Values | ICD-10-PCS Body Systems |
|--------|--------------------------|
| 0 | Central Nervous System |
| 1 | Peripheral Nervous System |
| 2 | Heart and Great Vessels |
| 3 | Upper Arteries |
| 4 | Lower Arteries |
| 5 | Upper Veins |
| 6 | Lower Veins |
| 7 | Lymphatic and Hemic System |
| 8 | Eye |
| 9 | Ear, Nose, Sinus |
| B | Respiratory System |
| C | Mouth and Throat |
| D | Gastrointestinal System |
| F | Hepatobiliary System and Pancreas |
| G | Endocrine System |
| H | Skin and Breast |
| J | Subcutaneous Tissue and Fascia |
| K | Muscles |
| L | Tendons |
| M | Bursae and Ligaments |
| N | Head and Facial Bones |
| P | Upper Bones |
| Q | Lower Bones |
| R | Upper Joints |
| S | Lower Joints |
| T | Urinary System |
| U | Female Reproductive System |
| V | Male Reproductive System |
| W | Anatomic Region, General |
| X | Anatomical Regions, Upper Extremities |
| Y | Anatomic Regions, Lower Extremities |

## Root Operations

The third character in the Medical and Surgical section is the root operation. There are a total of 31 root operations within this section, and when coding you must select the root operation that matches the specific objective of the procedure as documented in the medical record. These 31 root operations are divided into nine groups that share similar attributes.

The nine groups are:
1. Procedures that take out some/all of a body part
2. Procedures that take out solids/fluids/gases from a body part
3. Procedures involving cutting or separation only
4. Procedures that put in/put back or move some/all of a body part
5. Procedures that alter the diameter/route of a tubular body part
6. Procedures that always involve a device
7. Procedures involving examination only
8. Procedures that define other repairs
9. Procedures that define other objectives

The following table lists these nine groups and the root operations within each group.

| Root Operation | What Operation Does | Objective of Procedure | Procedure Site | Example |
|---|---|---|---|---|
| Root operations that take out some/all of a body part | | | | |
| Excision | Takes out some/ all of a body part | Cutting out/ off without replacement | Some of a body part | Breast lumpectomy |
| Resection | Takes out some/ all of a body part | Cutting out/ off without replacement | All of a body part | Total mastectomy |
| Detachment | Takes out some/ all of a body part | Cutting out/ off without replacement | Extremity only, any level | Amputation above elbow |
| Destruction | Takes out some/ all of a body part | Eradicating without replacement | Some/all of a body part | Fulguration of endometrium |
| Extraction | Takes out some/ all of a body part | Pulling out/ off without replacement | Some/all of a body part | Suction D&C |
| Root operations that take out solids/fluids/gases from a body part | | | | |
| Drainage | Takes out solids/ fluids/gases from a body part | Taking/letting out fluids/gases | Within a body part | Incision and drainage |
| Extirpation | Takes out solids/ fluids/gases from a body part | Taking/cutting out solid matter | Within a body part | Thrombectomy |
| Fragmentation | Takes out solids/ fluids/gases from a body part | Breaking solid matter into pieces | Within a body part | Lithotripsy |
| Root operations involving cutting or separation only | | | | |
| Division | Involves cutting or separation only | Cutting into/ separating a body part | Within a body part | Neurotomy |
| Release | Involves cutting or separation only | Freeing a body part from constraint | Around a body part | Adhesiolysis |

| Root operations that put in/put back or move some/all of a body part | | | | |
|---|---|---|---|---|
| Transplantation | Puts in/puts back or moves some/all of a body part | Putting in a living body part from a person/animal | Some/all of a body part | Kidney transplant |
| Reattachment | Puts in/puts back or moves some/all of a body part | Putting back a detached body part | Some/all of a body part | Reattach severed finger |
| Transfer | Puts in/puts back or moves some/all of a body part | Moving, to function for a similar body part | Some/all of a body part | Skin tissue transfer |
| Reposition | Puts in/puts back or moves some/all of a body part | Moving, to normal or other suitable location | Some/all of a body part | Move undescended testicle |
| Root operations that alter the diameter/route of a tubular body part | | | | |
| Restriction | Alters the diameter/route of a tubular body part | Partially closing orifice/lumen | Tubular body part | Gastroesophageal fundoplication |
| Occlusion | Alters the diameter/route of a tubular body part | Completely closing orifice/lumen — inner | Tubular body part | Fallopian tube ligation |
| Dilation | Alters the diameter/route of a tubular body part | Expanding orifice/lumen | Tubular body part | Percutaneous transluminal coronary angioplasty (PTCA) |
| Bypass | Alters the diameter/route of a tubular body part | Altering route of passage | Tubular body part | Coronary artery bypass graft (CABG) colostomy |

| Root operations that always involve a device | | | | |
|---|---|---|---|---|
| Insertion | Always involves a device | Putting in non-biological device | In/on a body part | Central line insertion |
| Replacement | Always involves a device | Putting in device that replaces a body part | Some/all of a body part | Total hip replacement |
| Supplement | Always involves a device | Putting in device that reinforces or augments a body part | In/on a body part | Abdominal wall herniorrhaphy using mesh |
| Change | Always involves a device | Exchanging a device without cutting/ puncturing | In/on a body part | Drainage tube change |
| Removal | Always involves a device | Taking out device | In/on a body part | Central line removal |
| Revision | Always involves a device | Correcting a malfunctioning/ displaced device | In/on a body part | Revision of pacemaker insertion |
| Root operations involving examination only | | | | |
| Inspection | Involves examination only | Visual/manual exploration | Some/all of a body part | Diagnostic cystoscopy |
| Map | Involves examination only | Locating electrical impulses/ functional areas | Brain/ cardiac conduction mechanism | Cardiac electrophysiological study |
| Root operations that include other repairs | | | | |
| Repair | Includes other repairs | Restoring body part to its normal structure | Some/all of a body part | Suture laceration |
| Control | Includes other repair | Stopping/ attempting to stop post- procedural bleed | Anatomical region | Post-prostatectomy bleeding |

| Root operations that include other objectives | | | | |
|---|---|---|---|---|
| Fusion | Includes other objectives | Rendering joint immobile | Joint | Spinal fusion |
| Alteration | Includes other objectives | Modifying body part for cosmetic purposes without affecting function | Some/all of a body part | Face lift |
| Creation | Includes other objectives | Making new structure for sex change operation | Perineum | Artificial vagina/penis |

**Activity 4: Root Operations**
Complete the following sentences with the correct root operation.

1. Cutting off all or a portion of an extremity is the definition of _____.

2. Cutting out or off, without replacement, a portion of a body part is the definition of _____.

3. Taking out or off a device from a body part is the definition of _____.

4. Correcting, to the extent possible, a malfunctioning or displaced device is the definition of _____.

5. Pulling or stripping out or off all or a portion of a body part by the use of force is the definition of _____.

# Code Components: Body Part, Approach, Device, and Qualifier

## Body Part

The meaning of the fourth character in the Medical and Surgical section is body part. The value chosen for this character represents the specific part of the body system (character 2) on which the surgery was performed. Body parts may specify laterality. Some examples of body parts and their body systems in ICD-10-PCS are:

| Body System | Body Part |
|---|---|
| Lower Extremities | Left Foot |
| Central Nervous | Trigeminal Nerve |
| Upper Veins | Right Cephalic Vein |
| Gastrointestinal | Stomach |

ICD-10-PCS does not provide a specific value for every body part. In those instances the body part value selected would be either the whole body part value (e.g., alveolar process is part of the mandible), or in the instance of nerves and vessels, the body part value is coded to the closest proximal branch.

Review the Alphabetic Index for a specific body part to locate the body part value character.

## Approach

ICD-10-PCS defines "approach" as the technique used to reach the site of the procedure. It is important to know the differences between the different approaches in order to correctly assign the fifth character value in the Medical and Surgical section.

There are seven different approaches. The approach is comprised of three components: the access location, method, and type of instrumentation.

**Access Location** – For procedures performed on an internal body part, the access location specifies the external site through which the site of the procedure is reached. There are two general types of access locations: skin or mucous membranes and external orifices. Every approach value, except External, includes one of these two access locations. The skin or mucous membrane can be cut or punctured to reach the procedure site and all Open and Percutaneous approach values use this access location. The site of a procedure can also be reached through an external opening which can be either natural (e.g., mouth) or artificial (e.g., colostomy stoma).

**Method** – For procedures performed on an internal body part, the method specifies how the external access location is entered. An open method specifies cutting through the skin or mucous membrane and any other intervening body layers necessary to expose the site of the procedure. An instrumental method specifies the entry of instrumentation through the access location to the internal procedure site. Instrumentation can be introduced by puncture or minor incision, or through an external opening.

**Type of Instrumentation** – For procedures performed on an internal body part, instrumentation refers to the specialized equipment used to perform the procedure. Instrumentation is used in all internal approaches other than the basic open approach. Instrumentation may or may not include the capacity to visualize the procedure site. For example, the instrumentation used to perform a sigmoidoscopy permits the internal site of the procedure to be visualized, while the instrumentation used to perform a needle biopsy of the liver does not. The term Endoscopic as used in approach values refers to instrumentation that permits a site to be visualized.

Procedures performed directly on the skin or mucous membrane are identified by the external approach. Procedures performed indirectly by the application of external force are also identified by the External approach (e.g., closed fracture reduction).

| Approach | Definition |
|---|---|
| Open | Cutting through the skin or mucous membrane and any other body layers necessary to expose the site of the procedure |
| Percutaneous | Entry, by puncture or minor incision, of instrumentation through the skin or mucous membrane and/or any other body layers necessary to reach the site of the procedure |
| Percutaneous Endoscopic | Entry, by puncture or minor incision, of instrumentation through the skin or mucous membrane and/or any other body layers necessary to reach and visualize the site of the procedure |
| Via Natural or Artificial Opening | Entry of instrumentation through a natural or artificial external opening to reach the site of the procedure |
| Via Natural or Artificial Opening Endoscopic | Entry of instrumentation through a natural or artificial external opening to reach and visualize the site of the procedure |
| Via Natural or Artificial Opening Endoscopic with Percutaneous Endoscopic Assistance | Entry of instrumentation through a natural or artificial external opening to reach and visualize the site of the procedure, and entry, by puncture or minor incision, of instrumentation through the skin or mucous membrane and any other body layers necessary to aid in the performance of the procedure |
| External | Procedures performed directly on the skin or mucous membrane and procedures performed indirectly by the application of external force through the skin or mucous membrane |

Source: CMS 2016a

```
APPROACH VALUES
    0        Open
    3        Percutaneous
    4        Percutaneous Endoscopic
    7        Via Natural or Artificial Opening
    8        Via Natural or Artificial Opening Endoscopic
    F        Via Natural or Artificial Opening with Percutaneous Endoscopic
             Assistance
    X        External
```

### Activity 5: Medical and Surgical Approaches

Answer the following questions.

1. The approach is comprised of three components: the access location, type of instrumentation, and _____.

2. External approaches are performed directly on the mucous membrane or _____.

3. What value is assigned for a Percutaneous approach?

4. What approach value would be used when instruments are introduced through a natural opening, without visualization, to reach the site of the procedure?

### Activity 6: Approach Definitions

For this activity you will select the correct approach value for each question.

1. Which approach value is defined as "entry, by puncture or minor incision, of instrumentation through the skin or mucous membrane and/or any other body layers necessary to reach the site of the procedure"?

2. Which approach value is defined as "entry of instrumentation through a natural or artificial external opening to reach and visualize the site of the procedure, and entry, by puncture or minor incision, of instrumentation through the skin or mucous membrane and any other body layers necessary to aid in the performance of the procedure"?

3. Which approach value is defined as "entry, by puncture or minor incision, of instrumentation through the skin or mucous membrane and/or any other body layers necessary to reach and visualize the site of the procedure"?

4. Which approach value is defined as "entry of instrumentation through a natural or artificial external opening to reach and visualize the site of the procedure"?

5. Which approach value is defined as "entry of instrumentation through a natural or artificial external opening to reach the site of the procedure"?

## *Device and Qualifier*

In the Medical and Surgical section, the sixth character specifies devices that remain after the procedure is completed. The seventh character, qualifier, is used with certain procedures to define an additional attribute of the procedure. The following lists illustrate examples of the sixth and seventh characters available in the urinary system.

**Device – Character 6**

| | |
|---|---|
| 0 | Drainage Device |
| 2 | Monitoring Device |
| 3 | Infusion Device |
| 7 | Autologous Tissue Substitute |
| C | Extraluminal Device |
| D | Intraluminal Device |
| J | Synthetic Substitute |
| K | Nonautologous Tissue Substitute |
| L | Artificial Sphincter |
| M | Stimulator Lead |
| Y | Other Device |
| Z | No Device |

**Qualifier – Character 7**

| | |
|---|---|
| 0 | Allogeneic |
| 1 | Syngeneic |
| 2 | Zooplastic |
| 3 | Kidney Pelvis, Right |
| 4 | Kidney Pelvis, Left |
| 6 | Ureter, Right |
| 7 | Ureter, Left |
| 8 | Colon |
| 9 | Colocutaneous |
| A | Ileum |
| B | Bladder |
| C | Ileocutaneous |
| D | Cutaneous |
| X | Diagnostic |
| Z | No Qualifier |

---

**Device** – As mentioned, the device is specified in the sixth character and is only used to specify devices that remain after the procedure is completed. There are four general types of devices:

- Biological or synthetic material that takes the place of all or a portion of a body part (i.e., skin graft, joint prosthesis)
- Biological or synthetic material that assists or prevents a physiological function (i.e., IUD)
- Therapeutic material that is not absorbed by, eliminated by, or incorporated into a body part (i.e., radioactive implant)
- Mechanical or electronic appliances used to assist, monitor, take the place of or prevent a physiological function (i.e., cardiac pacemaker, orthopedic pin)

Instrumentation used to visualize the procedure site is not specified in the device value. This information is specified in the approach value.

If the objective of the procedure is to put in a device, the root operation is Insertion. If the device is put in to meet an objective other than Insertion, the root operation defining the underlying objective of the procedure is used, with the device specified in the sixth character, device. For example, if a procedure to replace the hip joint is performed, the root operation Replacement is coded and the prosthetic device is specified as the sixth character. Materials incidental to a procedure such as clips, ligatures, and sutures are not specified in the device character.

**Qualifier** – The seventh character specifies the qualifier which contains unique values for individual procedures as needed. For example, the qualifier can be used to identify the destination site in a bypass.

Source: CMS 2016a

*Assigning Codes*

Now that all of the characters of a Medical and Surgical section code have been defined, it's time to practice assigning codes. The following case scenario will illustrate the process to follow in order to accurately assign an ICD-10-PCS code.

Procedure description: Open appendectomy

**Step 1:** Locate the main term (Appendectomy) in the Index.
**Step 2:** Appendectomy is followed by two subterms (Excision and Resection). From the procedure description, it is determined that this is a Resection procedure because the entire appendix is taken out.
**Step 3:** Follow the direction of the Index and go to Table 0DTJ for Resection, Appendix.
**Step 4:** After locating Table 0DT (see below), select characters 4-7.

| Section | 0 | Medical and Surgical |
| Body System | D | Gastrointestinal System |
| Operation | T | Resection: Cutting out or off, without replacement, all of a body part |

| Body Part | Approach | Device | Qualifier |
|---|---|---|---|
| 1 Esophagus, Upper<br>2 Esophagus, Middle<br>3 Esophagus, Lower<br>4 Esophagogastric Junction<br>5 Esophagus<br>6 Stomach<br>7 Stomach, Pylorus<br>8 Small Intestine<br>9 Duodenum<br>A Jejunum<br>B Ileum<br>C Ileocecal Valve<br>E Large Intestine<br>F Large Intestine, Right<br>G Large Intestine, Left<br>H Cecum<br>J Appendix<br>K Ascending Colon<br>L Transverse Colon<br>M Descending Colon<br>N Sigmoid Colon<br>P Rectum<br>Q Anus | 0 Open<br>4 Percutaneous Endoscopic<br>7 Via Natural or Artificial Opening<br>8 Via Natural or Artificial Opening Endoscopic | Z No Device | Z No Qualifier |

Source: 2016 ICD-10-PCS Tables and Index

**Step 5:** The Index indicated that character 4 is J for the body part Appendix; the approach is Open (0); there is No Device (Z); and No Qualifier (Z).

**Step 6:** The complete code for an open total appendectomy is 0DTJ0ZZ.

---

**Activity 7: Coding Exercise**

Using the ICD-10-PCS Index and Tables, assign the correct code for the following:

1. Diagnostic EGD with gastric biopsy

2. Laparoscopic total cholecystectomy

3. Left partial mastectomy, open

# Section 3 Review Questions

1. Which of the following body systems is assigned multiple body system values in ICD-10-PCS?
   a. Urinary system
   b. Respiratory system
   c. Musculoskeletal system
   d. Gastrointestinal system

2. Which of the following root operations does not share similar attributes with the other three root operations and therefore is not within the same group?
   a. Removal
   b. Excision
   c. Resection
   d. Destruction

3. True or false? The meaning of the second character in the Medical and Surgical section is body part.
   a. True
   b. False

4. The lumbar sympathetic nerve is a body part in which body system of ICD-10-PCS?
   a. Central Nervous System
   b. Anatomical Regions, General
   c. Peripheral Nervous System
   d. Anatomical Regions, Lower Extremities

5. True or false? In the ICD-10-PCS Body Part Key, the pterygoid muscle is classified as a Head Muscle.
   a. True
   b. False

6. True or false? The qualifier can be used to identify the destination site in a bypass.
   a. True
   b. False

7. If the objective of the procedure is to put in a device, the root operation is
   _____.
   a. Change
   b. Insertion
   c. Repair
   d. Replacement

8. True or false? The fifth character in an ICD-10-PCS code specifies the device.
   a. True
   b. False

9.    The root operation _____ in the Medical and Surgical section
      functions as a Not Elsewhere Classified option.
      a.    Inspection
      b.    Procedure
      c.    Repair
      d.    Revision

10.   Which approach value is assigned for an open liver biopsy utilizing a
      needle?
      a.    External
      b.    Open
      c.    Percutaneous
      d.    Percutaneous Endoscopic

# Section 4 – Review of the Medical and Surgical-related Sections – Section Values 1–9

## *Organization and Classification of Medical and Surgical-related Sections*

*General Overview of the Medical and Surgical-related Sections*

The Medical and Surgical-related procedure codes have a first character value of 1 through 9. For the remaining character definitions, some of those from the Medical and Surgical section apply but variations do exist.

To become familiar with the general differences, compare the code structure of the Obstetrics section, which carries the same meaning for all seven characters as those in the Medical and Surgical section, with the other Medical and Surgical-related sections.

> **Note:** Keep in mind while the general description may be the same, the actual detail may not be.

> *Example:* Ten of the 12 root operations found in the Obstetrics section are also in the Medical and Surgical section. There are also two additional root operations unique to Obstetrics: Abortion and Delivery.

### Obstetrics – Section Value 1

| Character 1 | Character 2 | Character 3 | Character 4 | Character 5 | Character 6 | Character 7 |
|---|---|---|---|---|---|---|
| Section | Body System | Root Operation | Body Part | Approach | Device | Qualifier |

### Placement – Section Value 2

| Character 1 | Character 2 | Character 3 | Character 4 | Character 5 | Character 6 | Character 7 |
|---|---|---|---|---|---|---|
| Section | Body System | Root Operation | Body Region | Approach | Device | Qualifier |

### Administration – Section Value 3

| Character 1 | Character 2 | Character 3 | Character 4 | Character 5 | Character 6 | Character 7 |
|---|---|---|---|---|---|---|
| Section | Body System | Root Operation | Body System/ Region | Approach | Substance | Qualifier |

## Measurement and Monitoring – Section Value 4

| Character 1 | Character 2 | Character 3 | Character 4 | Character 5 | Character 6 | Character 7 |
|---|---|---|---|---|---|---|
| Section | Body System | Root Operation | Body System | Approach | Function/ Device | Qualifier |

## Extracorporeal Assistance and Performance – Section Value 5

| Character 1 | Character 2 | Character 3 | Character 4 | Character 5 | Character 6 | Character 7 |
|---|---|---|---|---|---|---|
| Section | Body System | Root Operation | Body System | Duration | Function | Qualifier |

## Extracorporeal Therapies – Section Value 6

| Character 1 | Character 2 | Character 3 | Character 4 | Character 5 | Character 6 | Character 7 |
|---|---|---|---|---|---|---|
| Section | Body System | Root Operation | Body System | Duration | Qualifier | Qualifier |

## Osteopathic – Section Value 7

| Character 1 | Character 2 | Character 3 | Character 4 | Character 5 | Character 6 | Character 7 |
|---|---|---|---|---|---|---|
| Section | Body System | Root Operation | Body Region | Approach | Method | Qualifier |

## Other Procedures – Section Value 8

| Character 1 | Character 2 | Character 3 | Character 4 | Character 5 | Character 6 | Character 7 |
|---|---|---|---|---|---|---|
| Section | Body System | Root Operation | Body Region | Approach | Method | Qualifier |

## Chiropractic – Section Value 9

| Character 1 | Character 2 | Character 3 | Character 4 | Character 5 | Character 6 | Character 7 |
|---|---|---|---|---|---|---|
| Section | Body System | Root Operation | Body Region | Approach | Method | Qualifier |

*Examples of Procedures Found in the Medical and Surgical-related Sections*

Now that you have an idea of the character values for the various Medical and Surgical-related sections, the next step is to understand the types of procedures found in each section. To assist you, two examples from each section are presented next.

| Section | Examples |
|---|---|
| Obstetrics | Manually assisted delivery<br>Laparoscopy with total excision of tubal pregnancy |
| Placement | Application of sterile dressing to neck wound<br>Change of vaginal packing |
| Administration | Epidural injection of mixed steroid and local anesthetic for pain control<br>Peritoneal dialysis via indwelling catheter |
| Measurement and Monitoring | Holter monitoring<br>Fetal heart-rate monitoring, transvaginal |
| Extracorporeal Assistance and Performance | Controlled mechanical ventilation, 50 hours<br>Cardiopulmonary bypass in conjunction with CABG |
| Extracorporeal Therapies | Plasmapheresis, single treatment<br>Whole body hypothermia, single treatment |
| Osteopathic | Indirect osteopathic treatment of pelvis<br>Isotonic muscle energy treatment of left arm |
| Other Procedures | Robotic-assisted open prostatectomy<br>CT computer-assisted sinus surgery |
| Chiropractic | Chiropractic treatment of lumbar region using short lever specific contact<br>Chiropractic extra-articular treatment of knees |

# Code Components and Coding Tips – Section Values 1–9

*Obstetrics, Placement, and Administration Sections*

**Obstetrics Section** – The Obstetrics section follows the same conventions established in the Medical and Surgical section, with all seven characters retaining the same meaning. Obstetrics procedure codes have a first character value of 1 and the second character value for body system is Pregnancy. There are a total of 12 root operations in the Obstetrics section. Ten of these—Change, Drainage, Extraction, Insertion, Inspection, Removal, Repair, Reposition, Resection and Transplantation—are also found in the Medical and Surgical section.

The Obstetrics section also includes two additional root operations unique to this section:

| Value | Description | Definition |
|-------|-------------|------------|
| A | Abortion | Artificially terminating a pregnancy |
| E | Delivery | Assisting the passage of the products of conception from the genital canal |

Abortion is subdivided according to whether an additional device such as laminaria or abortifacient is used, or whether the abortion was performed by mechanical means.

Delivery applies only to manually assisted vaginal delivery and is defined as assisting the passage of the products of conception from the genital canal.

A cesarean section is not its own unique root operation, because the underlying objective is Extraction (pulling out all or a portion of a body part).

The body part values in the Obstetrics section are
- Products of conception
- Products of conception, retained
- Products of conception, ectopic

Only procedures performed on the products of conception are included in the Obstetrics section; procedures performed on the pregnant female are coded in the Medical and Surgical section (i.e., episiotomy). The phrase Products of Conception refers to all physical components of a pregnancy, including the fetus, amnion, umbilical cord and placenta.

The fifth character specifies approaches and the sixth character is used for devices such as fetal monitoring electrodes. Qualifier values are specific to root operation, and are used to specify the type of extraction (i.e., low forceps, low cervical cesarean, etc.), the type of fluid taken out during a drainage procedure (i.e., amniotic fluid, fetal blood, etc.), or the body system of the products of conception on which the repair was performed.

**Placement Section** – Placement section codes represent procedures for putting an externally placed device in or on a body region for the purpose of protection, immobilization, stretching, compression, or packing. Codes from this section have a first character value of 2. The second character value for body system is either anatomical regions or anatomical orifices. The root operations in the Placement section include only those procedures performed without making an incision or puncture. The root operations Change and Removal are contained in the Placement section, and retain the same meaning as in the

Medical and Surgical section. The Placement section also includes five additional root operations, defined as follows:

| Value | Description | Definition |
|-------|-------------|------------|
| 1 | Compression | Putting pressure on a body region |
| 2 | Dressing | Putting material on a body region for protection |
| 3 | Immobilization | Limiting or preventing motion of a body region |
| 4 | Packing | Putting material in a body region or orifice |
| 6 | Traction | Exerting a pulling force on a body region in a distal direction |

The fourth character values are either body regions (i.e., chest wall, face, left upper leg) or natural orifices (i.e., ear, mouth and pharynx, urethra). Since all placement procedures are performed directly on the skin or mucus membrane, or performed indirectly by the application of external force through the skin or mucous membrane, the approach value is always External, character value X.

The sixth character, the device character, always (except in the case of manual traction) specifies the device placed during the procedure (i.e., cast, splint, bandage, etc.). Except for casts, devices in the Placement section are off the shelf and do not require any extensive design, fabrication, or fitting. The placement of devices that require extensive design, fabrication, or fitting are coded in the Rehabilitation section of ICD-10-PCS. The qualifier character is not specified in this section; thus the qualifier value is always Z, No Qualifier.

**Administration Section** – The Administration section includes infusions, injections and transfusions, as well as other related procedures such as irrigation and tattooing. All codes in this section define procedures where a diagnostic or therapeutic substance is given to the patient.

Administration procedures have a first character value of 3. The body system character for this section contains three values: Circulatory System, Indwelling Device, and Physiological Systems and Anatomical Regions.

The three root operations in this section are classified according to the broad category of substance administered. If the substance given is a blood product or a cleansing substance, the procedure is coded to Transfusion and Irrigation, respectively. All other substances administered are coded to the root operation, Introduction. Following are the definitions for these three root operations:

| Value | Description | Definition |
|---|---|---|
| 0 | Introduction | Putting in or on a therapeutic, diagnostic, nutritional, physiological, or prophylactic substance except blood or blood products |
| 1 | Irrigation | Putting in or on a cleansing substance |
| 2 | Transfusion | Putting in blood or blood products |

The fourth character specifies the body system or region which identifies the site where the substance is administered, not the site where the substance administered takes effect. Sites include skin and mucous membrane, subcutaneous tissue and muscle which differentiate intradermal, subcutaneous and intramuscular injections respectively. Other sites include eye, respiratory tract, peritoneal cavity, and epidural space.

The fifth character specifies approach with the approach for intradermal, subcutaneous and intramuscular introductions (i.e., injections) being Percutaneous. If a catheter is placed to introduce a substance into an internal site within the circulatory system, the approach is also Percutaneous.

The body systems/regions for arteries and veins are peripheral artery, central artery, peripheral vein and central vein. The peripheral artery or vein is typically used when a substance is introduced locally into an artery or vein and in general, the substance introduced has a system effect.

The central artery or vein is typically used when the site where the substance is introduced is distant from the point of entry into the artery or vein and in general the substance introduced into a central artery or vein has a local effect.

The sixth character specifies the substance being introduced. Broad categories are defined such as anesthetic, contrast, dialysate, and blood products such as platelets. The seventh character, the qualifier, is used to indicate whether a substance transfused is autologous or nonautologous, or to further specify a substance introduced.

Source: CMS 2016a; CMS 2016b

*Measurement and Monitoring, Extracorporeal Assistance and Performance, and Extracorporeal Therapies Sections*

The Measurement and Monitoring, Extracorporeal Assistance and Performance, and Extracorporeal Therapies sections have similar general second through seventh character components, as shown here:

### Measurement and Monitoring – Section Value 4

| Character 1 | Character 2 | Character 3 | Character 4 | Character 5 | Character 6 | Character 7 |
|---|---|---|---|---|---|---|
| Section | Physiological System | Root Operation | Body System | Approach | Function/ Device | Qualifier |

### Extracorporeal Assistance and Performance – Section Value 5

| Character 1 | Character 2 | Character 3 | Character 4 | Character 5 | Character 6 | Character 7 |
|---|---|---|---|---|---|---|
| Section | Physiological System | Root Operation | Body System | Duration | Function | Qualifier |

### Extracorporeal Therapies – Section Value 6

| Character 1 | Character 2 | Character 3 | Character 4 | Character 5 | Character 6 | Character 7 |
|---|---|---|---|---|---|---|
| Section | Physiological System | Root Operation | Body System | Duration | Qualifier | Qualifier |

However, what the individual characters specify is dependent on the section from which you are coding.

> *Example:* The body system is shown as the meaning for character 4.

Looking further into the specific definitions for this term in each section reveals the following:

| Section | What the Fourth Character Specifies |
|---|---|
| Measurement and Monitoring | Body system measured or monitored |
| Extracorporeal Assistance and Performance | Body system to which extracorporeal assistance or performance is applied |
| Extracorporeal Therapies | Body system on which the extracorporeal therapy is performed |

**Measurement and Monitoring Section** – Measurement and Monitoring section codes represent procedures for determining the level of a physiological or physical function. Procedure codes from this section have a first character value of 4 and the second character value for body system is either physiological systems (A) or physiological devices (B). There are two root operations in this section, as defined here:

| Value | Description | Definition |
|-------|-------------|------------|
| 0 | Measurement | Determining the level of a physiological or physical function at a point in time |
| 1 | Monitoring | Determining the level of physiological or physical function repetitively over a period of time |

The fourth character defines the body system measured or monitored. The fifth character specifies approaches as defined in the Medical and Surgical section. The sixth character specifies the physiological or physical function being measured or monitored. Examples of sixth character values in this section are conductivity, metabolism, pulse, temperature, and volume. If a device used to perform the measurement or monitoring is inserted and left in, insertion of the device is coded as a separate procedure. The seventh character, qualifier, contains specific values as needed to further specify the body part or a variation of the procedure performed.

**Extracorporeal Assistance and Performance Section** – This section includes procedures performed in a critical care setting such as mechanical ventilation and cardioversion. Additionally, this section includes procedures such as hemodialysis and hyperbaric oxygen therapy. Procedures from this section use equipment to support a physiological function in some way, whether it is breathing, circulating the blood, or restoring the natural rhythm of the heart.

Extracorporeal Assistance and Performance codes have a first character value of 5. The second character of codes from this section is Physiological Systems.

There are three root operations in the Extracorporeal Assistance and Performance section, as specified here:

| Value | Description | Definition |
|-------|-------------|------------|
| 0 | Assistance | Taking over a portion of a physiological function by extracorporeal means |
| 1 | Performance | Completely taking over a physiological function by extracorporeal means |
| 2 | Restoration | Returning, or attempting to return, a physiological function to its original state by extracorporeal means |

The root operation Restoration contains a single procedure code that identifies extracorporeal cardioversion. The fourth character specifies the body system to which extracorporeal assistance or performance is applied and the fifth character specifies the duration of the procedure. For respiratory ventilation assistance or performance, the duration is specified in hours, i.e., <24 hours, 24–96 hours or >96 hours. The sixth character defines the physiological function assisted or performed (i.e., ventilation, oxygenation) and the seventh character defines the equipment used, if applicable.

**Extracorporeal Therapies Section** – The Extracorporeal Therapies section describes other extracorporeal procedures that are not defined by Assistance and Performance in section 5. Examples are bili-lite phototherapy and apheresis.

Codes from this section have a first character value of 6 and the second character value contains a single general body system, physiological systems. There are 10 root operations in this section, as defined here:

| Value | Description | Definition |
|---|---|---|
| 0 | Atmospheric Control | Extracorporeal control of atmospheric pressure and composition |
| 1 | Decompression | Extracorporeal elimination of undissolved gas from body fluids |
| 2 | Electromagnetic Therapy | Extracorporeal treatment by electromagnetic rays |
| 3 | Hyperthermia | Extracorporeal raising of body temperature |
| 4 | Hypothermia | Extracorporeal lowering of body temperature |
| 5 | Pheresis | Extracorporeal separation of blood products |
| 6 | Phototherapy | Extracorporeal treatment by light rays |
| 7 | Ultrasound Therapy | Extracorporeal treatment by ultrasound |
| 8 | Ultraviolet Light Therapy | Extracorporeal treatment by ultraviolet light |
| 9 | Shock Wave Therapy | Extracorporeal treatment by shock waves |

The fourth character of codes from this section specifies the body system on which the extracorporeal therapy is performed (i.e., skin, circulatory) and the fifth character defines the duration of the procedure (i.e., single, intermittent). The sixth character is not specified for extracorporeal therapies and always has a character value of Z, No Qualifier. The seventh character is used in the root operation Pheresis to specify the blood component on which the pheresis is performed.

Source: CMS 2016a; CMS 2016b

## Osteopathic, Other Procedures, and Chiropractic Sections

As illustrated here, the Osteopathic, Other Procedures, and Chiropractic sections also are very analogous at the general description level of the second through seventh character components.

### Osteopathic – Section Value 7

| Character 1 | Character 2 | Character 3 | Character 4 | Character 5 | Character 6 | Character 7 |
|---|---|---|---|---|---|---|
| Section | Anatomical Region | Root Operation | Body Region | Approach | Method | Qualifier |

### Other Procedures – Section Value 8

| Character 1 | Character 2 | Character 3 | Character 4 | Character 5 | Character 6 | Character 7 |
|---|---|---|---|---|---|---|
| Section | Body System | Root Operation | Body Region | Approach | Method | Qualifier |

### Chiropractic – Section Value 9

| Character 1 | Character 2 | Character 3 | Character 4 | Character 5 | Character 6 | Character 7 |
|---|---|---|---|---|---|---|
| Section | Anatomical Region | Root Operation | Body Region | Approach | Method | Qualifier |

**Osteopathic Section** – Section 7, Osteopathic, is one of the smallest sections in ICD-10-PCS. Procedures codes from this section have a first character value of 7 and a single body system, anatomical regions (W). Additionally, there is only one root operation in the Osteopathic section, Treatment.

| Value | Description | Definition |
|---|---|---|
| 0 | Treatment | Manual treatment to eliminate or alleviate somatic dysfunction and related disorders |

The fourth character defines the body region on which the osteopathic manipulation is performed. The fifth character value, approach, is always External in this section. The sixth character specifies the method by which the manipulation is accomplished. The seventh character is not specified in the Osteopathic section and always has the value, No Qualifier (Z).

**Other Procedures Section** – The Other Procedures section contains codes for procedures not included in the other Medical and Surgical-related sections such as suture removal, acupuncture and in vitro fertilization. Codes in this section have a first character value of 8. There is a single body system for this section, Physiological Systems and Anatomical Regions (E). A single root operation, Other Procedures, is found in this section, as defined here:

| Value | Description | Definition |
|---|---|---|
| 0 | Other Procedures | Methodologies which attempt to remediate or cure a disorder or disease |

The fourth character identifies specific body region values. The fifth character defines the approach used to perform the procedure. The sixth character specifies the method (i.e., robotic-assisted procedure) and the seventh character, qualifier, contains specific values as applicable.

**Chiropractic Section** – Chiropractic section procedure codes have a first character of 9. This section consists of a single body system, Anatomical Regions (W) for the second character value. Additionally, there is only one root operation in the Chiropractic section, as identified here:

| Value | Description | Definition |
|---|---|---|
| B | Manipulation | Manual procedure that involves a directed thrust to move a joint past the physiological range of motion, without exceeding the anatomical limit |

The fourth character specifies the body region on which the chiropractic manipulation is performed and the fifth character, approach, is always External (X). The sixth character is the method by which the manipulation is accomplished. The seventh character, qualifier, is not specified in the Chiropractic section, and always has the value No Qualifier (Z).

Source: CMS 2016a; CMS 2016b

**Activity 8: Coding Exercise**

Using the ICD-10-PCS Index and Tables, assign the correct code for the following:

1. Percutaneous irrigation of knee joint

2. Laparoscopy with total excision of tubal pregnancy

3. Peritoneal dialysis via indwelling catheter

4. Intermittent mechanical ventilation, 24 consecutive hours

**Activity 9: Root Operations in the Medical and Surgical-related Sections**

1. Complete the following sentence. Putting material on a body region for protection is the definition of _____.

2. Complete the following sentence. Determining the level of a physiological or physical function at a point in time is the definition of _____.

3. Complete the following sentence. Completely taking over a physiological function by extracorporeal means is the definition of _____.

4. Complete the following sentence. Extracorporeal lowering of body temperature is the definition of _____.

5. Complete the following sentence. Putting in or on a cleansing substance is the definition of _____.

# Section 4 Review Questions

1.  Which of the following procedures is assigned to the Medical and Surgical-related sections of ICD-10-PCS?
    a.  Central line insertion
    b.  Holter monitoring
    c.  Central line removal
    d.  Revision of pacemaker insertion

2.  Which of the following code components is found only in the Medical and Surgical-related sections?
    a.  Function
    b.  Body System
    c.  Qualifier
    d.  Root Operation

3.  True or false? Delivery is a root operation found in the Obstetrics section.
    a.  True
    b.  False

4.  The sixth character in the Measurement and Monitoring section describes the _____.
    a.  Approach
    b.  Function/Device
    c.  Method
    d.  Qualifier

5.  True or false? Mechanical ventilation is coded in the Extracorporeal Therapies section.
    a.  True
    b.  False

6.  True or false? Taking over a portion of a physiological function by extracorporeal means is the definition of the root operation Performance.
    a.  True
    b.  False

7.  Administrative section codes have a first character value of _____.
    a.  1
    b.  2
    c.  3
    d.  4

8.  True or false? The Obstetrics section includes two additional root operations: Cesarean Section and Delivery.
    a.  True
    b.  False

9.  Cesarean section is classified to which root operation?
    a.  Cesarean Section
    b.  Delivery
    c.  Extraction
    d.  Resection

10. True or false? Compression is defined as putting pressure on a body region.
    a.  True
    b.  False

# Section 5 – Review of Ancillary Sections – Section Values B–D, F–H, and New Technology X

## *Organization and Classification of Ancillary Sections*

### *General Overview of the Ancillary Sections*

The Ancillary procedure codes have a first character value of B through D or F through H. For the remaining character definitions, only a few of those from the Medical and Surgical section apply. There are six Ancillary sections of ICD-10-PCS, as illustrated in the following table:

| Section Value | Description |
|---|---|
| B | Imaging |
| C | Nuclear Medicine |
| D | Radiation Therapy |
| F | Physical Rehabilitation and Diagnostic Audiology |
| G | Mental Health |
| H | Substance Abuse Treatment |

To become familiar with the general differences, compare the code structure of the Medical and Surgical section with the Ancillary sections. Keep in mind, while the general description may be the same, the actual detail may not be. For example, the Imaging section includes the characters body system and body part as does the Medical and Surgical section. However, the Imaging section defines value 3 as circulatory system, upper arteries (above diaphragm), but the circulatory system in the Medical and Surgical section is assigned multiple body system values.

### Medical and Surgical – Section Value 0

| Character 1 | Character 2 | Character 3 | Character 4 | Character 5 | Character 6 | Character 7 |
|---|---|---|---|---|---|---|
| Section | Body System | Root Operation | Body Part | Approach | Device | Qualifier |

### Imaging – Section Value B

| Character 1 | Character 2 | Character 3 | Character 4 | Character 5 | Character 6 | Character 7 |
|---|---|---|---|---|---|---|
| Section | Body System | Root Type | Body Part | Contrast | Qualifier | Qualifier |

### Nuclear Medicine – Section Value C

| Character 1 | Character 2 | Character 3 | Character 4 | Character 5 | Character 6 | Character 7 |
|---|---|---|---|---|---|---|
| Section | Body System | Root Type | Body Part | Radionuclide | Qualifier | Qualifier |

## Radiation Therapy – Section Value D

| Character 1 | Character 2 | Character 3 | Character 4 | Character 5 | Character 6 | Character 7 |
|---|---|---|---|---|---|---|
| Section | Body System | Root Type | Treatment Site | Modality Qualifier | Isotope | Qualifier |

## Physical Rehabilitation and Diagnostic Audiology – Section Value F

| Character 1 | Character 2 | Character 3 | Character 4 | Character 5 | Character 6 | Character 7 |
|---|---|---|---|---|---|---|
| Section | Section Qualifier | Root Type | Body System/ Region | Type Qualifier | Equipment | Qualifier |

## Mental Health – Section Value G

| Character 1 | Character 2 | Character 3 | Character 4 | Character 5 | Character 6 | Character 7 |
|---|---|---|---|---|---|---|
| Section | Body System | Root Type | Type Qualifier | Qualifier | Qualifier | Qualifier |

## Substance Abuse Treatment – Section Value H

| Character 1 | Character 2 | Character 3 | Character 4 | Character 5 | Character 6 | Character 7 |
|---|---|---|---|---|---|---|
| Section | Body System | Root Type | Type Qualifier | Qualifier | Qualifier | Qualifier |

*Examples of Procedures Found in the Ancillary Sections*

Now that you have an idea of the character values for the various Ancillary sections, the next step is to understand the types of procedures found in each section. To assist you, the following list presents two examples from each section.

| Section | Examples |
|---|---|
| Imaging | Chest x-ray, AP/PA and lateral views<br>Transrectal ultrasound of prostate gland |
| Nuclear Medicine | PET scan of myocardium using rubidium with dobutamine<br>Gallium citrate scan of head and neck, single plane image |
| Radiation Therapy | Electron radiation treatment of right breast, dynamic 3-D with custom device<br>Heavy particle radiation treatment of pancreas, three ports, custom device, four risk sites |
| Physical Rehabilitation and Diagnostic Audiology | Wound care treatment of left calf ulcer using pulsatile lavage<br>Individual fitting of moveable brace, left knee |
| Mental Health | Crisis intervention, patient with severe mental disability<br>Family psychotherapy with patient present |
| Substance Abuse Treatment | Substance abuse treatment planning<br>Pharmacology treatment with Antabuse for drug addiction |

# Code Components and Coding Tips – Section Values B–D and F–H and New Technology X.

*Imaging, Nuclear Medicine, and Radiation Therapy Sections*

**Imaging Section** – Imaging procedure codes have a first character value of B. Codes from this section represent procedures including plain radiography, fluoroscopy, CT, MRI and ultrasound. The second character of codes in this section defines the body system and the fourth character defines the specific body part. The third character identifies the root type of the imaging procedure, as defined in the following table:

| Value | Description | Definition |
|---|---|---|
| 0 | Plain Radiography | Planar display of an image developed from the capture of external ionizing radiation on photographic or photoconductive plate |
| 1 | Fluoroscopy | Single plane or bi-plane real time display of an image developed from the capture of external ionizing radiation on a fluorescent screen. The image may also be stored by either digital or analog means. |
| 2 | Computerized Tomography (CT) | Computer reformatted digital display of multiplanar images developed from the capture of multiple exposures of external ionizing radiation |
| 3 | Magnetic Resonance Imaging (MRI) | Computer reformatted digital display of multiplanar images developed from the capture of radio-frequency signals emitted by nuclei in a body site excited within a magnetic field |
| 4 | Ultrasonography | Real time display of images of anatomy or flow information developed from the capture of reflected and attenuated high frequency sound waves |

The fifth character specifies whether the contrast material used in the imaging procedure is high or low osmolar, when applicable. The sixth character qualifier provides further detail as needed, such as unenhanced followed by enhanced (image taken without contrast followed by an image with contrast). Additionally, the sixth character occasionally specifies laser (1) or intravascular optical coherence (2). The seventh character for a majority of imaging codes has a value of Z but occasionally specifies either intraoperative (0), densitometry (1), intravascular (3), transesophageal (4) or guidance (A).

**Nuclear Medicine** – The Nuclear Medicine section is organized similar to the Imaging section. The only significant difference is in the character meaning of the fifth character. The codes in this section represent procedures that introduce radioactive material into the body in order to create an image, diagnosis and treat pathologic conditions, to assess metabolic functions.

Nuclear medicine procedure codes have a first character value of C and the second character specifies the body system on which the nuclear medicine procedure is performed. The third character, root type, indicates the type of nuclear medicine procedure, as defined in the following table:

| Value | Description | Definition |
|-------|-------------|------------|
| 1 | Planar Nuclear Medicine Imaging | Introduction of radioactive materials into the body for single plane display of images developed from the capture of radioactive emissions |
| 2 | Tomographic (Tomo) Nuclear Medicine Imaging | Introduction of radioactive materials into the body for three-dimensional display of images developed from the capture of radioactive emissions |
| 3 | Positron Emission Tomography (PET) | Introduction of radioactive materials into the body for three-dimensional display of images developed from the simultaneous capture, 180 degrees apart, of radioactive emissions |
| 4 | Nonimaging Nuclear Medicine Uptake | Introduction of radioactive materials into the body for measurements of organ function, from the detection of radioactive emissions |
| 5 | Nonimaging Nuclear Medicine Probe | Introduction of radioactive materials into the body for the study of distribution and fate of certain substances by the detection of radioactive emissions from an external source |

| Value | Description | Definition |
|-------|-------------|------------|
| 6 | Nonimaging Nuclear Medicine Assay | Introduction of radioactive materials into the body for the study of body fluids and blood elements, by the detection of radioactive emissions |
| 7 | Systemic Nuclear Medicine Therapy | Introduction of unsealed radioactive materials into the body for treatment |

The fourth character indicates the body part or body region studied with regional (i.e., lower extremity veins) and combination (i.e., liver and spleen) body part values being used. The fifth character defines the radionuclide, the radiation source. The sixth and seventh characters are not specified in this section, and always have the value Z, None.

**Radiation Therapy Section** – The Radiation Therapy section contains the radiation procedures performed for cancer treatment with the first character value of D. The second character of a code from this section specifies the body system. The third character defines the treatment modality as the root type. Four different root types are used in this section, as listed in this table:

| Value | Description |
|-------|-------------|
| 0 | Beam Radiation |
| 1 | Brachytherapy |
| 2 | Stereotactic Radiosurgery |
| Y | Other Radiation |

The fourth character specifies the treatment site that is the focus of the radiation therapy. The fifth character further specifies treatment modality and the sixth character defines the radioactive isotope introduced into the body, if applicable. The seventh character is not specified in the Radiation Therapy section, and always has the value Z, None.

Source: CMS 2016a; CMS 2016b

*Physical Rehabilitation and Diagnostic Audiology, Mental Health, and Substance Abuse Treatment Sections*

The Physical Rehabilitation and Diagnostic Audiology, Mental Health, and Substance Abuse Treatment sections have some similar general second through seventh character components, as shown here:

**Physical Rehabilitation and Diagnostic Audiology – Section Value F**

| Character 1 | Character 2 | Character 3 | Character 4 | Character 5 | Character 6 | Character 7 |
|---|---|---|---|---|---|---|
| Section | Section Qualifier | Root Type | Body System/ Region | Type Qualifier | Equipment | Qualifier |

**Mental Health – Section Value G**

| Character 1 | Character 2 | Character 3 | Character 4 | Character 5 | Character 6 | Character 7 |
|---|---|---|---|---|---|---|
| Section | Body System | Root Type | Type Qualifier | Qualifier | Qualifier | Qualifier |

**Substance Abuse Treatment – Section Value H**

| Character 1 | Character 2 | Character 3 | Character 4 | Character 5 | Character 6 | Character 7 |
|---|---|---|---|---|---|---|
| Section | Body System | Root Type | Type Qualifier | Qualifier | Qualifier | Qualifier |

*Example:* The procedure type is shown as the meaning for character 3 for each of these three Ancillary sections.

Looking further into the specific definitions for this term (root type) in each of these three sections reveals the following:

| Section | What the Character Named "Root Type" Specifies |
|---|---|
| Physical Rehabilitation and Diagnostic Audiology | One of 14 types – treatment, assessment, fitting(s), or caregiver training |
| Mental Health | One of 11 types – crisis intervention, family psychotherapy, biofeedback |
| Substance Abuse Treatment | One of 7 types – detoxification, counseling, pharmacotherapy |

**Physical Rehabilitation and Diagnostic Audiology Section** – Physical Rehabilitation section codes represent procedures including physical therapy, occupational therapy and speech-language pathology. Codes from this section have a first character value of F. The section qualifier rehabilitation or diagnostic audiology is specified in the second character. The third character specifies the 14 different root type values, as defined in this table:

| Value | Description | Definition |
|-------|-------------|------------|
| 0 | Speech Assessment | Measurement of speech and related functions |
| 1 | Motor and/or Nerve Function Assessment | Measurement of motor, nerve and related functions |
| 2 | Activities of Daily Living Assessment | Measurement of functional level for activities of daily living |
| 3 | Hearing Assessment | Measurement of hearing and related functions |
| 4 | Hearing Aid Assessment | Measurement of the appropriateness and/or effectiveness of a hearing device |
| 5 | Vestibular Assessment | Measurement of the vestibular system and related functions |
| 6 | Speech Treatment | Application of techniques to improve, augment, or compensate for speech and related functional impairment |
| 7 | Motor Treatment | Exercise or activities to increase or facilitate motor function |
| 8 | Activities of Daily Living Treatment | Exercise or activities to facilitate functional competence for activities of daily living |
| 9 | Hearing Treatment | Application of techniques to improve, augment or compensate for hearing and related functional impairment |
| B | Cochlear Implant Treatment | Application of techniques to improve the communication abilities of individuals with cochlear implant |
| C | Vestibular Treatment | Application of techniques to improve, augment, or compensate for vestibular and related functional impairment |
| D | Device Fitting | Fitting of a device designed to facilitate or support achievement of a higher level of function |
| F | Caregiver Training | Training in activities to support patient's optimal level of function |

The root type Treatment includes training as well as activities which restore function. Treatment procedures include swallowing dysfunction exercises, bathing and showering techniques, wound management, gait training, and a host of activities typically associated with rehabilitation. Assessments are further classified into more than 100 different tests or methods. The majority of these assessments focus on the faculties of hearing and speech, but others focus on various aspects of body function and on the patient's quality of life.

The fourth character of codes from this section specifies the body region and/or system on which the procedure is performed. The fifth character is a type qualifier that further specifies the procedure performed and the sixth character specifies the equipment used. Specific equipment is not defined in the equipment value instead broad categories of equipment are specified. The seventh character is not specified in this section and always has the value Z, None.

**Mental Health Section** – Mental Health procedure codes have a first character value of G. The second character, body system, does not apply in this section and always has the value Z, None. The third character specifies the 12 root types, as listed in this table:

| Value | Description |
| --- | --- |
| 1 | Psychological Tests |
| 2 | Crisis Intervention |
| 3 | Medication Management |
| 5 | Individual Psychotherapy |
| 6 | Counseling |
| 7 | Family Psychotherapy |
| B | Electroconvulsive Therapy |
| C | Biofeedback |
| F | Hypnosis |
| G | Narcosynthesis |
| H | Group Therapy |
| J | Light Therapy |

The fourth character for codes in this section is a type qualifier. The fifth, sixth and seventh characters are not specified and always have the value Z, None.

**Substance Abuse Treatment Section** – Substance Abuse Treatment codes have a first character value of H. The second character, body system, does not apply in this section and always has the value Z, None. The third character specifies the seven root types, as defined in this table:

| Value | Description |
|-------|-------------|
| 2 | Detoxification Services |
| 3 | Individual Counseling |
| 4 | Group Counseling |
| 5 | Individual Psychotherapy |
| 6 | Family Counseling |
| 8 | Medication Management |
| 9 | Pharmacotherapy |

The fourth character for codes in this section is a type qualifier. The fifth, sixth and seventh characters are not specified and always have the value Z, None.

Source: CMS 2016a; CMS 2016b

*New Technology – Section X*

New technology section codes represent procedures requested via the New Technology Application Process, and procedures that capture new technologies not currently classified in ICD-10-PCS. New technology procedure codes have a first character value of X. The second character values for body system combine the uses of body system, body region, and physiological system as specified in other sections in ICD-10-PCS. The two root operations use the same root operation values as their counterparts in other sections of ICD-10-PCS.

The fourth character specifies the same body part values as their closest counterparts in other sections of ICD-10-PCS. The fifth character specifies approaches as defined in the medical and surgical section. The sixth character specifies the key feature of the new technology procedure. It may be specified as a new device, a new substance, or other new technology. Examples of sixth character values are blinatumomab antineoplastic immunotherapy, orbital atherectomy technology, and intraoperative knee replacement sensor. The seventh character qualifier is used exclusively to specify the new technology group.

## New Technology - Section Value X

| Character 1 | Character 2 | Character 3 | Character 4 | Character 5 | Character 6 | Character 7 |
|---|---|---|---|---|---|---|
| Section | Body System | Root Operation | Body Part | Approach | Device/ Substance/ Technology | Qualifier |

*Coding note: Seventh Character New Technology Group*

In ICD-10-PCS, the type of information specified in the seventh character is called the qualifier, and the information specified depends on the section. In this section, the seventh character is used exclusively to indicate the new technology group.

The New Technology Group is a number or letter that changes each year that new technology codes are added to the system. For example, Section X codes added for the first year have the seventh character value 1, New Technology Group 1, and the next year that Section X codes are added have the seventh character value 2 New Technology Group 2, and so on.

Changing the seventh character New Technology Group to a unique value every year that there are new codes in this section allows the ICD-10-PCS to "recycle" the values in the third, fourth, and sixth characters as needed. This avoids the creation of duplicate codes, because the root operation, body part and device/substance/ technology values can specify a different meaning with every new technology group, if needed. Having a unique value for the New Technology Group maximizes the flexibility and capacity of section X over its lifespan, and allows it to evolve as medical technology evolves.

Source: CMS 2016a; CMS 2016b

# Section 5 Review Questions

1.  Which of the following procedures is assigned to the Ancillary sections of ICD-10-PCS?
    a.  Visual mobility test, single measurement
    b.  Intermittent mechanical ventilation
    c.  Routine fetal ultrasound, second trimester, twin gestation
    d.  Peritoneal dialysis via indwelling catheter

2.  Which of the following code components is found only in the Ancillary sections?
    a.  Body system
    b.  Qualifier
    c.  Body part
    d.  Isotope

3.  True or false? Procedure codes found in the Ancillary sections have a first character value of B through D, F through H, and X.
    a.  True
    b.  False

4.  True or false? Mental Health codes begin with the section value of M.
    a.  True
    b.  False

5.  All of the following sections are found in the Ancillary section, *except:*
    a.  Administration
    b.  Imaging
    c.  Mental Health
    d.  Nuclear Medicine

6.  True or false? Fetal ultrasound procedures are coded in the Imaging section of ICD-10-PCS.
    a.  True
    b.  False

7.  The fifth character in the Radiation Therapy section specifies the

    _____.
    a.  Qualifier
    b.  Isotope
    c.  Root type
    d.  Modality Qualifier

8.  True or false? Brachytherapy procedures are coded in the Nuclear Medicine section.
    a.  True
    b.  False

9.  All of the following are root types in the Mental Health section, *except:*
    a.  Electroconvulsive Therapy
    b.  Hypnosis
    c.  Pharmacotherapy
    d.  Psychological Tests

10.     True or false? Speech Treatment is coded in the Physical Rehabilitation and
        Diagnostic Audiology section.
        a.      True
        b.      False

# Section 6 – ICD-10-PCS Guidelines

With the development of a new classification comes the need to review content and decide what additional coding guidelines outside those available in the classification itself are necessary. CMS has published draft general coding guidelines for coding professionals to follow in order to properly select an ICD-10-PCS code.

There are four main sections of guidelines:
- A. Conventions
- B. Medical and Surgical Section Guidelines (Section 0)
- C. Obstetrics Section Guidelines (Section 1)
- Selection of Principal Procedure
- D. New Technology

### A. Conventions

**A1.** ICD-10-PCS codes are composed of seven characters. Each character is an axis of classification that specifies information about the procedure performed. Within a defined code range, a character specifies the same type of information in that axis of classification.

*Example:* The fifth axis of classification specifies the approach in sections 0 through 4 and 7 through 9 of the system.

**A2.** One of 34 possible values can be assigned to each axis of classification in the seven-character code: they are the numbers 0 through 9 and the alphabet (except I and O because they are easily confused with the numbers 1 and 0). The number of unique values used in an axis of classification differs as needed.

*Example:* Where the fifth axis of classification specifies the approach, seven different approach values are currently used to specify the approach.

**A3.** The valid values for an axis of classification can be added to as needed.

*Example:* If a significantly distinct type of device is used in a new procedure, a new device value can be added to the system.

**A4.** As with words in their context, the meaning of any single value is a combination of its axis of classification and any preceding values on which it may be dependent.

*Example:* The meaning of a body part value in the Medical and Surgical section is always dependent on the body system value. The body part value 0 in the Central Nervous body system specifies Brain and the body part value 0 in the Peripheral Nervous body system specifies Cervical Plexus.

**A5.** As the system is expanded to become increasingly detailed, over time more values will depend on preceding values for their meaning.

*Example:* In the Lower Joints body system, the device value 3 in the root operation Insertion specifies Infusion Device and the device value 3 in the root operation. Replacement specifies Ceramic Synthetic Substitute.

**A6.** The purpose of the Alphabetic Index is to locate the appropriate Table that contains all information necessary to construct a procedure code. The PCS Tables should always be consulted to find the most appropriate valid code.

**A7.** It is not required to consult the Index first before proceeding to the Tables to complete the code. A valid code may be chosen directly from the Tables.

**A8.** All seven characters must be specified to be a valid code. If the documentation is incomplete for coding purposes, the physician should be queried for the necessary information.

**A9.** Within a PCS Table, valid codes include all combinations of choices in characters 4 through 7 contained in the same row of the Table. In the following example, 0JHT3VZ is a valid code, and 0JHW3VZ is *not* a valid code.

| | |
|---|---|
| **Section:** | **0: Medical and Surgical** |
| **Body System:** | **J: Subcutaneous Tissue and Fascia** |
| **Operation:** | **H: Insertion:** Putting in a nonbiological appliance that monitors, assists, performs, or prevents a physiological function but does not physically take the place of a body part |

| Body Part | Approach | Device | Qualifier |
|---|---|---|---|
| **S** Subcutaneous Tissue and Fascia, Head and Neck<br>**V** Subcutaneous Tissue and Fascia, Upper Extremity<br>**W** Subcutaneous Tissue and Fascia, Lower Extremity | **0** Open<br>**3** Percutaneous | **1** Radioactive Element<br>**3** Infusion Device | **Z** No Qualifier |
| **T** Subcutaneous Tissue and Fascia, Trunk | **0** Open<br>**3** Percutaneous | **1** Radioactive Element<br>**3** Infusion Device<br>**V** Infusion Pump | **Z** No Qualifier |

**A10.** "And," when used in a code description, means "and/or."

*Example:* Lower Arm and Wrist Muscle means lower arm and/or wrist muscle.

**A11.** Many of the terms used to construct PCS codes are defined within the system. It is the coder's responsibility to determine what the documentation in the medical record equates to in the PCS definitions. The physician is not expected to use the terms used in PCS code descriptions, nor is the coder required to query the physician when the correlation between the documentation and the defined PCS terms is clear.

*Example:* When the physician documents "partial resection" the coder can independently correlate "partial resection" to the root operation Excision without querying the physician for clarification.

Source: CMS 2016c

# Section-Specific Coding Guidelines

In addition to the coding conventions, CMS has developed two section-specific guidelines: Medical and Surgical section guidelines and Obstetrics section guidelines.

### *Medical and Surgical Section (Section 0) Guidelines*

#### B2. Body System Guidelines

*General Guidelines*

**B2.1a.** The procedure codes in the general anatomical regions body systems should only be used when the procedure is performed on an anatomical region rather than a specific body part (e.g., root operations Control and Detachment, drainage of a body cavity) or on the rare occasion when no information is available to support assignment of a code to a specific body part.

*Example:* Control of postoperative hemorrhage is coded to the root operation Control found in the General Anatomical Regions body systems.

**B2.1b.** Where the general body part values Upper and Lower are provided as an option in the Upper Arteries, Lower Arteries, Upper Veins, Lower Veins, Muscles and Tendons body systems, Upper or Lower specifies body parts located above or below the diaphragm respectively.

*Example:* Vein body parts above the diaphragm are found in the Upper Veins body system; vein body parts below the diaphragm are found in the Lower Veins body system.

#### B3. Root Operation Guidelines

*General Guidelines*

**B3.1a.** In order to determine the appropriate root operation, the full definition of the root operation as contained in the PCS Tables must be applied.

**B3.1b.** Components of a procedure specified in the root operation definition and explanation are not coded separately. Procedural steps necessary to reach the operative site and close the operative site, including anastomosis of a tubular body part, are also not coded separately.

*Example:* Resection of a joint as part of a joint replacement procedure is included in the root operation definition of Replacement and is not coded separately. Laparotomy performed to reach the site of an open liver biopsy is not coded separately. In a Resection of sigmoid colon with anastomosis of descending colon to rectum, the anastomosis is not coded separately.

## Multiple Procedures

**B3.2.** During the same operative episode, multiple procedures are coded if

a. The same root operation is performed on different body parts as defined by distinct values of the body part character.

*Example:* Diagnostic excision of liver and pancreas are coded separately.

b. The same root operation is repeated at different body sites that are included in the same body part value.

*Example:* Excision of the sartorius muscle and excision of the gracilis muscle are both included in the Upper Leg Muscle body part value, and multiple procedures are coded.

c. Multiple root operations with distinct objectives are performed on the same body part.

*Example:* Destruction of sigmoid lesion and Bypass of sigmoid colon are coded separately.

d. The intended root operation is attempted using one approach, but is converted to a different approach.

*Example:* Laparoscopic cholecystectomy converted to an Open cholecystectomy is coded as Percutaneous Endoscopic Inspection and Open Resection.

## Discontinued Procedures

**B3.3.** If the intended procedure is discontinued, code the procedure to the root operation performed. If a procedure is discontinued before any other root operation is performed, code the root operation Inspection of the body part or anatomical region inspected.

*Example:* A planned aortic valve replacement procedure is discontinued after the initial thoracotomy and before any incision is made in the heart muscle, when the patient becomes hemodynamically unstable. This procedure is coded as an Open Inspection of the Mediastinum.

## Biopsy procedures

**B3.4a.** Biopsy procedures are coded using the root operations Excision, Extraction, or Drainage and the qualifier Diagnostic. The qualifier Diagnostic is used only for biopsies.

*Examples:* Fine needle aspiration biopsy of lung is coded to the root operation Drainage with the qualifier Diagnostic. Biopsy of bone marrow is coded to the root operation Extraction with the qualifier Diagnostic. Lymph node sampling for biopsy is coded to the root operation Excision with the qualifier Diagnostic.

### Biopsy Followed by More Definitive Treatment

**B3.4b.** If a diagnostic Excision, Extraction, or Drainage procedure (biopsy) is followed by a more definitive procedure, such as Destruction, Excision or Resection at the same procedure site, both the biopsy and the more definitive treatment are coded.

*Example:* Biopsy of breast followed by partial mastectomy at the same procedure site, both the biopsy and the partial mastectomy procedure are coded.

### Overlapping Body Layers

**B3.5.** If the root operations Excision, Repair or Inspection are performed on overlapping layers of the musculoskeletal system, the body part specifying the deepest layer is coded.

*Example:* Excisional debridement that includes skin and subcutaneous tissue and muscle is coded to the Muscle body part.

### Bypass Procedures

**B3.6a.** Bypass procedures are coded by identifying the body part bypassed "from" and the body part bypassed "to." The fourth character body part specifies the body part bypassed from, and the qualifier specifies the body part bypassed to.

*Example:* Bypass from stomach to jejunum, Stomach is the body part and Jejunum is the qualifier.

**B3.6b.** Coronary arteries are classified by number of distinct sites treated, rather than number of coronary arteries or anatomic name of a coronary artery (e.g., left anterior descending). Coronary artery bypass procedures are coded differently than other bypass procedures as described in the previous guideline. Rather than identifying the body part bypassed from, the body part identifies the number of coronary artery sites bypassed to, and the qualifier specifies the vessel bypassed from.

*Example:* Aortocoronary artery bypass of one site on the left anterior descending coronary artery and one site on the obtuse marginal coronary artery is classified in the body part axis of classification as two coronary artery sites and the qualifier specifies the aorta as the body part bypassed from.

**B3.6c.** If multiple coronary artery sites are bypassed, a separate procedure is coded for each coronary artery site that uses a different device and/or qualifier.

*Example:* Aortocoronary artery bypass and internal mammary coronary artery bypass are coded separately.

## Control vs. More Definitive Root Operations

**B3.7.** The root operation Control is defined as, "stopping, or attempting to stop, postprocedural bleeding." If an attempt to stop postprocedural bleeding is initially unsuccessful, and to stop the bleeding requires performing any of the definitive root operations Bypass, Detachment, Excision, Extraction, Reposition, Replacement, or Resection, that root operation is coded instead of Control.

*Example:* Resection of spleen to stop postprocedural bleeding is coded to Resection instead of Control.

## Excision vs. Resection

**B3.8.** PCS contains specific body parts for anatomical subdivisions of a body part, such as lobes of the lungs or liver and regions of the intestine. Resection of the specific body part is coded whenever all of the body part is cut out or off, rather than coding Excision of a less specific body part.

*Example:* Left upper lung lobectomy is coded to Resection of Upper Lung Lobe, Left rather than Excision of Lung, Left.

## Excision for Graft

**B3.9.** If an autograft is obtained from a different body part in order to complete the objective of the procedure, a separate procedure is coded.

*Example:* Coronary bypass with excision of saphenous vein graft, excision of saphenous vein is coded separately.

## Fusion Procedures of the Spine

**B3.10a.** The body part coded for a spinal vertebral joint(s) rendered immobile by a spinal fusion procedure is classified by the level of the spine (for example, thoracic). There are distinct body part values for a single vertebral joint and for multiple vertebral joints at each spinal level.

*Example:* Body part values specify Lumbar Vertebral Joint, Lumbar Vertebral Joints, 2 or More and Lumbosacral Vertebral Joint.

**B3.10b.** If multiple vertebral joints are fused, a separate procedure is coded for each vertebral joint that uses a different device and/or qualifier.

*Example:* Fusion of lumbar vertebral joint, posterior approach, anterior column and fusion of lumbar vertebral joint, posterior approach, posterior column are coded separately.

**B3.10c.** Combinations of devices and materials are often used on a vertebral joint to render the joint immobile. When combinations of devices are used on the same vertebral joint, the device value coded for the procedure is as follows:

- If an interbody fusion device is used to render the joint immobile (alone or containing other material like bone graft), the procedure is coded with the device value Interbody Fusion Device.

- If bone graft is the only device used to render the joint immobile, the procedure is coded with the device value Nonautologous Tissue Substitute or Autologous Tissue Substitute.
- If a mixture of autologous and nonautologous bone graft (with or without biological or synthetic extenders or binders) is used to render the joint immobile, code the procedure with the device value Autologous Tissue Substitute.

*Examples:* Fusion of a vertebral joint using a cage style interbody fusion device containing morsellized bone graft is coded to the device Interbody Fusion Device.

Fusion of a vertebral joint using a bone dowel interbody fusion device made of cadaver bone and packed with a mixture of local morsellized bone and demineralized bone matrix is coded to the device Interbody Fusion Device.

Fusion of a vertebral joint using both autologous bone graft and bone bank bone graft is coded to the device Autologous Tissue Substitute.

## Inspection Procedures

**B3.11a.** Inspection of a body part(s) performed in order to achieve the objective of a procedure is not coded separately.

*Example:* Fiberoptic bronchoscopy performed for irrigation of bronchus, only the irrigation procedure is coded.

**B3.11b.** If multiple tubular body parts are inspected, the most distal body part inspected is coded. If multiple non-tubular body parts in a region are inspected, the body part that specifies the entire area inspected is coded.

*Examples:* Cystoureteroscopy with inspection of bladder and ureters is coded to the Ureter body part value.

Exploratory laparotomy with general inspection of abdominal contents is coded to the Peritoneal Cavity body part value.

**B3.11c.** When both an Inspection procedure and another procedure are performed on the same body part during the same episode, if the Inspection procedure is performed using a different approach than the other procedure, the Inspection procedure is coded separately.

*Example:* Endoscopic Inspection of the duodenum is coded separately when open Excision of the duodenum is performed during the same procedural episode.

## Occlusion vs. Restriction for Vessel Embolization Procedures

**B3.12.** If the objective of an embolization procedure is to completely close a vessel, the root operation Occlusion is coded. If the objective of an embolization procedure is to narrow the lumen of a vessel, the root operation Restriction is coded.

*Examples:* Tumor embolization is coded to the root operation Occlusion, because the objective of the procedure is to cut off the blood supply to the vessel.

Embolization of a cerebral aneurysm is coded to the root operation Restriction, because the objective of the procedure is not to close off the vessel entirely, but to narrow the lumen of the vessel at the site of the aneurysm where it is abnormally wide.

### Release Procedures

**B3.13.** In the root operation Release, the body part value coded is the body part being freed and not the tissue being manipulated or cut to free the body part.

*Example:* Lysis of intestinal adhesions is coded to the specific Intestine body part value.

### Release vs. Division

**B3.14.** If the sole objective of the procedure is freeing a body part without cutting the body part, the root operation is Release. If the sole objective of the procedure is separating or transecting a body part, the root operation is Division.

*Examples:* Freeing a nerve root from surrounding scar tissue to relieve pain is coded to the root operation Release.

Severing a nerve root to relieve pain is coded to the root operation Division.

### Reposition for Fracture Treatment

**B3.15.** Reduction of a displaced fracture is coded to the root operation Reposition and the application of a cast or splint in conjunction with the Reposition procedure is not coded separately. Treatment of a nondisplaced fracture is coded to the procedure performed.

*Examples:* Putting a pin in a nondisplaced fracture is coded to the root operation Insertion.

Casting of a nondisplaced fracture is coded to the root operation Immobilization in the Placement section.

### Transplantation vs. Administration

**B3.16.** Putting in a mature and functioning living body part taken from another individual or animal is coded to the root operation Transplantation. Putting in autologous or nonautologous cells is coded to the Administration section.

*Example:* Putting in autologous or nonautologous bone marrow, pancreatic islet cells or stem cells is coded to the Administration section.

## B4. Body Part

### General Guidelines

**B4.1a.** If a procedure is performed on a portion of a body part that does not have a separate body part value, code the body part value corresponding to the whole body part.

*Example:* A procedure performed on the alveolar process of the mandible is coded to the mandible body part.

**B4.1b.** If the prefix *peri* is used with a body part to identify the site of the procedure, the body part value is defined as the body part named.

*Example:* A procedure site identified as perirenal is coded to the Kidney body part.

### Branches of Body Parts

**B4.2.** Where a specific branch of a body part does not have its own body part value in PCS, the body part is coded to the closest proximal branch that has a specific body part value.

*Example:* A procedure performed on the mandibular branch of the trigeminal nerve is coded to the Trigeminal Nerve body part value.

### Bilateral Body Part Values

**B4.3.** Bilateral body part values are available for a limited number of body parts. If the identical procedure is performed on contralateral body parts, and a bilateral body part value exists for that body part, a single procedure is coded using the bilateral body part value. If no bilateral body part value exists, each procedure is coded separately using the appropriate body part value.

*Example:* The identical procedure performed on both fallopian tubes is coded once using the body part value Fallopian Tube, Bilateral. The identical procedure performed on both knee joints is coded twice using the body part values Knee Joint, Right and Knee Joint, Left.

### Coronary Arteries

**B4.4.** The coronary arteries are classified as a single body part that is further specified by number of sites treated and not by name or number of arteries. Separate body part values are used to specify the number of sites treated when the same procedure is performed on multiple sites in the coronary arteries.

*Examples:* Angioplasty of two distinct sites in the left anterior descending coronary artery with placement of two stents is coded as Dilation of Coronary Arteries, Two Sites, with Intraluminal Device.

Angioplasty of two distinct sites in the left anterior descending coronary artery, one with stent placed and one without, is coded separately as

Dilation of Coronary Artery, One Site with Intraluminal Device, and Dilation of Coronary Artery, One Site with No Device.

### Tendons, Ligaments, Bursae and Fascia Near a Joint

**B4.5.** Procedures performed on tendons, ligaments, bursae and fascia supporting a joint are coded to the body part in the respective body system that is the focus of the procedure. Procedures performed on joint structures themselves are coded to the body part in the Joint body system.

*Example:* Repair of the anterior cruciate ligament of the knee is coded to the knee bursae and ligament body part in the bursae and ligaments body system. Knee arthroscopy with shaving of articular cartilage is coded to the Knee Joint body part in the Lower Joints body system.

### Skin, Subcutaneous Tissue and Fascia Overlying a Joint

**B4.6.** If a procedure is performed on the skin, subcutaneous tissue or fascia overlying a joint, the procedure is coded to the following body part:

- Shoulder is coded to Upper Arm
- Elbow is coded to Lower Arm
- Wrist is coded to Lower Arm
- Hip is coded to Upper Leg
- Knee is coded to Lower Leg
- Ankle is coded to Foot

### Fingers and Toes

**B4.7** If a body system does not contain a separate body part value for fingers, procedures performed on the fingers are coded to the body part value for the hand. If a body system does not contain a separate body part value for toes, procedures performed on the toes are coded to the body part value for the foot.

*Example:* Excision of finger muscle is coded to one of the hand muscle body part values in the Muscles body system.

### Upper and Lower Intestinal Tract

**B4.8** In the Gastrointestinal body system, the general body part values Upper Intestinal Tract and Lower Intestinal Tract are provided as an option for the root operations, Change, Inspection, Removal, and Revision. Upper Intestinal Tract includes the portion of the gastrointestinal tract from the esophagus down to and including the duodenum, and Lower Intestinal Tract includes the portion of the gastrointestinal tract from the jejunum down to and including the rectum and anus.

*Example:* In the root operation Change table, change of a device in the jejunum is coded using the body part Lower Intestinal Tract.

## B5. Approach Guidelines

*Open Approach with Percutaneous Endoscopic Assistance*
**B5.2.** Procedures performed using the open approach with percutaneous endoscopic assistance are coded to the approach Open.

*Example:* Laparoscopic-assisted sigmoidectomy is coded to the approach Open.

*External Approach*
**B5.3a.** Procedures performed within an orifice on structures that are visible without the aid of any instrumentation are coded to the approach External.

*Example:* Resection of tonsils is coded to the approach External.

**B5.3b.** Procedures performed indirectly by the application of external force through the intervening body layers are coded to the approach External.

*Example:* Closed reduction of fracture is coded to the approach External.

*Percutaneous Procedure via Device*
**B5.4.** Procedures performed percutaneously via a device placed for the procedure are coded to the approach Percutaneous.

*Example:* Fragmentation of kidney stone performed via percutaneous nephrostomy is coded to the approach Percutaneous.

## B6. Device Guidelines

*General Guidelines*
**B6.1a.** A device is coded only if a device remains after the procedure is completed. If no device remains, the device value No Device is coded.

**B6.1b.** Materials such as sutures, ligatures, radiological markers and temporary post-operative wound drains are considered integral to the performance of a procedure and are not coded as devices.

**B6.1c.** Procedures performed on a device only and not on a body part are specified in the root operations Change, Irrigation, Removal and Revision, and are coded to the procedure performed.

*Example:* Irrigation of percutaneous nephrostomy tube is coded to the root operation Irrigation of indwelling device in the Administration section.

*Drainage Device*

**B6.2.** A separate procedure to put in a drainage device is coded to the root operation Drainage with the device value Drainage Device.

### C. Obstetric Section Guidelines (Section 1)

*Products of Conception*

**C1.** Procedures performed on the products of conception are coded to the Obstetrics section. Procedures performed on the pregnant female other than the products of conception are coded to the appropriate root operation in the Medical and Surgical section.

*Example:* Amniocentesis is coded to the products of conception body part in the Obstetrics section. Repair of obstetric urethral laceration is coded to the urethra body part in the Medical and Surgical section.

*Procedures Following Delivery or Abortion*

**C2.** Procedures performed following a delivery or abortion for curettage of the endometrium or evacuation of retained products of conception are all coded in the Obstetrics section, to the root operation Extraction and the body part Products of Conception, Retained. Diagnostic or therapeutic dilation and curettage performed during times other than the postpartum or post-abortion period are all coded in the Medical and Surgical section, to the root operation Extraction and the body part Endometrium.

### D. New Technology Section

General guidelines

**D1** Section X codes are standalone codes. They are not supplemental codes. Section X codes fully represent the specific procedure described in the code title, and do not require any additional codes from other sections of ICD-10-PCS. When section X contains a code title which describes a specific new technology procedure, only that X code is reported for the procedure. There is no need to report a broader, non-specific code in another section of ICD-10-PCS. Example: XW04321 Introduction of Ceftazidime-Avibactam Anti-infective into Central Vein, Percutaneous Approach, New Technology Group 1, can be coded to indicate that Ceftazidime-Avibactam Anti-infective was administered via a central vein. A separate code from table 3E0 in the Administration section of ICD-10-PCS is not coded in addition to this code.

*Selection of Principal Procedure*

The following instructions should be applied in the selection of principal procedure and clarification on the importance of the relation to the principal diagnosis when more than one procedure is performed:

**1.** Procedure performed for definitive treatment of both principal diagnosis and secondary diagnosis

    **a.** Sequence procedure performed for definitive treatment most related to principal diagnosis as principal procedure.

2. Procedure performed for definitive treatment and diagnostic procedures performed for both principal diagnosis and secondary diagnosis

    a. Sequence procedure performed for definitive treatment most related to principal diagnosis as principal procedure

3. A diagnostic procedure was performed for the principal diagnosis and a procedure is performed for definitive treatment of a secondary diagnosis.

    a. Sequence diagnostic procedure as principal procedure, since the procedure most related to the principal diagnosis takes precedence.

4. No procedures performed that are related to principal diagnosis; procedures performed for definitive treatment and diagnostic procedures were performed for secondary diagnosis

    a. Sequence procedure performed for definitive treatment of secondary diagnosis as principal procedure, since there are no procedures (definitive or nondefinitive treatment) related to principal diagnosis.

Source: CMS 2016c

**Activity 10: ICD-10-PCS Coding Guidelines**
Select the guidelines to code the following procedures.

1. Laparoscopic cholecystectomy converted to an open cholecystectomy
   a. Diagnostic excision
   b. Approach
   c. Device
   d. Discontinued procedure
   e. Multiple procedures

2. Biopsy of breast followed by partial mastectomy at the same operative site
   a. Diagnostic excision
   b. Approach
   c. Biopsy followed by more definitive treatment
   d. Discontinued procedure
   e. Multiple procedures

3. Total excision of right lobe of liver
   a. Diagnostic excision
   b. Approach
   c. Device
   d. Excision vs. Resection
   e. Multiple procedures

4. Closed reduction of fracture
   a. Diagnostic excision
   b. Approach
   c. Device
   d. Control
   e. Multiple procedures

5. Coronary bypass with excision of saphenous vein graft
   a. Diagnostic excision
   b. Approach
   c. Excision for graft
   d. Inspection
   e. Multiple procedures

# Documentation Guidelines

## General Documentation Guidelines

The clinical detail found in many ICD-10-PCS codes is greater or, in some cases, different than that currently found in ICD-9-CM. In order to code in ICD-10-PCS, you will need to consider these differences.

---

*Example:*
- The Omit code is found in the Index of ICD-9-CM Volume 3. This means procedures performed only for the purpose of performing further surgery, namely, incisions, or those that represent operative approach are not coded.
- However, in the case of ICD-10-PCS, approach is one of the seven components that comprise a code from the Medical and Surgical section.

---

**Note:** Physician education on the various aspects of procedure classification will be necessary in order to code to the highest level of specificity in ICD-10-PCS. For Example:, note the additional detail in the following ICD-10-PCS codes in comparison to ICD-9-CM Volume 3 codes.

---

## Section-Specific Documentation Guidelines

In preparation for implementation of ICD-10-PCS, coding professionals should examine the most commonly assigned procedures in each ICD-10-PCS section and determine the necessary clinician education. Identifying where documentation improvement is needed most and focusing training in those areas will help ease the transition to the new system.

To provide a starting point for this education, a couple of Example:s from each ICD-10-PCS section have been selected for review and analysis. Take a look at each pair, compare the descriptions, and note what must be documented to support the ICD-10-PCS code assignment.

| Medical and Surgical Section – Example: 1 | | | |
|---|---|---|---|
| **ICD-10-PCS** | **Description** | **ICD-9-CM** | **Description** |
| 0V508ZZ | Transurethral endoscopic laser ablation of prostate | 60.21 | Transurethral guided laser induced prostatectomy |

| Medical and Surgical Section – Example: 2 | | | |
|---|---|---|---|
| **ICD-10-PCS** | **Description** | **ICD-9-CM** | **Description** |
| 0MN14ZZ | Right shoulder arthroscopy with coracoacromial ligament release | 80.41 | Release of ligament, shoulder |

| Medical and Surgical-related Section – Example: 1 | | | |
|---|---|---|---|
| **ICD-10-PCS** | **Description** | **ICD-9-CM** | **Description** |
| 3E0P7LZ | Transvaginal artificial insemination | 69.92 | Artificial insemination |

| Medical and Surgical-related Section – Example: 2 | | | |
|---|---|---|---|
| **ICD-10-PCS** | **Description** | **ICD-9-CM** | **Description** |
| 5A1945Z | Continuous mechanical ventilation, 40 consecutive hours | 96.71 | Continuous mechanical ventilation for less than 96 consecutive hours |

| Ancillary Section – Example: 1 | | | |
|---|---|---|---|
| **ICD-10-PCS** | **Description** | **ICD-9-CM** | **Description** |
| BP04ZZZ | Portable x-ray of right clavicle, limited study | 87.43 | X-ray of ribs, sternum, and clavicle |

| Ancillary Section – Example: 2 | | | |
|---|---|---|---|
| **ICD-10-PCS** | **Description** | **ICD-9-CM** | **Description** |
| GZB1ZZZ | ECT (electroconvulsive therapy), unilateral multiple seizure | 94.27 | Other electroshock therapy |

# Section 6 Review Questions

1.  True or false? If an intended procedure is discontinued, no code is assigned.
    a.  True
    b.  False

2.  Which of the following guidelines would you use when coding fiberoptic bronchoscopy with irrigation of bronchus?
    a.  Guideline B3.2c: During the same operative episode, multiple procedures are coded if multiple root operations with distinct objectives are performed on the same body part
    b.  Guideline B3.11a: Inspection of a body part(s) performed in order to achieve the objective of a procedure is not coded separately
    c.  Guideline B3.2a: During the same operative episode, multiple procedures are coded if the same root operation is performed on different body parts as defined by distinct values of the body part character
    d.  Guideline B3.4b: If a diagnostic excision, extraction, or drainage procedure (biopsy) is followed by a more definitive procedure, such as destruction, excision, or resection at the same procedure site, both the biopsy and the more definitive treatment are coded

3.  What would you need to look for in the documentation if you were coding in ICD-10-PCS rather than ICD-9-CM Volume 3 for the following procedure: Cryotherapy of wart on left hand?
    a.  The site, skin
    b.  The site, left hand
    c.  The root operation, destruction
    d.  The diagnosis, wart

4.  True or false? A device is coded only if a device remains after the procedure is completed. If no device remains the device value No Device is coded.
    a.  True
    b.  False

5.  Procedures performed within an orifice on structures that are visible without the aid of any instrumentation are coded to the approach _____.
    a.  External
    b.  Open
    c.  Percutaneous
    d.  Via Natural or Artificial Orifice

6.  True or false? If a body system does not contain a separate body part value for fingers, procedures performed on the fingers are coded to the body part value for the hand.
    a.  True
    b.  False

7. Where a specific branch of a body part does not have its own body part value in PCS, the body part is coded to the closest _____ branch that has a specific body part value.
   a. Distal
   b. Lower
   c. Proximal
   d. Upper

8. True or false? If the prefix "intra" is combined with a body part to identify the site of the procedure, the procedure is coded to the body part named.
   a. True
   b. False

9. All of the following are true regarding ICD-10-PCS codes, *except:*
   a. All ICD-10-PCS codes contain seven characters.
   b. It is required to consult the Index first before proceeding to the Tables to complete the code.
   c. If the intended root operation is discontinued, code the procedure to the root operation performed.
   d. In order to determine the appropriate root operation, the full definition of the root operation as contained in the PCS Tables must be applied.

10. True or false? "And," when used in a code description, means "and/or."
    a. True
    b. False

# Final Review Questions

1.  Which of the following characteristics was *not* identified as essential in the development of ICD-10-PCS?
    a.  Expandability
    b.  Completeness
    c.  Single axis
    d.  Standard terminology

2.  ICD-10-PCS codes are _____.
    a.  Three to four digits long with a decimal point placed after the second digit
    b.  Six characters long
    c.  Six characters long with a decimal point after the third digit
    d.  Seven characters long

3.  What are the seven spaces of an ICD-10-PCS code called?
    a.  Values
    b.  Characters
    c.  Sections
    d.  Qualifiers

4.  Which value represents an Ancillary section in ICD-10-PCS?
    a.  Section value 1
    b.  Section value D
    c.  Section value 0
    d.  Section value E

5.  Root operation tables within the Medical and Surgical section (first character 0) consist of _____.
    a.  Three columns and a single row
    b.  Three columns and a varying number of rows
    c.  Four columns and a single row
    d.  Four columns and a varying number of rows

6.  True or false? A combination of characters not in a single row of a Table is *not* a valid code.
    a.  True
    b.  False

7.  True or false? For the Medical and Surgical section, main terms in the Index are based on the third character value.
    a.  True
    b.  False

8.  True or false? One characteristic of the key attribute "completeness" is each code retains its unique definition.
    a.  True
    b.  False

9.  Which of the following ICD-10-PCS characteristics addresses the problematic ICD-9-CM code 28.11, Biopsy of tonsils and adenoids?
    a.  Diagnosis information excluded
    b.  Standardized terminology
    c.  NOS code options excluded
    d.  Limited NEC code options

10. Which of the following procedures would be classified to the root operation Resection?
    a.  Total mastectomy
    b.  Breast lumpectomy
    c.  Suction dilation and curettage
    d.  Fulguration of endometrium

11. Which of the following is the correct definition for a Percutaneous Endoscopic approach?
    a.  Entry, by puncture or minor incision, of instrumentation through the skin or mucous membrane and/or any other body layer necessary to reach the site of the procedure
    b.  Cutting through the skin or mucous membrane and any other body layers necessary to expose the site of the procedure, and entry, by puncture or minor incision, of instrumentation through the skin or mucous membrane and any other body layers necessary to aid in the performance of the procedure
    c.  Entry, by puncture or minor incision, of instrumentation through the skin or mucous membrane and/or any other body layers necessary to reach and visualize the site of the procedure
    d.  Entry of instrumentation through a natural or artificial opening to reach and visualize the site of the procedure

12. Which of the following is an Example: of a qualifier?
    a.  Excision
    b.  Orthopedic pins
    c.  Diagnostic
    d.  Resection

13. Which of the following codes is found in the Medical and Surgical-related section, Obstetrics, of ICD-10-PCS?
    a.  2W20X4Z
    b.  10E0XZZ
    c.  3E1U38Z
    d.  BW03ZZZ

14. Correcting, to the extent possible, a malfunctioning or displaced device is the definition of _____.
    a.  Replacement
    b.  Revision
    c.  Resection
    d.  Release

15. True or false? The following diagram represents the organizational structure of the Medical and Surgical section.

| Character 1 | Character 2 | Character 3 | Character 4 | Character 5 | Character 6 | Character 7 |
|---|---|---|---|---|---|---|
| Section | Body System | Root Operation | Body System | Approach | Substance | Qualifier |

    a.    True
    b.    False

16. Which of the following procedures is assigned to the Medical and Surgical-related sections of ICD-10-PCS?
    a.    Percutaneous ligation of esophageal vein
    b.    PTA of right brachial artery stenosis
    c.    Placement of intrathecal infusion pump for pain management, percutaneous
    d.    Epidural injection of mixed steroid and local anesthetic for pain control

17. True or false? The following diagram represents the organizational structure of the Obstetrics section found in the Medical and Surgical-related sections.

| Character 1 | Character 2 | Character 3 | Character 4 | Character 5 | Character 6 | Character 7 |
|---|---|---|---|---|---|---|
| Section | Body System | Root Operation | Body Part | Approach | Device | Qualifier |

    a.    True
    b.    False

18. Which of the following is *not* one of the Ancillary sections?
    a.    Radiation Therapy
    b.    Nuclear Medicine
    c.    Mental Health
    d.    Obstetrics

19. True or false? During the same operative episode, multiple procedures are coded if multiple root operations with distinct objectives are performed on the same body part.
    a.    True
    b.    False

20. True or false? All ICD-10-PCS alphanumeric codes begin with an alpha character.
    a.    True
    b.    False

# Part I: ICD-10-PCS Coding

## ICD-10-PCS Training—Day 1

## *ICD-10-PCS Resources – References*

2016 ICD-10-PCS available at www.cms.hhs.gov/ICD10

- 2016 Code Tables and Index
  - ICD-10-PCS 2016 Tables
  - Definitions
  - Body Part Key
  - Device Key
  - Device Aggregation Table
  - Index
- 2016 ICD-10-PCS Reference Manual
  - Chapter 1: ICD-10-PCS Overview
  - Chapter 2: Procedures in the Medical and Surgical Section
  - Chapter 3: Procedures in the Medical and Surgical-related Sections
  - Chapter 4: Procedures in the Ancillary Sections
  - Appendix A: ICD-10-PCS Definitions
  - Appendix B: ICD-10-PCS Device and Substance Classification
- 2016 ICD-10-PCS Official Guidelines for Coding and Reporting
  - Conventions
  - Medical and Surgical Section Guidelines
  - Obstetrics Section Guidelines
  - Selection of Principal Procedure
- 2016 ICD-10-PCS Slides
  - PCS 2016 Slides – PowerPoint Presentation
- 2016 Development of the ICD-10 Procedure Coding System
- 2016 Version—What's New
- 2016 Mapping ICD-10-PCS to ICD-9-CM and ICD-9-CM to ICD-10-PCS; and User Guide, Reimbursement Guide, Procedures
- 2016 Code Descriptions
- 2016 Addendum

# Discussion of ICD-10-PCS Definitions and Guidelines

## Guidelines

The ICD-10-PCS Draft Coding Guidelines (2016) are included in the *ICD-10-PCS 2016 Code Book*. There are four main sections of guidelines, not including New Technology X.:

> A. Conventions
> B. Medical and Surgical Section Guidelines
> C. Obstetrics Section Guidelines
>> Selection of Principal Procedure

Section B is by far the most extensive section. There are guidelines for

- Body System
- Root Operation
- Body Part
- Approach
- Device

An effort has been made to incorporate the various guidelines into the learning content of this training, but some of the guidelines have overarching principles that must be understood before proceeding.

## *Conventions*

**A1.** ICD-10-PCS codes are composed of seven characters. Each character is an axis of classification that specifies information about the procedure performed. Within a defined code range, a character specifies the same type of information in that axis of classification.

*Example*: The fifth axis of classification specifies the approach in sections 0 through 4 and 7 through 9 of the system.

**A2.** One of 34 possible values can be assigned to each axis of classification in the seven-character code: they are the numbers 0 through 9 and the alphabet (except I and O because they are easily confused with the numbers 1 and 0). The number of unique values used in an axis of classification differs as needed.

*Example*: Where the fifth axis of classification specifies the approach, seven different approach values are currently used to specify the approach.

**A3.** The valid values for an axis of classification can be added to as needed.

*Example*: If a significantly distinct type of device is used in a new procedure, a new device value can be added to the system.

**A4.** As with words in their context, the meaning of any single value is a combination of its axis of classification and any preceding values on which it may be dependent.

*Example*: The meaning of a body part value in the Medical and Surgical section is always dependent on the body system value. The body part value 0 in the Central Nervous body system specifies Brain, and the body part value 0 in the Peripheral Nervous body system specifies Cervical Plexus.

**A5.** As the system is expanded to become increasingly detailed, over time more values will depend on preceding values for their meaning.

*Example*: In the Lower Joints body system, the device value 3 in the root operation Insertion specifies Infusion Device, and the device value 3 in the root operation Replacement specifies Ceramic Synthetic Substitute.

**A6.** The purpose of the Alphabetic Index is to locate the appropriate table that contains all information necessary to construct a procedure code. The PCS Tables should always be consulted to find the most appropriate valid code.

**A7.** It is not required to consult the Index first before proceeding to the Tables to complete the code. A valid code may be chosen directly from the Tables.

**A8.** All seven characters must be specified to be a valid code. If the documentation is incomplete for coding purposes, the physician should be queried for the necessary information.

**A9.** Within a PCS Table, valid codes include all combinations of choices in characters 4 through 7 contained in the same row of the table. In the following example, 0JHT3VZ is a valid code, and 0JHW3VZ is *not* a valid code.

| Section: | 0: Medical and Surgical |
| Body System: | J: Subcutaneous Tissue and Fascia |
| Operation: | H: Insertion: Putting in a nonbiological appliance that monitors, assists, performs, or prevents a physiological function but does not physically take the place of a body part. |

| Body Part | Approach | Device | Qualifier |
|---|---|---|---|
| **S** Subcutaneous Tissue and Fascia, Head and Neck<br>**V** Subcutaneous Tissue and Fascia, Upper Extremity<br>**W** Subcutaneous Tissue and Fascia, Lower Extremity | **0** Open<br>**3** Percutaneous | **1** Radioactive Element<br>**3** Infusion Device | **Z** No Qualifier |
| **T** Subcutaneous Tissue and Fascia, Trunk | **0** Open<br>**3** Percutaneous | **1** Radioactive Element<br>**3** Infusion Device<br>**V** Infusion Pump | **Z** No Qualifier |

**A10.** "And," when used in a code description, means "and/or."

*Example*: Lower Arm and Wrist Muscle means lower arm and/or wrist muscle.

**A11.** Many of the terms used to construct PCS codes are defined within the system. It is the coder's responsibility to determine what the documentation in the medical record equates to in the PCS definitions. The physician is not expected to use the terms used in PCS code descriptions, nor is the coder required to query the physician when the correlation between the documentation and the defined PCS terms is clear.

*Example*: When the physician documents "partial resection," the coder can independently correlate "partial resection" to the root operation Excision without querying the physician for clarification.

---

**Coding Note:** Main Index term is a root operation, root procedure type, or common procedure name. Examples are
- Resection (root operation)
- Fluoroscopy (root type)
- Prostatectomy (common procedure name)

---

**Coding Note:** When reviewing Tables, sometimes there are multiple tables for the first three characters and they may cover multiple pages in the code book.

---

## Discussion of ICD-10-PCS Definitions and Guidelines in the Medical and Surgical Section – Section 0

### *ICD-10-PCS Section*

All codes in ICD-10-PCS are seven characters. The letters O and I are not used in PCS so as not to be confused with the numbers 0 and 1. Each character has a meaning and the meanings change by sections, or the broad procedure category.

The section provides the first character value. The sections of ICD-10-PCS are

| Section Value | Description |
| --- | --- |
| 0 | Medical and Surgical |
| 1 | Obstetrics |
| 2 | Placement |
| 3 | Administration |
| 4 | Measurement and Monitoring |
| 5 | Extracorporeal Assistance and Performance |
| 6 | Extracorporeal Therapies |
| 7 | Osteopathic |
| 8 | Other Procedures |
| 9 | Chiropractic |
| B | Imaging |
| C | Nuclear Medicine |
| D | Radiation Oncology |
| F | Physical Rehabilitation and Diagnostic Audiology |
| G | Mental Health |
| H | Substance Abuse Treatment |

## ICD-10-PCS Body System

The second character defines the body system, or the general physiological system or anatomical region involved. This way of categorizing into larger groupings makes the Tables easier to navigate and also provides information quickly about the procedure. All procedures with the same second character would be of the same anatomical region or system.

### Medical and Surgical Section Body Systems

(Note: The following table illustrates the 31 body systems within the Medical and Surgical section, along with the body system's respective character value)

| Body System | Value | Body System | Value |
|---|---|---|---|
| Central Nervous | 0 | Subcutaneous Tissue and Fascia | J |
| Peripheral Nervous | 1 | Muscles | K |
| Heart and Great Vessels | 2 | Tendons – Includes synovial membrane | L |
| Upper Arteries | 3 | Bursae and Ligaments – Includes synovial membrane | M |
| Lower Arteries | 4 | Head and Facial Bones | N |
| Upper Veins | 5 | Upper Bones | P |
| Lower Veins | 6 | Lower Bones | Q |
| Lymphatic and Hemic – Includes lymph vessels and lymph nodes | 7 | Upper Joints – Includes synovial membrane | R |
| Eye | 8 | Lower Joints – Includes synovial membrane | S |
| Ear, Nose, Sinus – Includes sinus ducts | 9 | Urinary | T |
| Respiratory | B | Female Reproductive | U |
| Mouth and Throat | C | Male Reproductive | V |
| Gastrointestinal | D | Anatomical Regions, General | W |
| Hepatobiliary and Pancreas | F | Anatomical Regions, Upper Extremities | X |
| Endocrine | G | Anatomical Regions, Lower Extremities | Y |
| Skin and Breast – Includes skin and breast glands and ducts | H | | |

### Body System Guidelines

#### General Guidelines

**B2.1a.** The procedure codes in the General Anatomical Regions body systems should only be used when the procedure is performed on an anatomical region rather than a specific body part (e.g., root operations Control and Detachment, drainage of a body cavity) or on the rare occasion when no information is available to support assignment of a code to a specific body part.

*Example*: Control of postoperative hemorrhage is coded to the root operation Control found in the General Anatomical Regions body systems.

**B2.1b.** Where the general body part values Upper and Lower are provided as an option in the Upper Arteries, Lower Arteries, Upper Veins, Lower Veins, Muscles and Tendons body systems, Upper or Lower specifies body parts located above or below the diaphragm respectively.

*Example*: Vein body parts above the diaphragm are found in the Upper Veins body system; vein body parts below the diaphragm are found in the Lower Veins body system.

### ICD-10-PCS Root Operations

The third character defines the root operation, or the **objective** of the procedure. There are 31 root operations and they are arranged by groups with similar attributes. If multiple procedures as defined by distinct objectives are performed, multiple codes are assigned.

Examples of Root Operations are
- Bypass
- Drainage
- Reattachment
- Resection
- Inspection

Refer to the *ICD-10-PCS 2016 Code Book* Root Operation Definitions.

**List of Root Operations for the Medical and Surgical Section**

| Medical and Surgical Section Root Operations | | | |
|---|---|---|---|
| Alteration | Division | Inspection | Reposition |
| Bypass | Drainage | Map | Resection |
| Change | Excision | Occlusion | Restriction |
| Control | Extirpation | Reattachment | Revision |
| Creation | Extraction | Release | Supplement |
| Destruction | Fragmentation | Removal | Transfer |
| Detachment | Fusion | Repair | Transplantation |
| Dilation | Insertion | Replacement | |

## Root Operation Guidelines

### General Guidelines
**B3.1a.** In order to determine the appropriate root operation, the full definition of the root operation, as contained in the PCS Tables, must be applied.

**B3.1b.** Components of a procedure specified in the root operation definition and explanation are not coded separately. Procedural steps necessary to reach the operative site and close the operative site, including anastomosis of a tubular body part, are also not coded separately.

*Example*: Resection of a joint as part of a joint replacement procedure is included in the root operation definition of Replacement and is not coded separately. Laparotomy performed to reach the site of an open liver biopsy is not coded separately. In a Resection of sigmoid colon with anastomosis of descending colon to rectum, the anastomosis is not coded separately.

### Multiple Procedures
**B3.2.** During the same operative episode, multiple procedures are coded if

a. The same root operation is performed on different body parts as defined by distinct values of the body part character.

   *Example*: Diagnostic excision of liver and pancreas are coded separately.

b. The same root operation is repeated at different body sites that are included in the same body part value.

   *Example*: Excision of the sartorius muscle and excision of the gracilis muscle are both included in the Upper Leg Muscle body part value, and multiple procedures are coded.

c. Multiple root operations with distinct objectives are performed on the same body part.

   *Example*: Destruction of sigmoid lesion and bypass of sigmoid colon are coded separately.

d. The intended root operation is attempted using one approach, but is converted to a different approach.

   *Example*: Laparoscopic cholecystectomy converted to an open cholecystectomy is coded as Percutaneous Endoscopic Inspection and Open Resection.

### Discontinued Procedures
**B3.3.** If the intended procedure is discontinued, code the procedure to the root operation performed. If a procedure is discontinued before any other root operation is performed, code the root operation Inspection of the body part or anatomical region inspected.

*Example*: A planned aortic valve replacement procedure is discontinued after the initial thoracotomy and before any incision is made in the heart muscle, when the patient becomes hemodynamically unstable. This procedure is coded as an Open Inspection of the Mediastinum.

### Biopsy Procedures

**B3.4a.** Biopsy procedures are coded using the root operations Excision, Extraction, or Drainage and the qualifier Diagnostic. The qualifier Diagnostic is used only for biopsies.

*Examples:* Fine needle aspiration biopsy of lung is coded to the root operation Drainage with the qualifier Diagnostic. Biopsy of bone marrow is coded to the root operation Extraction with the qualifier Diagnostic. Lymph node sampling for biopsy is coded to the root operation Excision with the qualifier Diagnostic.

### Biopsy Followed by More Definitive Treatment

**B3.4b.** If a diagnostic Excision, Extraction, or Drainage procedure (biopsy) is followed by a more definitive procedure such as Destruction, Excision, or Resection at the same procedure site, both the biopsy and the more definitive treatment are coded.

*Example*: Biopsy of breast followed by partial mastectomy at the same procedure site, both the biopsy and the partial mastectomy procedure are coded.

### Overlapping Body Layers

**B3.5.** If the root operations Excision, Repair, or Inspection are performed on overlapping layers of the musculoskeletal system, the body part specifying the

---

**Coding Note:** The specific Root Operation Guidelines (B3.6a–B3.16) are presented in the appropriate section of training.

---

deepest layer is coded.

*Example*: Excisional debridement that includes skin and subcutaneous tissue and muscle is coded to the Muscle body part.

## ICD-10-PCS Body Part

The fourth character defines the body part or specific anatomical site where the procedure was performed. This is the specific site, different from the second character that provided the general body system. There are 34 possible body part values in each body system.

Examples of Body Parts are
- Liver
- Kidney
- Thalamus
- Ascending Colon

- Optic Nerve
- Tonsil

## Body Part Guidelines

### General Guidelines

**B4.1a.** If a procedure is performed on a portion of a body part that does not have a separate body part value, code the body part value corresponding to the whole body part.

*Example*: A procedure performed on the alveolar process of the mandible is coded to the mandible body part.

**B4.1b.** If the prefix *peri* is combined with a body part to identify the site of the procedure, the body part value is defined as the body part named.

*Example*: A procedure site identified as perirenal is coded to the Kidney body part.

### Branches of Body Parts

**B4.2.** Where a specific branch of a body part does not have its own body part value in PCS, the body part is coded to the closest proximal branch that has a specific body part value.

*Example*: A procedure performed on the mandibular branch of the trigeminal nerve is coded to the Trigeminal Nerve body part value.

### Bilateral Body Part Values

**B4.3.** Bilateral body part values are available for a limited number of body parts. If the identical procedure is performed on contralateral body parts, and a bilateral body part value exists for that body part, a single procedure is coded using the bilateral body part value. If no bilateral body part value exists, each procedure is coded separately using the appropriate body part value.

*Example*: The identical procedure performed on both fallopian tubes is coded once using the body part value Fallopian Tube, Bilateral. The identical procedure performed on both knee joints is coded twice using the body part values Knee Joint, Right and Knee Joint, Left.

### Coronary Arteries

**B4.4.** The coronary arteries are classified as a single body part that is further specified by number of sites treated and not by name or number of arteries. Separate body part values are used to specify the number of sites treated when the same procedure is performed on multiple sites in the coronary arteries.

*Examples*:
Angioplasty of two distinct sites in the left anterior descending coronary artery with placement of two stents is coded as Dilation of Coronary Arteries, Two Sites, with Intraluminal Device.

Angioplasty of two distinct sites in the left anterior descending coronary artery, one with stent placed and one without, is coded separately as Dilation of Coronary Artery, One Site with Intraluminal Device, and Dilation of Coronary Artery, One Site with No Device.

### Tendons, Ligaments, Bursae and Fascia Near a Joint

**B4.5.** Procedures performed on tendons, ligaments, bursae and fascia supporting a joint are coded to the body part in the respective body system that is the focus of the procedure. Procedures performed on joint structures themselves are coded to the body part in the Joint body system.

*Example*: Repair of the anterior cruciate ligament of the knee is coded to the Knee Bursae and Ligament body part in the Bursae and Ligaments body system. Knee arthroscopy with shaving of articular cartilage is coded to the Knee Joint body part in the Lower Joints body system.

### Skin, Subcutaneous Tissue, and Fascia Overlying a Joint

**B4.6.** If a procedure is performed on the skin, subcutaneous tissue, or fascia overlying a joint, the procedure is coded to the following body part:
- Shoulder is coded to Upper Arm
- Elbow is coded to Lower Arm
- Wrist is coded to Lower Arm
- Hip is coded to Upper Leg
- Knee is coded to Lower Leg
- Ankle is coded to Foot

### Fingers and Toes

**B4.7.** If a body system does not contain a separate body part value for fingers, procedures performed on the fingers are coded to the body part value for the hand. If a body system does not contain a separate body part value for toes, procedures performed on the toes are coded to the body part value for the foot.

### Upper and Lower Intestinal Tract

**B4.8.** In the Gastrointestinal body system, the general body part values Upper Intestinal Tract and Lower Intestinal Tract are provided as an option for the root operations, Change, Inspection, Removal and Revision. Upper Intestinal Tract includes the portion of the gastrointestinal tract from the esophagus down to and including the duodenum, and Lower Intestinal Tract includes the portion of the gastrointestinal tract from the jejunum down to and including the rectum and anus.

*Example*: In the root operation Change table, change of a device in the jejunum is coded using the body part Lower Intestinal Tract.

> **Coding Note: Central Nervous System (0) vs. Peripheral Nervous System (1)**
> It is important to review anatomy regarding nerves
> - Examples of Central Nervous System: brain, optic nerve, trigeminal nerve, vagus nerve, spinal meninges
> - Examples of Peripheral Nervous System: cervical nerve, ulnar nerve, radial nerve, thoracic nerve, tibial nerve, sciatic nerve, sacral plexus

*Example*: Excision of finger muscle is coded to one of the hand muscle body part values in the Muscles body system.

## ICD-10-PCS Approaches

The fifth character defines the approach or the technique used to reach the procedure site. There are seven different approach values in the Medical and

> Approaches through the skin or mucous membranes:
> - Open
> - Percutaneous
> - Percutaneous Endoscopic
>
> Approaches through an orifice:
> - Via Natural or Artificial Opening
> - Via Natural or Artificial Opening Endoscopic
> - Via Natural or Artificial Opening with Percutaneous Endoscopic Assistance

Surgical section.

Approaches may be through the skin or mucous membrane, an orifice, or external.

When assigning the approach value, remember that the approach defines the technique used to reach the procedure site, not necessarily the instruments used.

## ICD-10-PCS Approaches

| Value | Approach | Definition | Applicable Guidelines | Examples |
|---|---|---|---|---|
| 0 | Open | Cutting through the skin or mucous membrane and any other body layers necessary to expose the site of the procedure. | B5.2 | Open CABG<br>Open endarterectomy<br>Open resection cecum<br>Abdominal hysterectomy |
| 3 | Percutaneous | Entry, by puncture or minor incision, of instrumentation through the skin or mucous membrane and any other body layers necessary to reach the site of the procedure. | B5.4 | Percutaneous needle core biopsy of kidney<br>Liposuction<br>Percutaneous drainage of ascites<br>Needle biopsy of liver |
| 4 | Percutaneous Endoscopic | Entry, by puncture or minor incision, of instrumentation through the skin or mucous membrane and any other body layers necessary to reach and visualize the site of the procedure. | | Laparoscopic cholecystectomy<br>Laparoscopy with destruction of endometriosis<br>Endoscopic drainage of sinus<br>Arthroscopy |
| 7 | Via Natural or Artificial Opening | Entry of instrumentation through a natural or artificial external opening to reach the site of the procedure. | | Foley catheter placement<br>Transvaginal intraluminal cervical cerclage<br>Digital rectal exam<br>Endotracheal intubation |
| 8 | Via Natural or Artificial Opening Endoscopic | Entry of instrumentation through a natural or artificial external opening to reach and visualize the site of the procedure. | | Transurethral cystoscopy with removal bladder stone<br>Endoscopic ERCP<br>Hysteroscopy<br>Colonoscopy<br>EGD<br>Sigmoidoscopy |
| F | Via Natural or Artificial Opening with Percutaneous Endoscopic Assistance | Entry of instrumentation through a natural or artificial external opening and entry, by puncture or minor incision, of instrumentation through the skin or mucous membrane and any other body layers necessary to aid in the performance of the procedure. | | Laparoscopic-assisted vaginal hysterectomy (LAVH) |
| X | External | Procedures performed directly on the skin or mucous membrane and procedures performed indirectly by the application of external force through the skin or mucous membrane. | B5.3a<br>B5.3b | Resection of tonsils<br>Closed reduction of fracture<br>Excision of skin lesion<br>Cautery nosebleed<br>Manual rupture joint adhesions<br>Reattachment severed ear |

For additional information, refer to Approach Definitions in the *ICD-10-PCS 2016 Code Book.*

## *Approach Guidelines*

### *Open Approach with Percutaneous Endoscopic Assistance*

**B5.2.** Procedures performed using the open approach with percutaneous endoscopic assistance are coded to the approach Open.

*Example*: Laparoscopic-assisted sigmoidectomy is coded to the approach Open.

### *External Approach*

**B5.3a.** Procedures performed within an orifice on structures that are visible without the aid of any instrumentation are coded to the approach External.

*Example*: Resection of tonsils is coded to the approach External.

**B5.3b.** Procedures performed indirectly by the application of external force through the intervening body layers are coded to the approach External.

*Example*: Closed reduction of fracture is coded to the approach External.

### *Percutaneous Procedure via Device*

**B5.4.** Procedures performed percutaneously via a device placed for the procedure are coded to the approach Percutaneous.

*Example*: Fragmentation of kidney stone performed via percutaneous nephrostomy is coded to the approach Percutaneous.

## *ICD-10-PCS Devices*

There may be a device left in place, depending on the procedure performed. The sixth character identifies these devices. Device values fall into four basic groups:
- Grafts and Prostheses
- Implants
- Simple or Mechanical Appliances
- Electronic Appliances

The four general types of devices are
- Biological or synthetic material that takes the place of all or a portion of a body part (e.g., skin graft, joint prosthesis).
- Biological or synthetic material that assists or prevents a physiological function (e.g., urinary catheter, IUD).
- Therapeutic material that is not absorbed by, eliminated by, or incorporated into a body part (e.g., radioactive implant). Therapeutic materials that are considered devices can be removed.
- Mechanical or electronic appliances used to assist, monitor, take the place of, or prevent a physiological function (e.g., diaphragmatic pacemaker, hearing device, cardiac pacemaker, orthopedic pins).

---

**Coding Note: Devices**
Only procedures that have a device that remains after the procedure is completed will have a specific device value assigned. Remember that all codes require seven characters. The default value to indicate that no device was involved is **Z**.

---

Examples of Device values:
- Drainage device
- Radioactive element
- Autologous tissue substitute
- Extraluminal device
- Intraluminal device
- Synthetic substitute
- Nonautologous tissue substitute

Refer to the *ICD-10-PCS 2016 Code Book* Index for the specific brand of a device. Additional information on device types is available in the Device Key and Device Aggregation Table.

In the Medical and Surgical section, two significant Not Elsewhere Classified options are the root operation value Q, Repair and the device value Y, Other Device. Other Device is intended to be used to temporarily define new devices that do not have a specific value assigned, until one can be added to the system. No categories of medical or surgical devices are permanently classified to Other Device.

---

**Coding Note:** Materials incidental to a procedure such as clips and sutures are not considered devices.

---

**Coding Note: Appendix B ICD-10-PCS Device and Substance Classification**
This ICD-10-PCS Reference Manual Appendix B discusses the distinguishing features of device, substance, and equipment as classified in ICD-10-PCS, to provide further guidance for correct identification and coding. This information also appears as Appendix D in this training manual.

---

### *Device Guidelines*

#### *General Guidelines*

**B6.1a.** A device is coded only if a device remains after the procedure is completed. If no device remains, the device value No Device is coded.

**B6.1b.** Materials such as sutures, ligatures, radiological markers and temporary postoperative wound drains are considered integral to the performance of a procedure and are not coded as devices.

**B6.1c.** Procedures performed on a device only and not on a body part are specified in the root operations Change, Irrigation, Removal, and Revision, and are coded to the procedure performed.

*Example*: Irrigation of percutaneous nephrostomy tube is coded to the root operation Irrigation of indwelling device in the Administration section.

*Drainage Device*

**B6.2.** A separate procedure to put in a drainage device is coded to the root operation Drainage with the device value Drainage Device.

## *ICD-10-PCS Qualifier*

The seventh character defines a qualifier for the code that provides additional information about a specific attribute of the procedure. These qualifiers may have a narrow application, to a specific root operation, body system, or body part. There are no specific guidelines for qualifiers.

Examples of Qualifiers:
- Type of transplant
- Second site for a bypass
- Diagnostic excision (biopsy)

---

**Coding Note: Qualifiers**

Most procedures will not have an applicable qualifier. The default value to indicate that no qualifier is needed is **Z**.

---

### *Selection of Principal Procedure*

The following instructions should be applied in the selection of principal procedure and clarification on the importance of the relation to the principal diagnosis when more than one procedure is performed.

1. Procedure performed for definitive treatment of both principal diagnosis and secondary diagnosis
   a. Sequence procedure performed for definitive treatment most related to principal diagnosis as principal procedure.
2. Procedure performed for definitive treatment and diagnostic procedures performed for both principal diagnosis and secondary diagnosis.
   a. Sequence procedure performed for definitive treatment most related to principal diagnosis as principal procedure
3. A diagnostic procedure was performed for the principal diagnosis and a procedure is performed for definitive treatment of a secondary diagnosis.
   a. Sequence diagnostic procedure as principal procedure, since the procedure most related to the principal diagnosis takes precedence.
4. No procedures performed that are related to principal diagnosis; procedures performed for definitive treatment and diagnostic procedures were performed for secondary diagnosis.
   a. Sequence procedure performed for definitive treatment of secondary diagnosis as principal procedure, since there are no procedures (definitive or nondefinitive treatment) related to principal diagnosis.

# ICD-10-PCS Guidelines and Root Operations Review

## ICD-10-PCS Guidelines

1. True or false? A biological or synthetic material that takes the place of all or a portion of a body part such as a joint prosthesis would qualify as a device in ICD-10-PCS.
   a. True
   b. False

2. True or false? According to ICD-10-PCS Coding Guidelines, if a diagnostic biopsy is followed by a therapeutic definitive procedure at the same site, code only the therapeutic excision or resection.
   a. True
   b. False

3. True or false? When coding in ICD-10-PCS, it is necessary to consult the Alphabetic Index and then proceed to the Tables.
   a. True
   b. False

4. True or false? Lower arm and wrist muscle means lower arm and wrist muscle according to the definition of "and."
   a. True
   b. False

5. True or false? In the root operation Release, the body part character is defined as the body part being freed and not the tissue that is being cut to free the body part.
   a. True
   b. False

6. True or false? Two codes would be assigned for this procedure: Resection of a joint with joint replacement.
   a. True
   b. False

7. True or false? If the prefix *peri* is used with a body part to identify the site of the procedure, the procedure is coded to the body part named.
   a. True
   b. False

8. True or false? Materials such as sutures, ligatures, radiological markers, and temporary postop wound drains should be coded separately using ICD-10-PCS device codes.
   a. True
   b. False

9. True or false? Irrigation of a percutaneous nephrostomy tube is coded to the root operation Irrigation of indwelling device in the Administration section.
   a. True
   b. False

10. True or false? Body systems designated as upper or lower contain the body parts that are above or below the diaphragm respectively.
    a. True
    b. False

## Root Operations

11. True or false? In ICD-10-PCS, when an entire lymph node chain is cut out, the appropriate root operation is Resection.
    a. True
    b. False

12. True or false? The root operation Detachment is used exclusively for amputation procedures.
    a. True
    b. False

13. True or false? Forceps removal of a foreign body is an example of an Extirpation procedure.
    a. True
    b. False

14. True or false? The root operation Division is coded when the objective is to cut or separate the area around a body part, the attachments to a body part, or between subdivisions of a body that are causing abnormal constraint.
    a. True
    b. False

15. True or false? Adhesiolysis is an example of a Release procedure.
    a. True
    b. False

16. True or false? The root operation Restriction is coded when the objective of the procedure is to close off a tubular body part or orifice.
    a. True
    b. False

17. True or false? The root operation Dilation is coded when the objective of the procedure is to enlarge the diameter of a tubular body part or orifice.
    a. True
    b. False

18. True or false? Typical Change procedures include exchange of drainage devices and feeding devices.
    a. True
    b. False

19. True or false? All codes in the ICD-10-PCS Administration section define procedures where a diagnostic or therapeutic substance is given to the patient, such as a platelet transfusion.
    a. True
    b. False

20. True or false? In ICD-10-PCS, the term *measurement* refers to a series of levels obtained at intervals, while *monitoring* describes a single level taken.
    a. True
    b. False

# Coding Procedures in the Medical and Surgical Section – Section 0

The seven characters in the Medical and Surgical section are

| Character 1 | Character 2 | Character 3 | Character 4 | Character 5 | Character 6 | Character 7 |
|---|---|---|---|---|---|---|
| Section | Body System | Root Operation | Body Part | Approach | Device | Qualifier |

1. Character 1 refers to the broad procedure category where the code is found (0) for Medical and Surgical.
2. Character 2 defines the body system or general physiological system or anatomical region.
3. Character 3 defines the root operation, or the objective of the procedure.
4. Character 4 defines the body part or anatomical site where the procedure was performed.
5. Character 5 defines the approach, or the technique used to reach the procedure site.
6. Character 6 defines the device (if any) left in place at the end of the procedure.
7. Character 7 defines the qualifier for the code.

## Root Operation Groupings

There are nine groups of root operations, arranged by similar attributes:
- Root Operations That Take Out Some or All of a Body Part
- Root Operations That Take Out Solids/Fluids/Gases from a Body Part
- Root Operations Involving Cutting or Separation Only
- Root Operations That Put in/Put Back or Move Some/All of a Body Part
- Root Operations That Alter the Diameter/Route of a Tubular Body Part
- Root Operations That Always Involve a Device
- Root Operations Involving Examination Only
- Root Operations That Define Other Repairs
- Root Operations That Define Other Objectives

## Root Operations That Take Out Some or All of a Body Part

Refer to *ICD-10-PCS 2016 Code Book* Root Operation Definitions.

The five root operations belonging to this group are
- Excision (B)
- Resection (T)
- Detachment (6)
- Destruction (5)
- Extraction (D)

## Excision – Root Operation B

| Excision B | Definition | Cutting out or off, without replacement, a portion of a body part |
| --- | --- | --- |
| | Explanation | The qualifier **Diagnostic** is used to identify excision procedures that are biopsies |
| | Examples | Partial nephrectomy, liver biopsy, breast lumpectomy, breast reduction for medical reasons (for cosmetic reasons is Alteration), Excisional debridement (non-excisional debridement is Extraction) |

**Excision** is coded when a portion of a body part is cut out or off using a sharp instrument. All root operations that employ cutting to accomplish the objective allow the use of any sharp instrument, including but not limited to

- Scalpel
- Wire
- Scissors
- Bone saw
- Electrocautery tip

---

**Coding Note: Bone Marrow and Endometrial Biopsies**
Bone marrow and endometrial biopsies are not coded to **Excision**. They are coded to **Extraction**, with the qualifier **Diagnostic**.

---

**Coding Guideline B3.9. Excision for Graft**
If an autograft is obtained from a different body part in order to complete the objective of the procedure, a separate procedure is coded.

*Example*: Coronary bypass with excision of saphenous vein graft, excision of saphenous vein is coded separately.

### *Resection – Root Operation T*

| Resection T | Definition | Cutting out or off, without replacement, all of a body part |
|---|---|---|
| | Explanation | N/A |
| | Examples | Total nephrectomy, total lobectomy of lung, total mastectomy |

**Resection** is similar to **Excision** except **Resection** includes all of a body part, or any subdivision of a body part that has its own body part value in ICD-10-PCS, while **Excision** includes only a portion of a body part.

---

**Coding Note: Lymph Nodes**

When an entire lymph node chain is cut out, the appropriate root operation is **Resection**. When a lymph node(s) is cut out, the root operation is **Excision**.

---

**Coding Note: Documentation**

There is an opportunity to provide physician education on the need for more complete documentation in the medical record on the following:
- Lymph node(s) versus the complete chain
- The complete body part removal versus a portion

---

**Coding Guideline B3.8 Excision vs. Resection**

PCS contains specific body parts for anatomical subdivisions of a body part, such as lobes of the lungs or liver and regions of the intestine. Resection of the specific body part is coded whenever all of the body part is cut out or off, rather than coding Excision of a less specific body part.

*Example*: Left upper lung lobectomy is coded to Resection of Upper Lung Lobe, Left rather than Excision of Lung, Left.

## Detachment – Root Operation 6

| Detachment 6 | Definition | Cutting off all or part of the upper or lower extremities |
|---|---|---|
| | Explanation | The body part value is the site of the detachment, with a qualifier, if applicable, to further specify the level where the extremity was detached |
| | Examples | Below-knee amputation, disarticulation of shoulder, amputation above elbow |

**Detachment** represents a narrow range of procedures; it is used exclusively for amputation procedures. **Detachment** procedure codes are found only in body systems X, Anatomical Regions, Upper Extremities and Y, Anatomical Regions, Lower Extremities because amputations are performed on extremities across overlapping body layers and so could not be coded to a specific musculoskeletal body system such as the Bones or Joints.

---

**Coding Note: Detachment Qualifiers**
The specific qualifiers used for **Detachment** are dependent on the body part value in the upper and lower extremities body systems.

---

The following definitions have been developed for these qualifiers. (These definitions are only available in the *ICD-10-PCS Reference Manual*.)

| Body Part | Qualifier | Definition |
|---|---|---|
| Upper arm and upper leg | 1 | **High:** Amputation at the proximal portion of the shaft of the humerus or femur |
| | 2 | **Mid:** Amputation at the middle portion of the shaft of the humerus or femur |
| | 3 | **Low:** Amputation at the distal portion of the shaft of the humerus or femur |

Note: The same definitions would be utilized for lower arm and leg.

---

**Coding Note: Documentation**
There is an opportunity to provide physician education on the need for more complete documentation in the medical record on the actual location of the amputation. According to the definition the coding professional needs to know if the amputation is at the proximal, middle, or distal portion of the *shaft* of the humerus, femur, radius/ulna, or tibia/fibula.

---

| Body Part | Qualifier | Definition |
|---|---|---|
| Hand and foot | 0 | Complete |
| | 4 | Complete 1st Ray |
| | 5 | Complete 2nd Ray |
| | 6 | Complete 3rd Ray |
| | 7 | Complete 4th Ray |
| | 8 | Complete 5th Ray |
| | 9 | Partial 1st Ray |
| | B | Partial 2nd Ray |
| | C | Partial 3rd Ray |
| | D | Partial 4th Ray |
| | F | Partial 5th Ray |

When coding amputation of Hand and Foot, the following definitions are followed:
- Complete: Amputation through the carpometacarpal joint of the hand, or through the tarsal-metatarsal joint of the foot.
- Partial: Amputation anywhere along the shaft or head of the metacarpal bone of the hand, or of the metatarsal bone of the foot.

| Body Part | Qualifier | Definition |
|---|---|---|
| Thumb, finger, or toe | 0 | **Complete:** Amputation at the metacarpophalangeal/metatarsal-phalangeal joint |
| | 1 | **High:** Amputation anywhere along the proximal phalanx |
| | 2 | **Mid:** Amputation through the proximal interphalangeal joint or anywhere along the middle phalanx |
| | 3 | **Low:** Amputation through the distal interphalangeal joint or anywhere along the distal phalanx |

**Coding Note: Qualifier Value**
When a surgeon uses the word "toe" to describe the amputation, but the operative report says he extends the amputation to the midshaft of the fifth metatarsal, which is the foot, the qualifier is Partial 5th Ray.

## Destruction – Root Operation 5

| Destruction 5 | Definition | Physical eradication of all or a portion of a body part by the direct use of energy, force, or a destructive agent |
|---|---|---|
| | Explanation | None of the body part is physically taken out |
| | Examples | Fulguration of rectal polyp, cautery of skin lesion, fulguration of endometrium |

**Destruction** "takes out" a body part in the sense that it obliterates the body part so it is no longer there. This root operation defines a broad range of common procedures, since it can be used anywhere in the body to treat a variety of conditions, including

- Skin and genital warts
- Nasal and colon polyps
- Esophageal varices
- Endometrial implants
- Nerve lesions

**Coding Note:** Usually there would be no pathology report present for Destruction procedures because it is destroyed or obliterated. Occasionally, tissue remains in an instrument, and may be sent to pathology.

### *Extraction – Root Operation D*

| Extraction D | Definition | Pulling or stripping out or off all or a portion of a body part by the use of force |
|---|---|---|
| | Explanation | The qualifier **Diagnostic** is used to identify extraction procedures that are biopsies |
| | Examples | Dilation and curettage, vein stripping, phacoemulsification without IOL implant (phacoemulsification with IOL implant is Replacement), non-excisional debridement (excisional debridement is Excision), liposuction for medical reasons (liposuction for cosmetic reasons is Alteration) |

**Extraction** is coded when the method employed to take out the body part is pulling or stripping. Minor cutting, such as that used in vein stripping procedures, is included in **Extraction** if the objective of the procedure is nevertheless met by pulling or stripping. As with all applicable ICD-10-PCS codes, cutting used to reach the procedure site is specified in the approach value.

To completely understand the intent of Extraction, it is necessary to understand how these surgical procedures are performed. The following Teaching Tips are included to help, but certainly additional research is recommended.

---

**Coding Note: Documentation**

Be careful of documentation. It is important to convert common terminology to the appropriate root operation according to the intent of the procedure. For example, the procedure documentation may *say* removal, but in actuality, using PCS definitions, an extraction was performed. Removal of a thumbnail would be coded to Extraction. The root operation of Removal is not correct because by definition a *removal* in ICD-10-PCS is defined as taking out or off a device from a body part.

---

---

**Coding Guideline B3.4b. Biopsy Followed by More Definitive Treatment**
If a diagnostic Excision, Extraction, or Drainage procedure (biopsy) is followed by a more definitive procedure, such as Destruction, Excision, or Resection at the same procedure site, both the biopsy and the more definitive treatment are coded.

---

2.1. Percutaneous needle biopsy of upper quadrant of right breast. Biopsy specimen was sent for frozen section with adenocarcinoma of right breast being diagnosed. An open total right mastectomy was then performed.

Code(s): _____

2.2. The patient sustained an injury while working at the factory. Due to the unsustainability of the limb, an amputation of the left arm was performed at the mid shaft of the humerus.

Code(s): _____

---

**Coding Guideline B3.2a. Multiple Procedures**
During the same operative episode, multiple procedures are coded if the same root operation is performed on different body parts as defined by distinct values of the body part character.

---

2.3. The patient has condylomas of the cervix, vagina and vulva. Laser speculum was inserted via the vagina and using Xener on 20-watt setting, the laser was used to obliterate the condyloma in both the vagina and cervix. The laser speculum was then removed. The laser was then used to obliterate the third condyloma in the vulva area.

Code(s): _____

2.4. A scope with instrumentation was inserted via small incisions in the left neck region and the left lobe of the thyroid gland was removed in total. Biopsies were then taken from surrounding lymph nodes and the scope and instrumentation were then removed.

Code(s): OGTG4ZZ, 07B24ZX

*[handwritten: ① Root operation Resection Thyroid gland left node ② Excision: Lymphatic, Neck, Left]*

2.5. Percutaneous denervation by neurolytic agent, common fibular nerve

Code(s): _____

2.6. The patient is admitted for a vertical sleeve gastrectomy for weight loss. The greater curvature of the stomach is removed laparoscopically.

Code(s): ODB64Z3

*[handwritten: Excision Stomach]*

2.7. The patient underwent a dilation and curettage. A bivalve speculum was placed in the vagina and the cervix was prepped with Betadine solution. The uterine cavity was sounded at 7 cm. The endometrial cavity was curetted for tissue sampling.

Code (s): OUDB7ZX

*[handwritten: Extraction Endometrium]*

> **Coding Guideline B3.11a. Inspection Procedures**
> Inspection of a body part(s) performed in order to achieve the objective of a procedure is not coded separately.

> **Coding Guideline B3.2b. Multiple Procedures**
> During the same operative episode, multiple procedures are coded if the same root operation is repeated at different body sites that are included in the same body part value.

**2.8.** The patient underwent a bronchoscopy with transbronchial biopsies of the right lower lobe. The bronchoscope was passed through the right nasal cavity into the trachea. Two transbronchial biopsies were obtained from different sites in the right lower lobe. The trachea, carina, left and right-sided airways were all within normal limits.

Code(s): _____

**2.9.** A rigid bronchoscope is inserted and advanced through the larynx to the main bronchus. The carcinoma in situ lesion in the right main bronchus was treated with Nd:YAG laser photoresection.

Code(s): 0B538Z2

*[handwritten left margin: Destruction HW Bronchus Main Right]*

**2.10.** The patient has a herniated lumbar disc at the L4 level. A partial discectomy is performed by incision, with loose fragments of disc material removed.

Code(s): _____

**2.11.** The patient has an ingrown toenail of the right great toe. A nail elevator is slid under the cuticle and the nail plate is identified. The right piece of nail is grasped with a hemostat and removed in one piece, pulling straight out. The left piece of nail is grasped and removed in a similar manner. Next, electrocautery ablation is used to destroy the nail matrix where the nail was removed.

Code(s): _____

**2.12.** The patient is admitted for an open removal of the left lower lobe of the lung due to adenocarcinoma.

Code(s): 0BTJ0ZZ

*[handwritten left margin: Resection Lung, Lower Lobe HW Left]*

**2.13.** A LEEP conization procedure was performed for moderate dysplasia of the cervix. A laser speculum was placed in the vaginal vault. Using the 2 cm loop electrosurgical electrode excision, the endocervical canal tissue was excised with bipolar cautery. The speculum was removed.

Code(s): _____

> **Coding Guideline B3.2d. Multiple Procedures**
> During the same operative episode, multiple procedures are coded if the intended root operation is attempted using one approach, but is converted to a different approach.

**2.14.** Laparoscopic cholecystectomy converted to open cholecystectomy. The gallbladder was removed in total.

Code(s): _____

**2.15.** The patient's left leg was prepped and draped. Using a fishmouth incision, the distal aspect of the thigh was entered. Using the scalpel, the skin and subcutaneous tissue were incised. The muscle groups were separated and the vessels were secured and doubly ligated using free ties of 0-Vicryl. The femoral nerve was secured. The distal femur was transected using a saw, and the edges were rasped smooth. Hemostasis was achieved, and the muscle groups, the hamstrings, and the quadriceps were approximat ed. The subcutaneous tissue was then reapproximated, and the skin was closed with staples.

Code(s): _____

> **Coding Guideline B3.2a. Multiple Procedures**
> During the same operative episode, multiple procedures are coded if the same root operation is performed on different body parts as defined by distinct values of the body part character.

> **Coding Guideline B3.2b. Multiple Procedures**
> During the same operative episode, multiple procedures are coded if the same root operation is repeated at different body sites that are included in the same body part value.

**2.16.** An adult colonoscope was placed in the rectum and successfully advanced to the cecum. The colonscope was then slowly withdrawn with the entire colon being inspected. Biopsies were obtained in the descending and sigmoid colon. There were also two hyperplastic appearing polyps in the rectum which were resected using cold forceps.

Code(s): _____

## Root Operations That Take Out Solids, Fluids, or Gases from a Body Part

Refer to *ICD-10-PCS 2016 Code Book* Root Operation Definitions.

The three root operations belonging to this group are
- Drainage (9)
- Extirpation (C)
- Fragmentation (F)

### Drainage – Root Operation 9

| Drainage 9 | Definition | Taking or letting out fluids and/or gases from a body part |
|---|---|---|
| | Explanation | The qualifier **Diagnostic** is used to identify drainage procedures that are biopsies |
| | Examples | Thoracentesis, Incision and Drainage, Aspiration, Lumbar puncture |

The root operation **Drainage** is coded for both diagnostic and therapeutic drainage procedures. When drainage is accomplished by putting in a catheter, the device value **Drainage Device** is coded in the sixth character.

## Extirpation – Root Operation C

| Extirpation C | Definition | Taking or cutting out solid matter from a body part. |
|---|---|---|
| | Explanation | The solid matter may be an abnormal byproduct of a biological function or a foreign body; it may be imbedded in a body part, or in the lumen of a tubular body part. The solid matter may or may not have been previously broken into pieces. |
| | Examples | Thrombectomy, endarterectomy, choledocholithotomy, excision foreign body. |

**Extirpation** represents a range of procedures where the body part itself is not the focus of the procedure. Instead, the objective is to remove solid material such as a foreign body, thrombus, or calculus from the body part.

## Fragmentation – Root Operation F

| Fragmentation F | Definition | Breaking solid matter in a body part into pieces. |
|---|---|---|
| | Explanation | The physical force (e.g., manual, ultrasonic) applied directly or indirectly is used to break the solid matter into pieces. The solid matter may be an abnormal byproduct of a biological function or a foreign body. The pieces of solid matter are not taken out. |
| | Examples | Extracorporeal shockwave lithotripsy, transurethral lithotripsy. |

**Fragmentation** is coded for procedures to break up, but not remove, solid material such as a calculus or foreign body. This root operation includes both direct and extracorporeal **Fragmentation** procedures.

**2.17.** The patient is being evaluated for septic arthritis of the right knee. A needle arthrocentesis was performed on the right knee with 15 cc of fluid being removed.

Code(s): _____

**2.18.** A staghorn calculus of the right renal pelvis was treated five days ago by lithotripsy. During this encounter the calculus pieces are removed via a percutaneous nephrostomy tube.

Code(s): _____

**2.19.** The patient was placed in the supine position and in the F2 focus of the MSL 5000 lithotriptor. Shock wave lithotripsy was begun at 17 kV and progressed to 23. A total of 3,000 shocks were given to the stone with resultant fragmentation of the calculus in the left renal pelvis.

Code(s): _____

**2.20.** A minor stab incision was made in the patient's left chest wall. Using a hemostat, the chest cavity is entered percutaneously through the skin and fluid returned. Next, using the trocar, the chest tube is placed in the left pleural cavity. There was approximately 1,000 ml of fluid returned. The chest tube was sewn into place.

Code(s): _____

**2.21.** Endoscopic retrograde cholangiopancreatography (ERCP) with lithotripsy of common bile duct stone

Code(s): _____

**2.22.** A 21-French ACMI panendoscope is inserted into the patient's bladder without difficulty. Inspection of the left ureter reveals a large stone is obstructing the middle third of the ureter. A guide wire is passed into the left ureter orifice and the cystoscope is removed and a ureteroscope is passed alongside the guide wire up to the mid-ureter. The large stone is fragmented with lithotripsy. A total of only about 80 shocks were needed. At this point, the large remaining fragments were removed via basket extraction.

Code(s): _____

**2.23.** The patient presents with an abscess overlying his left buttock. An 18-gauge needle was placed in the area of induration on the buttock. Purulent material was obtained. An elliptical incision was made excising a segment of skin and the abscess cavity was bluntly opened, drained and digitally explored to break up loculations. It was then irrigated and packed with iodoform gauze.

Code(s): _____

**2.24.** Percutaneous mechanical thrombectomy, right common interosseous artery

Code(s): _____

**2.25.** The patient has acute panophthalmitis of the right eye and a sclerotomy and drainage of the right eye vitreous was performed. A lid speculum was placed in the right eye and Betadine dripped on the conjunctival surface. A needle was placed through the temporal pars plana into the mid vitreous cavity and 0.5 cc of liquid vitreous was aspirated without difficulty.

Code(s): _____

**2.26.** The patient has acute dysphagia following ingestion of egg roll and chicken earlier today. The Olympus Video Endoscope was inserted by mouth and advanced into the esophagus. In the distal esophagus, a foreign body was identified. This appeared to be meat. The endoscope was advanced to the area and the foreign body was gently pushed into the stomach without difficulty. Inspection of the stomach revealed florid erosions in the gastric antrum. A biopsy was taken in the stomach from an erosive appearing lesion. The duodenum appeared normal. The endoscope was then withdrawn.

Code(s): _____

# Root Operations Involving Cutting or Separation Only

Refer to *ICD-10-PCS 2016 Code Book* Root Operation Definitions.

The two root operations belonging to this group are
- Division (8)
- Release (N)

## *Division – Root Operation 8*

| Division 8 | Definition | Cutting into a body part without draining fluids and/or gases from the body part in order to separate or transect a body part |
| --- | --- | --- |
| | Explanation | All or a portion of the body part is separated into two or more portions |
| | Examples | Spinal cordotomy, osteotomy, neurotomy, episiotomy |

The root operation **Division** is coded when the objective of the procedure is to cut into, transect, or otherwise separate all or a portion of a body part. When the objective is to cut or separate the area around a body part, the attachments to a body part, or between subdivisions of a body part that are causing abnormal constraint, the root operation **Release** is coded instead.

---

**Coding Guideline B3.14. Release vs. Division**

If the sole objective of the procedure is freeing a body part without cutting the body part, the root operation is Release. If the sole objective of the procedure is separating or transecting a body part, the root operation is Division.

*Examples:* Freeing a nerve root from surrounding scar tissue to relieve pain is coded to the root operation Release. Severing a nerve root to relieve pain is coded to the root operation Division.

---

## *Release – Root Operation N*

| Release N | Definition | Freeing a body part from an abnormal physical constraint by cutting or by use of force |
| --- | --- | --- |
| | Explanation | Some of the restraining tissue may be taken out but none of the body part is taken out |
| | Examples | Adhesiolysis, carpal tunnel release, manipulation of joint adhesions |

The objective of procedures represented in the root operation **Release** is to free a body part from abnormal constraint. **Release** procedures are coded to the body part being freed. The procedure can be performed on the area around a body part, on the attachments to a body part, or between subdivisions of a body part that are causing the abnormal constraint.

---

**Coding Guideline B3.13. Release Procedures**
In the root operation Release, the body part value coded is the body part being freed and not the tissue being manipulated or cut to free the body part.

*Example:* Lysis of intestinal adhesions is coded to the specific intestine body part value.

---

2.27.   A patient is being treated for a cumulative injury resulting in a frozen left shoulder. The patient has been unresponsive to exercise and medication. An arthroscopic manipulation is performed to release the frozen shoulder.

Code(s): _____

2.28.   The patient has bilateral flexion contractures of the knees at 45 degrees. Posterior capsulotomy via incision was performed on both knees.

Code(s): _____

2.29    In preparation for an impending delivery, the physician performs a midline episiotomy.

Code(s): _____

2.30.   The patient is several weeks status post right knee total knee arthroplasty, with tissue adhesions not allowing more than 70 degrees of flexion. During this encounter, the patient undergoes manipulation under general anesthesia. During the surgery the right knee was gently manipulated to 110–120 degrees with a solid end point being reached.

Code(s): _____

---

**Coding Guideline B4.1a. Body Part Guideline**
If a procedure is performed on a portion of a body part that does not have a separate body part value, code the body part value corresponding to the whole body part.

---

**Coding Guideline B.3.2b. Multiple Procedures**
During the same operative episode, multiple procedures are coded if the same root operation is repeated at different body sites that are included in the same body part value.

---

**2.31.** Percutaneous osteotomy of the capitate and lunate bones, right hand

Code(s): _____

# Root Operations That Put In/Put Back or Move Some/All of a Body Part

Refer to *ICD-10-PCS 2016 Code Book* Root Operation Definitions.

The four root operations belonging to this group are
- Transplantation (Y)
- Reattachment (M)
- Transfer (X)
- Reposition (S)

## *Transplantation – Root Operation Y*

| Transplantation Y | Definition | Putting in or on all or a portion of a living body part taken from another individual or animal to physically take the place and/or function of all or a portion of a similar body part |
|---|---|---|
| | Explanation | The native body part may or may not be taken out, and the transplanted body part may take over all or a portion of its function |
| | Examples | Kidney transplant, heart transplant |

A small number of procedures is represented in the root operation **Transplantation** and includes only the body parts currently being transplanted. Qualifier values specify the genetic compatibility of the body part transplanted.

---

**Coding Guideline B3.16. Transplantation vs. Administration**

Putting in a mature and functioning living body part taken from another individual or animal is coded to the root operation Transplantation. Putting in autologous or nonautologous cells is coded to the Administration section.

*Example:* Putting in autologous or nonautologous bone marrow, pancreatic islet cells, or stem cells is coded to the Administration section.

---

**Coding Note: Bone Marrow Transplant**

Bone marrow transplant procedures are coded in section 3, Administration, to the root operation 2, Transfusion.

---

In the Tables for Transplant Procedures, the Qualifier values are
- Allogeneic
- Syngeneic
- Zooplastic

The following table provides definitions of these terms:

**Qualifier Choices**

| Type of Transplant | Qualifier Character | Definition |
|---|---|---|
| Allogeneic | 0 | Taken from different individuals of the same species |
| Syngeneic | 1 | Having to do with individuals or tissues that have identical genes, such as identical twins |
| Zooplastic | 2 | Tissue from an animal to a human |

## *Reattachment – Root Operation M*

| Reattachment M | Definition | Putting back in or on all or a portion of a separated body part to its normal location or other suitable location |
| --- | --- | --- |
| | Explanation | Vascular circulation and nervous pathways may or may not be reestablished |
| | Examples | Reattachment of hand, reattachment of avulsed kidney, reattachment of finger |

Procedures coded to **Reattachment** include putting back a body part that has been cut off or avulsed. Nerves and blood vessels may or may not be reconnected in a **Reattachment** procedure.

### Transfer – Root Operation X

| Transfer X | Definition | Moving, without taking out, all or a portion of a body part to another location to take over the function of all or a portion of a body part |
| --- | --- | --- |
| | Explanation | The body part transferred remains connected to its vascular and nervous supply |
| | Examples | Tendon transfer, skin pedicle flap transfer, skin transfer flap |

**Coding Note:** Free grafts are coded to the root operation of Replacement.

The root operation **Transfer** is used to represent procedures where a body part is moved to another location without disrupting its vascular and nervous supply.
In the body systems that classify the subcutaneous tissue, fascia, and muscle body parts, a qualifier is used to specify when more than one tissue layer was used in the transfer procedure, such as musculocutaneus flap transfer.

**Coding Note: Body System Value**
For procedures involving transfer of tissue layers such as skin, fascia and muscle, the procedure is coded to the body system value that describes the deepest tissue layer in the flap. When the tissue transferred is composed of more than one tissue layer, the qualifier can be used to describe the other tissue layers, if any, being transferred.
For transfer procedures classified to other body systems such as peripheral nervous system, the body part value specifies the body part that is the source of the transfer ("from"). Where qualifiers are available, they specify the destination of the transfer ("to").

## Reposition – Root Operation S

| Reposition S | Definition | Moving to its normal location or other suitable location all or a portion of a body part. |
|---|---|---|
| | Explanation | The body part is moved to a new location from an abnormal location, or from a normal location where it is not functioning correctly. The body part may or may not be cut out or off to be moved to the new location. |
| | Examples | Reposition of undescended testicle, fracture reduction. |

**Reposition** represents procedures for moving a body part to a new location. The range of **Reposition** procedures includes moving a body part to its normal location, or moving a body part to a new location to enhance its ability to function.

---

**Coding Guideline B3.15. Reposition for Fracture Treatment**
Reduction of a displaced fracture is coded to the root operation Reposition and the application of a cast or splint in conjunction with the Reposition procedure is not coded separately. Treatment of a nondisplaced fracture is coded to the procedure performed.

*Examples:* 1. Putting in a pin in a nondisplaced fracture is coded to the root operation Insertion.
2. Casting of a nondisplaced fracture is coded to the root operation Immobilization in the Placement section.

---

**Coding Note:** The diagnosis code in ICD-10-CM would reflect that a displaced fracture is being reduced when the root operation of Reposition is used.

---

2.32. A 20-year-old patient with cystic fibrosis is admitted for a double lung transplant from a cadaver donor.

Code(s): _____

2.33. The patient undergoes nerve surgery to prevent a residual claw-hand injury after injuring his left hand. An anterior interosseous to ulnar nerve graft is accomplished via incision using an operative microscope and the interosseous and ulnar nerve are brought together without dissection.

Code(s): _____

2.34 The patient was involved in a farm injury and his left arm was severed to the elbow. The arm was reconnected, with full revascularization and nerve attachment.

Code(s): _____

**2.35.** A 46-year-old male was admitted after being involved in a motor vehicle accident. The patient was found to have a fracture of the left femoral shaft and a fracture of the right fibula and tibia. The patient underwent an open reduction with intramedullary fixation device of the left femoral shaft and an open reduction and ring external fixation of the right tibia and fibula.

Code(s): _____

**2.36.** The patient underwent a donor-matched right kidney transplant due to end-stage renal disease.

Code(s): _____

**2.37.** The patient presents for an open reconstruction procedure involving a pedicle flap of the transverse rectus muscle to the left mastectomy site. The patient had a mastectomy of the left breast previously.

Code(s): _____

---

**Coding Guideline B3.15. Reposition for Fracture Treatment**
Reduction of a displaced fracture is coded to the root operation Reposition and the application of a cast or splint in conjunction with the Reposition procedure is not coded separately. Treatment of a nondisplaced fracture is coded to the procedure performed.

*Examples:* 1. Putting a pin in a nondisplaced fracture is coded to the root operation Insertion.
2. Casting of a nondisplaced fracture is coded to the root operation Immobilization in the Placement section.

---

**Coding Note:** The diagnosis code in ICD-10-CM would reflect that a displaced fracture is being reduced when the root operation of Reposition is used.

---

**2.38.** The patient underwent a closed reduction and percutaneous pinning of a right distal radius fracture and closed reduction of right distal ulnar fracture. At the beginning of the procedure, the splint was removed from the right upper extremity and a closed reduction of both fractures was performed. Two K wires were then placed across the fracture site in the radius. After assuring that the pins were in good position, they were cut and bent. Sterile dressing followed by sugar tong type of splint were then applied.

Code(s): _____

**2.39.** Endoscopic radial to median nerve transfer

Code(s): _____

**2.40.** Open transplantation of both testes to inner thigh space due to scrotal destruction.

Code(s): _____

**2.41.**   Left foot flexor digitorum brevis tendon transfer, open approach

Code(s): _____

**2.42.**   The patient underwent a recess of the right superior rectus muscle to repair hypertrophia of the right eye. A lid speculum was placed in the right eye and traction sutures placed with the eye rotated down and out. The right superior rectus muscle was isolated. A double-armed 6-0 Vicryl suture was then woven through the distal muscle tendon in locking fashion and the muscle disinserted from the globe. The needles were then passed through superficial sclera, 5.0 mm posterior to the original insertion and the muscle tied down firmly into this position.

Code (s): _____

**2.43.**   The procedure performed is a repair of a left quadriceps tendon due to rupture of the left quadriceps tendon. A midline incision was made and centered over the patella and carried down to the quadriceps mechanism. Medial and lateral dissection was carried out to expose the retinaculum, which was torn approximately 2 cm laterally and medially. There was a direct avulsion of the quadriceps tendon off the patella. The quadriceps tendon was freshened and then repaired by reattaching to the patella.

Code(s): _____

**2.44.**   The patient underwent an open reduction with internal fixation to repair an open fracture of the head of the right proximal thumb. An incision was made and the entire fracture site was opened. The proximal fracture was stabilized with 0.35 crossed K-wires, resulting in excellent bony fixation. The fracture was then anatomically reduced and transfixed with transverse 0.35 K-wires to the distal phalanx.

Code(s): _____

### Root Operations That Alter the Diameter/Route of a Tubular Body Part

Refer to *ICD-10-PCS 2016 Code Book* Root Operation Definitions.

The four root operations belonging to this group are
- Restriction (V)
- Occlusion (L)
- Dilation (7)
- Bypass (1)

### *Restriction – Root Operation V*

| Restriction V | Definition | Partially closing an orifice or the lumen of a tubular body part |
|---|---|---|
| | Explanation | The orifice can be a natural orifice or an artificially created orifice |
| | Examples | Esophagogastric fundoplication, cervical cerclage |

The root operation **Restriction** is coded when the objective of the procedure is to narrow the diameter of a tubular body part or orifice. **Restriction** includes either intraluminal or extraluminal methods for narrowing the diameter.

**Coding Note:** Since intraluminal or extraluminal clips are frequently used to accomplish the objectives of Restriction and Occlusion procedures, careful review of the operative report is required. Research on the procedure technique may also be helpful.

## Occlusion – Root Operation L

| Occlusion L | Definition | Completely closing an orifice or the lumen of a tubular body part |
|---|---|---|
| | Explanation | The orifice can be a natural orifice or an artificially created orifice |
| | Examples | Fallopian tube ligation, ligation of inferior vena cava |

The root operation **Occlusion** is coded when the objective of the procedure is to close off a tubular body part or orifice. **Occlusion** includes both intraluminal and extraluminal methods of closing off the body part. Division of the tubular body part prior to closing it is an integral part of the **Occlusion** procedure.

---

**Coding Guideline B3.12. Occlusion vs. Restriction for Vessel Embolization Procedures**

If the objective of an embolization procedure is to completely close a vessel, the root operation Occlusion is coded. If the objective of an embolization procedure is to narrow the lumen of a vessel, the root operation Restriction is coded.

*Examples:* 1. Tumor embolization is coded to the root operation Occlusion, because the objective of the procedure is to cut off the blood supply to the vessel. 2. Embolization of a cerebral aneurysm is coded to the root operation Restriction, because the objective of the procedure is not to close off the vessel entirely, but to narrow the lumen of the vessel at the site of the aneurysm where it is abnormally wide.

---

Research on embolizations may be required to gain additional information about how the procedure is performed. The purpose of an embolization is to prevent blood flow to an area of the body. It is used during hemorrhage (e.g., arteriovenous [AV] malformation, cerebral aneurysms, GI bleeding, epistaxis, post-partum hemorrhage). However, the procedure has other uses, such as in the treatment of tumors and disorders of the portal vein. An artificial embolus is introduced (coils, particles, foam, plugs). Some of the common agents used to do this are sclerosing agents, ethanol, or Gelfoam. In order to code occlusions and restrictions correctly, the coder must know if it is complete or partial, and physician documentation or additional physician query is essential.

## *Dilation – Root Operation 7*

| Dilation 7 | Definition | Expanding an orifice or the lumen of a tubular body part. |
|---|---|---|
| | Explanation | The orifice can be a natural orifice or an artificially created orifice. Accomplished by stretching a tubular body part using intraluminal pressure or by cutting part of the orifice or wall of the tubular body part. |
| | Examples | Percutaneous transluminal angioplasty, percutaneous transluminal coronary angioplasty (PTCA), laryngeal stenosis dilation, dilation common bile duct. |

The root operation **Dilation** is coded when the objective of the procedure is to enlarge the diameter of a tubular body part or orifice. **Dilation** includes both intraluminal and extraluminal methods of enlarging the diameter. A device placed to maintain the new diameter is an integral part of the **Dilation** procedure, and is coded to a sixth-character device value in the **Dilation** procedure code.

---

**Coding Guideline B4.4. Coronary Arteries**
The coronary arteries are classified as a single body part that is further specified by number of sites treated and not by name or number of arteries. Separate body part values are used to specify the number of sites treated when the same procedure is performed on multiple sites in the coronary arteries.

*Examples*: 1. Angioplasty of two distinct sites in the left anterior descending coronary artery with placement of two stents is coded as Dilation of Coronary Arteries, Two Sites, with Intraluminal Device.
2. Angioplasty of two distinct sites in the left anterior descending coronary artery, one with stent placed and one without, is coded separately as Dilation of Coronary Artery, One Site with Intraluminal Device, and Dilation of Coronary Artery, One Site with No Device.

---

**Coding Note:** In ICD-10-PCS, the classification of the coronary arteries is as a single body part. It doesn't matter what the number of arteries treated is (that is, right coronary artery, left anterior descending, or left circumflex, or the branches). The distinguishing factor is the **number of sites treated**.

---

During PTAs and PTCAs the narrowed or obstructed blood vessel is mechanically widened. Typically, a collapsed balloon on a guide wire (balloon catheter) is passed into the narrowed locations and then inflated. The balloon crushes the fatty deposits, and then the balloon is collapsed and withdrawn. When a device is placed, it is identified by the sixth character. The device values are
- Drug-eluting intraluminal device
- Intraluminal device
- Radioactive intraluminal device

## Bypass – Root Operation 1

| Bypass 1 | Definition | Altering the route of passage of the content of a tubular body part |
|---|---|---|
| | Explanation | Rerouting content of a body part to a downstream area of the normal route, to a similar route and body part, or to an abnormal route and dissimilar body part. Includes one or more anastomoses, with or without the use of a device |
| | Examples | Coronary artery bypass graft (CABG), colostomy formation |

**Bypass** is coded when the objective of the procedure is to reroute the contents of a tubular body part. The range of **Bypass** procedures includes normal routes such as those made in coronary artery bypass procedures, and abnormal routes such as those made in colostomy formation procedures.

---

**Coding Guideline B3.6a. Bypass Procedures**

Bypass procedures are coded by identifying the body part bypassed "from" and the body part bypassed "to." The fourth character body part specifies the body part bypassed from, and the qualifier specifies the body part bypassed to.

*Example*: Bypass from stomach to jejunum, Stomach is the body part and Jejunum is the qualifier.

---

**Coding Guideline B3.6b. Bypass Procedures**

Coronary arteries are classified by number of distinct sites treated, rather than number of coronary arteries or anatomic name of a coronary artery (e.g., left anterior descending). Coronary artery bypass procedures are coded differently than other bypass procedures as described in the previous guideline. Rather than identifying the body part bypassed from, the body part identifies the number of coronary artery sites bypassed to, and the qualifier specifies the vessel bypassed from.

*Example*: Aortocoronary artery bypass of one site on the left anterior descending coronary artery and one site on the obtuse marginal coronary artery is classified in the body part axis of classification as Two Coronary Artery Sites and the qualifier specifies the Aorta as the body part bypassed from.

---

**Coding Guideline B3.6c. Bypass Procedures**

If multiple coronary artery sites are bypassed, a separate procedure is coded for each coronary artery site that uses a different device and/or qualifier.

*Example*: Aortocoronary artery bypass and internal mammary coronary artery bypass are coded separately.

---

**Coding Guideline B3.9. Excision for Graft**

If an autograft is obtained from a different body part in order to complete the objective of the procedure, a separate procedure is coded.

*Example*: Coronary bypass with excision of saphenous vein graft, excision of saphenous vein is coded separately.

---

**Coding Note: Autograft**

An autograft is tissue or organ transferred into a new position in the body of the same individual. Synonyms are autotransplant, autogeneic graft, autologous graft, autoplastic graft (*Stedman's* 2006).

---

The choices for devices are autologous, synthetic substitute, or nonautologous tissue substitute. The definitions for each are listed here:

| Type of Tissue | Device Character | Definition |
|---|---|---|
| Autologous (vein or artery) | 9 or A | Referring to a graft in which the donor and recipient areas are in the same individual |
| Synthetic Substitute | J | Any type of synthetic substitute |
| Nonautologous Tissue Substitute | K | Nonautologous allogeneic donor tissue implanted from one human to another |

---

**Coding Note: Bypass with Free Graft**

| Non-Coronary | | Coronary Artery | |
|---|---|---|---|
| *Downstream Route* | | | |
| **Body Part** | **Qualifier** | **Body Part** | **Qualifier** |
| FROM | TO | NUMBER OF SITES | FROM |

---

**Coding Note:** When assigning the device value, the key to remember is that to be considered a device, it needs to be material used as a graft (separated) and not moved over. For example, when the internal mammary is loosened from one side and brought around to the occluded coronary artery, the artery is not used as free graft material—this would be considered No Device.

---

2.45. An osteotomy was performed to enlarge the right lacrimal fossa. The stenotic puncta was dilated with increasingly larger lacrimal probes in both superior and inferior canaliculi. A silicone tube was passed through the superior and inferior canaliculi through the osteotomy into the nose and secured.

Code(s): _____

**2.46.** The patient has respiratory failure and multiple attempts to wean from the ventilator have been unsuccessful; therefore, the decision to perform a tracheostomy was made. A 3-cm incision was made approximately two fingerbreadths above the sterna notch. Subcutaneous fat was dissected and removed. The strap muscles were identified and divided and an incision was made between the second and third tracheal ring with an inferior based tracheal flap being created. The inferior tracheal flap was sewn to the inferior skin edge, creating a skin flap with 3-0 Vicryl in order to secure the stoma. The ET tube was slowly withdrawn to just above the tracheostomy site. An 8.0 XLT Shiley trach was inserted with no difficulties.

Code(s): _____

**2.47.** The patient underwent an exploratory laparotomy after presentation with severe urinary hemorrhage. During the procedure, an extensive adenocarcinoma of the left kidney with metastasis to the left lower lobe of the lung, great vessels, and lateral diaphragm was discovered. The tumor could not be removed; therefore, the left ureter was surgically ligated to prevent further urinary hemorrhage.

Code(s): _____

**2.48.** The patient underwent a transabdominal cervical cerclage for cervical incompetence. The abdomen was opened using a transverse suprapubic incision. The vesical peritoneum overlying the lower uterine segment was divided transversely. The needle was passed anteroposteriorly through the paracervical vessels immediately adjacent to the cervix at the level of the cervicoisthmic junction superior to the medial insertions of the uterosacral ligaments. Before being pulled through completely, the band width of the tape was verified as being flush with the anterior cervicoisthmic tissues. The knot was then tied in the posterior.

Code(s): _____

**2.49.** Laparoscopic placement of a gastric band for morbid obesity.

Code(s): _____

**2.50.** The procedure performed is an embolization of the anterior cerebral artery aneurysm. The surgeon made a very small nick in the skin and using image-guidance, the catheter is inserted through the skin and advanced to the anterior cerebral artery. Next the detachable coated platinum coils are inserted through the catheter and placed within the aneurysm for embolization.

Code(s): _____

---

**Coding Guideline B3.9. Excision for Graft**

If an autograft is obtained from a different body part in order to complete the objective of the procedure, a separate procedure is coded.

*Example:* Coronary bypass with excision of saphenous vein graft, excision of saphenous vein is coded separately.

---

**2.51.** CABG x 3, the diagonal and obtuse marginal arteries are bypassed from the aorta utilizing graft material from the patient's left greater saphenous vein and the left descending artery was bypassed using the left internal mammary artery. The left internal mammary artery was dissected as a pedicle using electrocautery and small hemoclips at the same time that the greater saphenous vein was harvested endoscopically from the left lower extremity. Cardiopulmonary bypass was then instituted. (Do not code the cardiopulmonary bypass portion of the procedure).

Code(s): _____

*[handwritten: 2 Answers]*

*[handwritten: Dilation, Artery, coronary One site / Dilation, Artery, coronary, One Site]*

**2.52.** The patient, with known coronary artery disease, underwent a PTCA of two coronary artery sites. Angioplasty was carried out on both the right coronary artery and the left anterior descending coronary artery. A CYPHER drug-eluting stent was placed in proximal-mid left anterior descending coronary artery.

Code(s): _____

*[handwritten: Occulusion - Fallopian tubes. Bilateral]*

**2.53.** Bilateral tubal ligation using Fallope Ring, laparoscopic

Code(s): _____

*[handwritten: Dilation Esophagus, Lower]*

**2.54** The patient underwent an upper endoscopy with balloon dilation of the esophagus for treatment of stricture of the distal esophagus. An Olympus video upper endoscope was passed into the upper esophagus and there was a stricture in the distal esophagus. Balloon dilation was performed in gradations from 36 French to 45 French. The balloon was inflated for 60 seconds. Visualization showed appropriate mucosal dilation. The stomach and duodenum were otherwise normal on endoscopic exam.

Code (s): _____

*[handwritten: Bypass / colon, descending]*

**2.55.** Colostomy formation, open, descending colon to abdominal wall

Code(s): *[handwritten: 0D1M0Z4]* _____

**2.56.** Uterine artery embolization is performed for treatment of uterine fibroids. Utilizing imaging-guidance, a catheter is inserted into the femoral artery and is maneuvered into the uterine arteries. The embolic particles are released into both the right and left uterine artery.

Code (s): _____

**2.57.** The patient has an obstruction of the common bile duct. An ERCP with balloon dilation of the common bile duct is performed to treat the obstruction. During the procedure a scope is passed via the mouth to the biliary system via the duodenum. Once the instrumentation reaches the common bile duct, the dilation is performed. (A fluoroscopy code from the Medical and Surgical Related section would be appropriate if the facility reports this imaging procedure. The fluoroscopy code will be discussed in the Imaging Section.)

Code(s): _____

**2.58.** A patient with obliterative arterial disease with an ischemic right foot undergoes a right femoral to posterior tibial bypass using autologous saphenous graft. The patient's right groin was incised and opened. An excellent portion of the patient's greater saphenous vein was dissected for graft material. A femoral to posterior tibial bypass was then performed.

Code(s): _____

**2.59.** A morbidly obese patient undergoes an open gastric bypass with Roux-en-Y to the jejunum

Code(s): _____

**2.60.** Laryngoscopy with Intraluminal dilation of laryngeal stenosis.

Code(s): _0C7S8ZZ_____

Dilation
Layrnt

# Root Operations That Always Involve a Device

Refer to *ICD-10-PCS 2016 Code Book* Root Operation Definitions.

The six root operations belonging to this group are
- Insertion (H)
- Replacement (R)
- Supplement (U)
- Change (2)
- Removal (P)
- Revision (W)

## *Insertion – Root Operation H*

| Insertion H | Definition | Putting in a non-biological device that monitors, assists, performs, or prevents a physiological function but does not physically take the place of a body part |
|---|---|---|
| | Explanation | N/A |
| | Examples | Insertion of radioactive implant, insertion of central venous catheter |

The root operation **Insertion** represents those procedures where the sole objective is to put in a device without doing anything else to a body part. Procedures typical of those coded to **Insertion** include putting in a vascular catheter, a pacemaker lead, or a tissue expander.

## *Replacement – Root Operation R*

| Replacement R | Definition | Putting in or on biological or synthetic material that physically takes the place and/or function of all or a portion of a body part. |
|---|---|---|
| | Explanation | The body part may have been taken out or replaced, or may be taken out, physically eradicated, or rendered nonfunctional during the **Replacement** procedure. **A Removal procedure is coded for taking out the device used in a previous replacement procedure.** |
| | Examples | Total hip replacement, bone graft, free skin graft, phacoemulsification with IOL implant (phaco without IOL implant is Extraction), heart valve replacement, replacement cornea, free TRAM. |

The objective of procedures coded to the root operation **Replacement** is to put in a device that takes the place of some or all of a body part. **Replacement** encompasses a wide range of procedures, from joint replacements to grafts of all kinds.

**Coding Note:** Replacement includes taking out the body part.

### Supplement – Root Operation U

| Supplement U | Definition | Putting in or on biologic or synthetic material that physically reinforces and/or augments the function of a portion of a body part. |
|---|---|---|
| | Explanation | The biological material is non-living, or is living and from the same individual. The body part may have been previously replaced, and the **Supplement** procedure is performed to physically reinforce and/or augment the function of the replaced body part. |
| | Examples | Herniorrhaphy using mesh (herniorrhaphy without mesh is Repair), free nerve graft, mitral valve ring annuloplasty, put a new acetabular liner in a previous hip replacement, abdominal wall herniorrhaphy using mesh. |

The objective of procedures coded to the root operation **Supplement** is to put in a device that reinforces or augments the functions of some or all of a body part. The body part may have been taken out during a previous procedure, but is not taken out as part of the **Supplement** procedure. **Supplement** includes a wide range of procedures, from hernia repairs using mesh reinforcement to heart valve annuloplasties and grafts such as nerve grafts that supplement but do not physically take the place of the existing body part.

## Change – Root Operation 2

| Change 2 | Definition | Taking out or off a device from a body part and putting back an identical or similar device in or on the same body part without cutting or puncturing the skin or a mucous membrane |
| --- | --- | --- |
| | Explanation | All **Change** procedures are coded using the approach External |
| | Examples | Urinary catheter change, gastrostomy tube change, drainage tube change |

The root operation **Change** represents only those procedures where a similar device is exchanged without making a new incision or puncture. Typical **Change** procedures include exchange of drainage devices and feeding devices.

**Coding Note: Change**
In the root operation Change, general body part values are used when the *specific* body part value is not in the Table.

## Removal – Root Operation P

| Removal P | Definition | Taking out or off a device from a body part. |
|---|---|---|
| | Explanation | If the device is taken out and a similar device is put in without cutting or puncturing the skin or mucous membrane, the procedure is coded to the root operation Change. Otherwise, the procedure for taking out the device is coded to the root operation **Removal**. |
| | Examples | Drainage tube removal, cardiac pacemaker removal, central line removal. |

**Removal** represents a much broader range of procedures than those for removing the devices contained in the root operation **Insertion**. A procedure to remove a device is coded to **Removal** if it is not an integral part of another root operation and regardless of the approach or the original root operation by which the device was put in.

**Coding Note: Removal**
In the root operation Removal, general body part values are used when the specific body part value is not in the Table.

## Revision – Root Operation W

| Revision W | Definition | Correcting, to the extent possible, a malfunctioning or displaced device |
|---|---|---|
| | Explanation | Revision can include correcting a malfunctioning device by taking out and/or putting in part of the device |
| | Examples | Adjustment of pacemaker lead, adjustment of hip prosthesis, revision of pacemaker insertion |

**Revision** is coded when the objective of the procedure is to correct the positioning or function of a previously placed device, without taking the entire device out and putting a whole new device in its place. A complete re-do of the original root operation is coded to the root operation that is performed.

---

**Coding Note: Revision**

In the root operation Revision, general body part values are used when the specific body part value is not in the Table.

---

2.61.  A patient who has a history of compartment syndrome has a tissue expander inserted in the subcutaneous tissue of the right lower leg in preparation for future surgery. The procedure was performed via open incision.

Code(s): _____

2.62.  The patient underwent a left inguinal hernia repair with Marlex mesh for a left inguinal hernia. An inguinal incision was made and carried down through the subcutaneous tissues until the external oblique fascia was reached. A piece of 3x5 mesh was obtained and trimmed to fit. It was placed in the inguinal canal.

Code(s): _____

2.63.  The patient has a chest tube in the right pleural cavity for a right pneumothorax. The chest tube was exchanged for a new similar chest tube.

Code(s): _____

2.64.  The patient underwent percutaneous lamellar keratoplasty, with donor corneal tissue, bilateral.

Code(s): _____

---

**Coding Guideline B3.2b. Multiple Procedures**

During the same root operation, multiple procedures are coded if the same root operation is repeated at different body sites that are included in the same body part value.

*Example:* Excision of the Sartorius muscle and excision of the gracilis muscle are both included in the upper leg muscle body part value, and multiple procedures are coded.

---

**2.65.** Percutaneous replacement of transvenous right atrial and ventricular leads of a dual chambered pacemaker. The pacemaker was initially placed four years ago. The generator remains intact and is not replaced.

Code(s): _____

**2.66.** Open heart surgery for repair of atrial septal defect with mesh.

Code(s): _____

**2.67.** The patient undergoes a placement of a dual chamber pacemaker for treatment of symptomatic sick sinus syndrome. An incision was made and a subcutaneous pocket in the chest wall area was created. The generator was placed in the subcutaneous pocket and the incision was closed. Both the right atrial and right ventricle leads were placed percutaneously.

Code(s): _____

**2.68.** A patient with critical aortic valvular stenosis undergoes aortic valve replacement with a 21 mm St. Jude Medical Biocor bioprosthetic porcine valve. At the beginning of the procedure a median sternotomy incision was made and the sternum was split along the midline using a sternal saw.

Code(s): _____

**2.69.** Adjustment of position, pacemaker lead in right atrium, percutaneous

Code(s): _____

**2.70.** The patient has full-thickness burn injuries to the left buttock and left thigh. Application of cultured epidermal graft to the full-thickness burn injuries of the left buttock and left thigh was performed. The patient had previously undergone preparation with excision and removal of allograft and granulation tissue in preparation for application of cultured epidermal graft today.

Code(s): _____

**2.71.** Cystoscopy with retrieval of right ureteral stent

Code(s): _____

**2.72.** Tracheostomy tube exchange

Code(s): _____

**2.73.** Left reverse shoulder replacement, metal on polyethylene

Code (s): _____

**2.74.** Insertion of PICC line. Under ultrasound guidance, a #21 gauge needle was placed into the right subclavian vein. A wire was passed percutaneously into the superior vena cava. The catheter was then placed down to the superior vena cava.

Code(s): _____

**2.75.** The patient underwent removal of hardware of the right distal humerus due to excessive pain from the hardware. An incision was made directly over the prominent screws going up into the humerus both medially and laterally. Dissection was carried down bluntly to the screw head and the screw head was delivered through the incision. Both screws were removed.

Code(s): _____

**2.76.** Percutaneous insertion of posterior spinous process decompression device (spinal stabilization device), L2-L3.

Code(s): _____

**2.77.** Right tibia and fibula Z osteotomy with insertion of external limb lengthening devices on each bone.

Code(s): _____

**2.78.** Placement of a dual chamber implantable pacing cardioverter-defibrillator. An incision was made under the left clavicle. A pocket was made in the subcutaneous tissue and the ICD generator was placed into the pocket. Leads were percutaneously inserted to both the right ventricle and right atrial appendage. The leads were then attached to the generator, which was tested and sutured down in the pocket. Wounds closed in layers.

Code(s): _____

**2.79.** The patient underwent a right hip hemiarthroplasty for a right femoral neck fracture. An anterolateral incision of the right hip was made and carried down through skin, subcutaneous tissue, IT bland and gluteus maximus. The capsule was identified and opened in an H-fashion. The femoral head was removed and sized to a size 47 metal implant. A 9 press-fit stem was placed, put through a trial range of motion and found to be adequate. The stem was cemented.

Code(s): _____

**2.80.** Percutaneous insertion of bone growth stimulator, left femoral shaft.

Code(s): _____

## Root Operations Involving Examination Only

Refer to *ICD-10-PCS 2016 Code Book* Root Operation Definitions.

The two root operations belonging to this group are
- Inspection (J)
- Map (K)

## *Inspection – Root Operation J*

| Inspection J | Definition | Visually and/or manually exploring a body part |
|---|---|---|
| | Explanation | Visual exploration may be performed with or without optical instrumentation. Manual exploration may be performed directly or through intervening body layers |
| | Examples | Diagnostic arthroscopy, exploratory laparotomy, diagnostic cystoscopy |

The root operation **Inspection** represents procedures where the sole objective is to examine a body part. Procedures that are discontinued without any other root operation being performed are also coded to **Inspection**.

---

**Coding Guideline B3.11a. Inspection Procedures**

Inspection of a body part(s) performed in order to achieve the objective of a procedure is not coded separately.

*Example*: Fiberoptic bronchoscopy performed for irrigation of bronchus, only the irrigation procedure is coded.

---

**Coding Guideline B3.11b. Inspection Procedures**

If multiple tubular body parts are inspected, the most distal body part inspected is coded. If multiple non-tubular body parts in a region are inspected, the body part that specifies the entire area inspected is coded.

*Examples*: 1. Cystourethroscopy with inspection of bladder and ureters is coded to the Ureter body part value. 2. Exploratory laparotomy with general inspection of abdominal contents is coded to the Peritoneal Cavity body part value.

---

**Coding Guideline B3.11c. Inspection Procedures**

When both an Inspection procedure and another procedure are performed on the same body part during the same episode, if the Inspection procedure is performed using a different approach than the other procedure, the Inspection procedure is coded separately.

*Example*: Endoscopic inspection of the duodenum is coded separately when open Excision of the duodenum is performed during the same procedural episode.

**Coding Note:** Procedures that are discontinued without any other root operation being performed are coded to Inspection.

**Coding Guideline B4.8 Upper and Lower Intestinal Tract**
In the Gastrointestinal body system, the general body part values Upper Intestinal Tract and Lower Intestinal Tract are provided as an option for the root operations Change, Inspection, Removal, and Revision. Upper Intestinal Tract includes the portion of the gastrointestinal tract from the esophagus down to and including the duodenum, and Lower Intestinal Tract includes the portion of the gastrointestinal tract from the jejunum down to and including the rectum and anus.

*Example:* In the root operation Change table, change of a device in the jejunum is coded using the body part Lower Intestinal Tract.

## Map – Root Operation K

| Map K | Definition | Locating the route of passage of electrical impulses and/or locating functional areas in a body part |
| --- | --- | --- |
| | Explanation | Applicable only to the cardiac conduction mechanism and the central nervous system |
| | Examples | Cardiac mapping, cortical mapping, cardiac electrophysiological study |

The root operation **Map** represents a very narrow range of procedures. Procedures include only cardiac mapping and cortical mapping.

---

**Coding Note:** The only two body systems under Map Procedures are the Central Nervous System (00K) and Heart and Great Vessels (02K).

---

**2.81.** An elderly patient is seen after a syncope incident and is suspected to be suffering from bowel ischemia. An open exploratory laparotomy of the gastrointestinal tract is performed with no evidence of transmural ischemia or necrosis.

Codes(s): _____

**2.82.** Mapping of right hemisphere of the brain, percutaneous

Code(s): _____

---

**Coding Guideline B3.2d Multiple Procedures**
During the same operative episode, multiple procedures are coded if the intended root operation is attempted using one approach, but is converted to a different approach.

*Example:* Laparoscopic cholecystectomy converted to an open cholecystectomy is coded as percutaneous endoscopic Inspection and open Resection.

---

**2.83.** The patient was admitted to have a thoracoscopic lobectomy performed. The patient has a malignant neoplasm of the right middle lobe of the lung. Being unable to advance through the entire right lung because of extensive pleural effusion, the surgeon was unable to complete the procedure endoscopically. The procedure was then converted to an open technique, and a successful lobectomy was performed.

Code(s): _____

**2.84.** Diagnostic bronchoscopy of the left bronchus

Code(s): _____

**2.85.** Colonoscopy to the descending colon

Code(s): _____

**2.86.** Heart catheterization with cardiac mapping

Code(s): _____

**2.87.** The patient underwent a flexible cystoscopy to recheck a previous bladder lesion removal. The flexible scope was inserted per urethra into bladder and landmarks noted. Bladder was grossly normal. Urethroscopic examination revealed a trilobar obstructive prostate.

Code(s): _____

# Root Operations That Define Other Repairs

Refer to *ICD-10-PCS 2016 Code Book* Root Operation Definitions.

The two root operations belonging to this group are
- Control (3)
- Repair (Q)

## *Control – Root Operation 3*

| Control 3 | Definition | Stopping, or attempting to stop, postprocedural bleeding |
|---|---|---|
| | Explanation | The site of the bleeding is coded as an anatomical region and not to a specific body part |
| | Examples | Control of post-prostatectomy hemorrhage, control of post-tonsillectomy hemorrhage |

**Control** is used to represent a small range of procedures performed to treat postprocedural bleeding. If the following procedures are required to stop the bleeding, **Control** is not coded separately.
- Bypass
- Detachment
- Excision
- Extraction
- Reposition
- Replacement
- Resection

---

**Coding Guideline B3.7. Control vs. More Definitive Root Operations**

The root operation Control is defined as, "stopping, or attempting to stop, postprocedural bleeding." If an attempt to stop postprocedural bleeding is initially unsuccessful, and to stop the bleeding requires performing any of the definitive root operations Bypass, Detachment, Excision, Extraction, Reposition, Replacement, or Resection, that root operation is coded instead of Control.

*Example*: Resection of spleen to stop postprocedural bleeding is coded to Resection instead of Control.

---

**Coding Note: Control**

Control includes irrigation or evacuation of hematoma done at the operative site. Both irrigation and evacuation may be necessary to clear the operative field and effectively stop the bleeding.

## *Repair – Root Operation Q*

| Repair Q | Definition | Restoring, to the extent possible, a body part to its normal anatomic structure and function |
|---|---|---|
| | Explanation | Used only when the method to accomplish the repair is not one of the other root operations |
| | Examples | Herniorrhaphy, suture of laceration |

The root operation **Repair** represents a broad range of procedures for restoring the anatomic structure of a body part such as suture of lacerations. Repair also functions as the Not Elsewhere Classified (NEC) root operation, to be used when the procedure performed does not meet the definition of one of the other root operations. Fixation devices are included for procedures to repair the bones and joints.

---

**Coding Note: Limited NEC Code Options**
- ICD-9-CM often designates codes as Not Elsewhere Classified or Other Specified versions of a procedure throughout the code set. NEC options are also provided in ICD-10-PCS, but only for specific, limited use.
- In the Medical and Surgical section, two significant NEC options are the root operations value Q, Repair and the device value Y, Other Device.
- The root operation Repair is a true NEC value. It is used only when the procedure performed is not one of the other root operations in the Medical and Surgical section.

---

2.88. The patient presents for surgical repair of a rotator cuff tear of the left shoulder and undergoes arthroscopic investigation and repair of the glenoid labrum ligament.

Code(s): _____

2.89. A patient is returned to the operating room after open heart surgery to investigate post operative hemorrhage. An incision is made at the original operative site and the source of the bleeding is identified in the pericardial cavity and repaired.

Code(s): _____

2.90. Arthroscopy with drainage of hemarthrosis at site of previous repair, left shoulder

Code(s): _____

2.91. The patient underwent an umbilical hernia repair. The incision from a previous surgery was opened and sharp dissection lead to identification of the hernia, which was dissected free from surrounding tissues. The contents were reduced into the abdominal cavity and the edges were reapproximated with sutures.

Code(s): _____

**2.92.** Suture of laceration of subcutaneous tissue and fascia of the left foot with layered closure.

Code(s): _____

---

**Coding Guideline B5.3a External Approach**

Procedures performed within an orifice on structures that are visible without the aid of any instrumentation are coded to the approach External.

*Example:* Resection of tonsils is coded to the approach External

---

**2.93.** The patient experienced post-tonsillectomy bleeding. The patient had an arterial bleeder from the right tonsillar fossa. A Crowe-Davis mouth gag was placed, and clots were suctioned from the pharynx. An arterial bleeder was noted and was controlled with suction cautery.

Code(s): _____

---

**Coding Guideline B4.7 Fingers and Toes**

If a body system does not contain a separate body part value for fingers, procedures performed on the fingers are coded to the body part value for the hand. If a body system does not contain a separate body part value for toes, procedures performed on the toes are coded to the body part value for the foot.

*Example:* Excision of finger muscle is coded to one of the hand muscle body part values in the Muscles body system.

---

**2.94.** The patient underwent a suture repair of the left extensor tendon to repair a complex laceration of the dorsal aspect of the left index finger with laceration of the extensor tendon.

Code(s): _____

# Root Operations That Define Other Objectives

Refer to *ICD-10-PCS 2016 Code Book* Root Operation Definitions.

The three root operations belonging to this group are
- Fusion (G)
- Alteration (0)
- Creation (4)

## *Fusion – Root Operation G*

| Fusion G | Definition | Joining together portions of an articular body part rendering the articular body part immobile |
|---|---|---|
| | Explanation | The body part is joined together by fixation device, bone graft, or other means |
| | Examples | Spinal fusion, ankle arthrodesis |

A limited range of procedures is represented in the root operation **Fusion**, because fusion procedures are by definition only performed on the joints. Qualifier values are used to specify whether a vertebral joint fusion uses an anterior or posterior approach, and whether the anterior or posterior column of the spine is fused.

---

**Coding Guideline B3.10a. Fusion Procedures of the Spine**
The body part coded for a spinal vertebral joint(s) rendered immobile by a spinal fusion procedure is classified by the level of the spine (e.g., Thoracic). There are distinct body part values for a single vertebral joint and for multiple joints at each spinal level.

*Example:* Body part values specify Lumbar Vertebral Joint, Lumbar Vertebral Joints, 2 or More, and Lumbosacral Vertebral Joint.

---

**Coding Guideline B3.10b. Fusion Procedures of the Spine**
If multiple vertebral joints are fused, a separate procedure is coded for each vertebral joint that uses a different device and/or qualifier.

*Example:* Fusion of lumbar vertebral joint, Posterior approach, Anterior column and Fusion of lumbar vertebral joint, Posterior approach, Posterior column are coded separately.

---

**Coding Guideline B3.10c. Fusion Procedures of the Spine**
Combinations of devices and materials are often used on a vertebral joint to render the joint immobile. When combinations of devices are used on the same vertebral joint, the device value coded for the procedure is as follows:

- If an interbody fusion device is used to render the joint immobile (alone or containing other material like bone graft), the procedure is coded with the device value Interbody Fusions Device
- If bone graft is the only device used to render the joint immobile, the procedure is coded with the device value Nonautologous Tissue Substitute or Autologous Tissue Substitute
- If a mixture of autologous and nonautologous bone graft (with or without biological or synthetic extenders or binders) is used to render the joint immobile, code the procedure with the device value Autologous Tissue Substitute.

*Examples*:

- Fusion of a vertebral joint using a cage style interbody fusion device containing morselized bone graft is coded to the device Interbody Fusion Device.
- Fusion of a vertebral joint using a bone dowel interbody fusion device made of cadaver bone and packed with a mixture of local morselized bone and demineralized bone matrix is coded to the device Interbody Fusion Device.
- Fusion of a vertebral joint using both autologous bone graft and bone bank bone graft is coded to the device Autologous Tissue Substitute.

**Coding Note:** When coding fusions, it is important to understand that PCS body part values are classified as joints and not vertebra. For example, if a fusion is done at L1-L2, this is value 0, Lumbar vertebral joint (single), or one joint. If a fusion is done on L1-L3, this is value 1, Lumbar Vertebral Joints, 2 or more, for 2 joints.

## *Alteration – Root Operation 0*

| Alteration 0 | Definition | Modifying the natural anatomic structure of a body part without affecting the function of the body part |
|---|---|---|
| | Explanation | Principal purpose is to improve appearance |
| | Examples | Face lift, breast augmentation, cosmetic liposuction (Liposuction for medical reasons is Extraction.) |

**Alteration** is coded for all procedures performed solely to improve appearance. All methods, approaches, and devices used for the objective of improving appearance are coded here.

---

**Coding Note: Alteration**

Because some surgical procedures can be performed for either medical or cosmetic purposes, coding for Alteration requires diagnostic confirmation that the surgery is in fact performed to improve appearance. If the procedure is done for medical conditions, the appropriate root operation is assigned such as Extraction, Reposition, Resection, Repair, Replacement, and such.

---

## Creation – Root Operation 4

| Creation 4 | Definition | Making a new genital structure that does not physically take the place of a body part |
| --- | --- | --- |
| | Explanation | Used only for sex change operations |
| | Examples | Creation of vagina in a male, creation of penis in a female |

**Creation** is used to represent a very narrow range of procedures. Only the procedures performed for sex change operations are included here.

---

**Coding Note: Harvesting Autograft Tissue**

If a separate procedure is performed to harvest autograft tissue, it is coded to the appropriate root operation in addition to the primary procedure.

---

The qualifier identifies the body part being created, either vagina or penis. The body part values are **M**, Perineum, Male or **N**, Perineum, Female and pertain to the current sex of the patient.

---

**Coding Note: Creation**

| Body Part . . . | Started As . . . | Female |
| --- | --- | --- |
| Qualifier . . . | Going To . . . | Male |

---

2.95. Open posterior lumbar interbody fusion, anterior column at L2-L4 levels, using BAK threaded fusion cages and Danek pedicle screws with nonautologous bone graft.

Code(s): _____

2.96. A patient presents for a cosmetic rhinoplasty in which a Goretex implant is placed via an incision.

Code(s): _____

2.97. The patient underwent a percutaneous arthrodesis of the carpometacarpal joint of the right thumb using a cannulated screw and threaded washer.

Code(s): _____

2.98. The patient undergoes male to female gender-reassignment surgery in which a vagina is formed using an autograft that was previously harvested.

Code(s): _____

**2.99.** The patient undergoes a female to male sex-change operation in which a penis is created using synthetic material.

Code(s): _____

**2.100.** Anterior lumbar arthrodesis of L1-L3 through a posterior approach, posterior lumbar segmental instrumentation (pedicle-based) of L1-L3 and local bone graft from right rib, open approach.

Code(s): _____

**2.101.** Bilateral breast augmentation with silicone implants, open

Code(s): _____

**2.102.** Abdominoplasty, open (tummy tuck)

Code(s): _____

# Part II: ICD-10-PCS Coding

## ICD-10-PCS Training—Day 2

# Case Studies from Inpatient Health Records

## Detailed and/or Complex Cases and Scenarios Using ICD-10-PCS Procedure Codes

---

**Coding Guideline B3.2a. Multiple Procedures**
During the same operative episode, multiple procedures are coded if the same root operation is performed on different body parts as defined by distinct values of the body part character.

---

**Coding Guideline B4.3. Bilateral Body Part Values**
Bilateral body part values are available for a limited number of body parts. If the identical procedure is performed on contralateral body parts, and a bilateral body part value exists for that body part, a single procedure is coded using the bilateral body part value. If no bilateral body part value exists, each procedure is coded separately using the appropriate body part value.

---

**3.1.**

**Preoperative Diagnosis:** Abnormal bleeding; pelvic pain; uterine retroversion and malposition; uterine descensus; abnormal liver function studies; status-postop ovarian cystectomies; status-postop cesarean section, tubal ligation

**Postoperative Diagnosis:** Same

**Operation:** Total abdominal hysterectomy; bilateral salpingo-oophorectomy; liver biopsy

**Procedure:** With the patient in the supine position under general anesthesia, the abdomen was prepped and draped in the usual sterile fashion. A Pfannenstiel incision was made in the area of the patient's previous Pfannenstiel incision and this was carried down through the subcutaneous fat to the fascia, which was incised transversely. The fascia was dissected off of the underlying rectus muscles. Bleeders were coagulated. The rectus muscles were separated from the fascia above. There was some scarring of the fascia, particularly on the patient's left side. The rectus muscles were parted. The peritoneum was identified. Entry was made into the peritoneal cavity without difficulty. The peritoneal incision was carried inferiorly to superiorly. At this point, I explored the upper abdomen and performed a Tru-Cut needle biopsy of the left lobe of the liver without difficulty.

Coagulation was utilized to control bleeding. Hemostasis was established and at the end of the procedure, the area of the biopsy site was re-evaluated and was noted to be hemostatic. A moist lap was used against this area for compression during the remaining portion of the case, and this lap was removed prior to closing the abdomen.

At this time, the O'Conner-O'Sullivan retractor was put in place. A series of moist laps were used to pack the bowel out of the operative field. The uterus was noted to be markedly retroverted with marked pelvic congestion and the large infundibulopelvic vessels were noted, as well as the broad ligament. The round ligaments were bilaterally doubly Heaney clamped, cut, and suture ligated with 0 Vicryl. The anterior leaf of the broad ligament and posterior leaf of the broad ligament were sharply dissected. Hemostasis was accomplished by coagulation. The quadrangular space was bluntly penetrated bilaterally. Two ligatures of 0 Vicryl were put in place along the infundibulopelvic vessels after taking care to assure the location of the ureters was out of the operative field. This area was then clamped and cut. Hemostasis along the infundibulopelvic pedicle was noted to be good. The ovaries and fallopian tubes were bilaterally removed. There was a right ovarian cyst with multiple smaller cysts noted on the right ovary. The left ovary appeared to be somewhat scarred and was small and reflective of a previous partial oophorectomy, which was performed many years ago on this ovary. The anterior leaf of the broad ligament was sharply dissected. The bladder was sharply dissected off the anterior aspect of the lower uterine segment.

The uterine vessels were bilaterally doubly Heaney clamped, cut, and suture ligated with 0 Vicryl. The remaining portions of the uterine vessels and cardinal ligaments were singularly Ochsner clamped, cut, and suture ligated with 0 Vicryl. The bladder was further dissected off of the anterior aspect of the lower uterine segment. The uterosacral ligaments were singularly Ochsner clamped, cut, and suture ligated with 0 Vicryl, which was held. Entrance was made into the lateral aspects of the vagina. The cervix was sharply dissected away from the vaginal mucosa and the uterine body (uterus and cervix) were removed in total. Aldrich angle sutures were put in place bilaterally. The anterior and posterior vaginal cuffs were approximated with a series of interrupted figure-of-eight sutures utilizing 0 Vicryl. Hemostasis was noted to be good. Copious irrigation was carried out with good evidence of hemostasis in the pelvis. At this time, the O'Conner-O'Sullivan and lap squares were removed. Further visualization of the liver biopsy site was noted and found to be hemostatic.

At this point, the abdomen was closed in a series of layers. The peritoneum was closed with 0 Vicryl in a running fashion. The rectus muscles were reapproximated with 0 Vicryl interrupted mattress sutures. The fascia was closed with #1 Vicryl in a running fashion. Small bleeders were coagulated in the subcutaneous fat. The skin was closed with staples. A sterile dressing was applied. The patient will be sent to Recovery following the procedure. Sponge, lap, and instrument counts were correct times two.

Code(s): _____

> **Coding Guideline B3.15. Reposition for Fracture Treatment**
> Reduction of a displaced fracture is coded to the root operation Reposition and the application of a cast or splint in conjunction with the Reposition procedure is not coded separately. Treatment of a nondisplaced fracture is coded to the procedure performed.

> **Coding Guideline B4.7. Fingers and Toes**
> If a body system does not contain a separate body part value for fingers, procedures performed on the fingers are coded to the body part value for the hand. If a body system does not contain a separate body part value for toes, procedures performed on the toes are coded to the body part value for the foot.

### 3.2.

**Preoperative Diagnosis:** Extensive laceration of distal left index finger with partial severance of distal phalanx

**Postoperative Diagnosis:** Same

**Operation:** Open reduction internal fixation distal phalanx left index finger with Kirschner wire stabilization; nonexcisional debridement of laceration of left index finger; repair laceration left middle finger

**Procedure:** The patient was prepped and draped in the usual manner after an axillary block had been administered. The patient had a Miter saw go into his index finger, lacerating the dorsal radial aspect of the index finger at the distal phalangeal phalanx level. The saw went into the base of the nail. We used the C-arm fluoroscopy to thoroughly evaluate the area and then inflated the tourniquet to 280 mm of Mercury after the arm had been exsanguinated. The wound was thoroughly irrigated with saline solution to which antibiotics had been added and the subcutaneous tissue was debrided of all devitalized tissue, trash, and foreign bodies that were present in the tissue. I then used a Kirschner wire of 0.045 inches in diameter and drilled across the fracture site in the joint to totally stabilize the area. Once this was in place, I then very carefully closed the skin with interrupted running 5-0 Ethibond suture. The area of laceration on the middle finger was just distal to the insertion of the extensor tendon. It looks like the bulk of the nail bed would be viable, but he had some damage to the base of the nail bed. The laceration of the left middle finger, which extended into the subcutaneous tissue, was then repaired with 4-0 Vicryl sutures. A large compression dressing was applied.
(Note: Code only the Medical and Surgical section procedures.)

Code(s): _____

> **Coding Guideline B4.1a. Body Part Guideline**
> If a procedure is performed on a portion of a body part that does not have a separate body part value, code the body part value corresponding to the whole body part.

**3.3.**

**Preoperative Diagnosis:** Left upper eyelid laceration and chin laceration

**Postoperative Diagnosis:** Same

**Operation:** Repair of left upper eyelid and chin lacerations

**Procedure:** After the patient was suitably prepared under general anesthesia, the left upper eyelid and chin were dressed and draped with Betadine. The left upper eyelid laceration (3 cm) was inspected. It did appear to go through the left upper eyelid canaliculus. The distal end could be seen, the proximal end could not. It was elected not to try to repair the canaliculus. One interrupted 6-0 silk suture was placed through the lid margin and then three interrupted 5-0 Vicryl sutures were placed through the deep tissue. A running 6-0 silk suture was then placed through the skin.

The 2.0 cm chin laceration of the skin was closed with three interrupted 6-0 silk sutures. Gentamicin ointment was applied to the lacerations and a dressing was placed over the left eye. The patient tolerated the procedure well and left the operating room in stable condition.

Code(s): _____

> **Coding Guideline B3.1b. General Guidelines for Root Operation**
> Components of a procedure specified in the root operation definition and explanation are not coded separately. Procedural steps necessary to reach the operative site and close the operative site, including anastomosis of a tubular body part, are also not coded separately.

**3.4.**

**Operation:** Transurethral resection of the prostate

**Anesthesia:** Spinal

**Procedure:** After operative consent, the patient was brought to the operating room and placed on the table in the supine position. With spinal anesthesia induced, the patient was converted to the dorsolithotomy position. The genital area was prepped and draped in the usual and sterile fashion. A 26 French continuous flow resectoscope sheath was inserted per urethra into the bladder with the obturator in place. The obturator was removed and the resectoscope was seated within its sheath. The bladder was visualized. The ureteral orifices were identified. The resectoscope was pulled to the distal portion of the verumontanum and turned to the 12 o'clock position, and resection of the posterior lobe was begun. Resection of the posterior lobe was carried circumferentially around the glans, channeling a large channel. Hemostasis was obtained by means of electrocoagulation. There were no major venous sinuses or capsular perforations encountered. The verumontanum was left intact. After completion of resection of the posterior lobe, the bladder was evacuated of residual prostatic chips using the Ellik evacuator. The bladder was then visualized. There were no residual chips identified. Ureteral orifices were intact and uninjured. The bladder neck and prostatic fossa were widely patent. Final hemostasis was obtained by means of electrocoagulation, and the resectoscope was removed. A 22 French, 3-way, 30-cc Foley catheter was inserted per urethra into the bladder with ease. It was irrigated until clear. It was placed on light traction with continuous bladder irrigation with sterile water, and the patient was transported to the recovery room in stable condition.

Code(s): _____

---

**Coding Guideline B3.1b. General Guidelines for Root Operation**
Components of a procedure specified in the root operation definition and explanation are not coded separately. Procedural steps necessary to reach the operative site and close the operative site, including anastomosis of a tubular body part, are also not coded separately.

---

---

**Coding Guideline B3.8. Excision vs. Resection**
PCS contains specific body parts for anatomical subdivisions of a body part, such as lobes of the lungs or liver and regions of the intestine. Resection of the specific body part is coded whenever all of the body part is cut out or off, rather than coding Excision of a less specific body part.

---

### 3.5

**Preoperative Diagnosis:** Bronchial alveolar cell carcinoma of the left lung

**Postoperative Diagnosis:** Same

**Operation:** Exploratory left thoracotomy; left total pneumonectomy

**Procedure:** This patient was operated on under general endotracheal anesthesia. We used a double lumen tube where we could selectively ventilate both lungs. He was in the lateral decubitus position. A standard posterior lateral left thoracotomy incision was made and the chest was opened. There was a large diffuse lesion in the left upper lobe periphery. The lesion had previously been biopsied, and we thought we were dealing with a bronchial alveolar cell carcinoma. The man did have a past history of non-Hodgkin's lymphoma years ago, which was presumably cured. I began dissecting on the pulmonary artery to look at things to see what kind of fissure I had developed, but the inner lobar branches were just too dense; that is, there was basically no fissure. I knew if I did a lobectomy, it was really entering the tumor area peripherally. I therefore went ahead and elected to do a left pneumonectomy since his pulmonary function studies were satisfactory preop. The main pulmonary artery was divided between a vascular staple gun. Dissection was a little tenuous. The artery seemed quite friable, but it held nicely. I then reinforced this with a large Chromic tie. We divided the superior and inferior pulmonary vein and prepared for clamping of the bronchus. This completed the pneumonectomy. He tolerated the procedure well. He had some hypotension, but he was hypotensive on induction throughout the entire procedure. Blood gases were satisfactory during clamping of the mainstem bronchus, and he seemed to be reacting well. We closed the chest in layers with Dexon pericostal sutures, approximated clips on the skin.

Code(s): _____

**3.6.**

**Preoperative Diagnosis:** Localized area of extensive fibrocystic mastitis, upper outer quadrant, right breast

**Postoperative Diagnosis:** Same

**Operation:** Partial mastectomy (quadrectomy), upper outer quadrant, right breast

**Procedure:** The patient was prepped and draped in the usual manner after general anesthesia had been achieved. Local anesthesia with Xylocaine and Marcaine, to which Epinephrine had been added, was infiltrated around the breast to lessen the postoperative pain. This patient had a localized area of extensive fibrocystic mastitis in the upper outer quadrant of the right breast, which was persistently tender. We made an infra-areolar incision around the upper outer quadrant of the right breast and then undermined the skin to the upper outer quadrant. We were able then to carry out a wedge excision of the right breast, removing the full thickness of the breast in a traditional quadrectomy and partial mastectomy type. The specimen was then sent to the laboratory for histological frozen section. This revealed it to be a benign fibrocystic mastitis without any evidence of malignancy. Hemostasis was secured with electrocoagulation, and then the breast parenchyma was secured with electrocoagulation. The breast parenchyma was then reconstructed with 2-0 Dexon suture, followed by 4-0 chromic, and finally 4-0 subcuticular Prolene. A large compression dressing and Jobst mammary support were applied.

Code(s): _____

---

**Coding Guideline C2. Procedures Following Delivery or Abortion**
Procedures performed following a delivery or abortion for curettage of the endometrium or evacuation of retained products of conception are all coded in the Obstetrics section, to the root operation Extraction and the body part Products of Conception, Retained. Diagnostic or therapeutic dilation and curettage performed during times other than the postpartum or post-abortion period are all coded in the Medical and Surgical section, to the root operation Extraction and the body part Endometrium.

---

**3.7.**

**Preoperative Diagnosis:** Retained placenta

**Postoperative Diagnosis:** Same

**Operation:** Manual extraction of placenta

**Procedure:** The patient was brought to the operating room, where anesthesia was administered. The patient was then placed in the dorsal lithotomy position, prepped and draped in the usual fashion. Exam under anesthesia at this time revealed a dilated cervix and placenta was palpated secondary to previous vaginal delivery. At this time, the placenta was then gently extracted via manual extraction. The placenta appeared to be completely intact.

Code(s): _____

Code(s): _____

> **Coding Guideline B3.2c. Multiple Procedures**
> During the same operative episode, multiple procedures are coded if multiple root operations with distinct objectives are performed on the same body part.

> **Coding Guideline B3.6a. Bypass Procedures**
> Bypass procedures are coded by identifying the body part bypassed "from" and the body part bypassed "to." The fourth character body part specifies the body part bypassed "from," and the qualifier specifies the body part bypassed "to."

### 3.8.

**Procedure Performed:** Subtotal gastrectomy with Billroth II anastomosis

The patient is a 56-year-old male who was admitted with a history of hematemesis for the past 36 hours. He also had some tarry black stools and was noted to have a giant gastric ulcer which was actively bleeding. Patient was subsequently referred for surgical intervention.

**Operative Procedure:** The patient was brought to the operating room and placed on the table in a supine position, at which time general anesthesia was administered without difficulty. His abdomen was then prepped and draped in the usual sterile fashion. An upper midline incision was made. The peritoneum was then entered using the Metzenbaum scissors and hemostats. A retractor was placed, and he was noted to have a cirrhotic liver with micronodular cirrhosis. The left lobe of the liver was mobilized at that point, and the retractors were placed. On palpation of the stomach along the lesser curvature at approximately the mid portion, there was a large gastric ulcer located in the body of the stomach. At this point, the gastrocolic omentum was taken off the greater curvature of the stomach to the level just above the pylorus. Additionally, the lesser omentum was taken down off the lesser curvature of the stomach to the level just above the pylorus. The body of the stomach was then transected approximately 3 cm above the ulcer. At that point, the stomach was reconstructed in a Billroth II fashion by bringing the jejunum through the transverse colon mesentery. Two stay sutures were placed to align the jejunum along the posterior wall of the stomach, and a GIA stapler was used to create the anastomosis without difficulty. The stomach and jejunum were then pulled below the transverse colon mesentery, and this was tacked in several places using 3-0 silk sutures. A feeding tube was then placed in the jejunum using the feeding tube kit without difficulty. The abdomen was then irrigated thoroughly using normal saline solution. Hemostasis was achieved using Bovie electrocautery. The midline incision was then closed using #1 PDS in a running fashion. The skin was closed using skin staples. A sterile dressing was applied. The patient was extubated in the operating room and returned to the intensive care unit in guarded condition.

Code(s): _____

> **Coding Guideline B 3.9. Excision for Graft**
> If an autograft is obtained from a different body part in order to complete the objective of the procedure, a separate procedure is coded.

**3.9.**

**Preoperative Diagnosis:** Full thickness burn to right foot

**Postoperative Diagnosis:** Same

**Operation:** Split thickness skin graft from right thigh to right foot

**Indications:** The patient is a 33-year-old male who suffered a full thickness burn to his right foot. The patient has a history of cardiac disease and hypertension. The patient is a 40-pack-a-year smoker who quit 10 years ago. The patient presents for elective debridement of wound and split thickness skin graft.

**Operative Description:** The patient was taken to the operating room and placed supine on the operating table. After adequate IV sedation was provided, the right lower extremity was prepped and draped in the standard sterile fashion. Sharp debridement of the ulcer was carried out. The ulcer was approximately 4 × 5 cm in area in the lateral dorsum of the right foot. Debridement was carried down to viable tissue. A 4 × 5 cm split thickness skin graft was harvested from the upper aspect of the right thigh. The graft was then meshed and applied to the right foot wound. The graft was secured with a running locked #3-0 chromic suture. Two centrally located chromic sutures were placed for further support. Attention was placed to the donor site, which was dressed with Xeroform and 4 × 4 gauze. The right lower extremity was then wrapped in Kerlix dressing. Sponge and instrument counts were correct at the end of the case. The patient tolerated the procedure well and was transported to the recovery room.

Code(s): _____

> **Coding Guideline B3.6a. Bypass Procedures**
> Bypass procedures are coded by identifying the body part bypassed "from" and
> the body part bypassed "to." The fourth character body part specifies the body part
> bypassed "from," and the qualifier specifies the body part bypassed "to."

## 3.10.
**Pre- and Postoperative Diagnoses:** Arterial insufficiency of the legs

**Operation:** Aorto-bifemoral bypass graft

**Procedure:** The patient was prepped and draped, and groin incisions were opened.
The common femoral vein and its branches were isolated, and rubber loops were
placed around the vessels. At the completion of this, the abdomen was opened
and explored. The patient was found to have evidence of radiation changes in
the abdominal wall and some of the small bowel. The remainder of the abdominal
exploration was unremarkable.

After the abdomen was explored, a Balfour retractor was put in place. The aorta
and iliacs were mobilized. Bleeding points were controlled with electrocoagulation.
The tapes were placed around the vessel. The vessel was measured, and the aorta
was found to be a 12-mm vessel. An 11 × 6 bifurcated microvelour graft was then
preclotted with the patient's own blood.

An end-to-end anastomosis was made on the aorta and the graft, using a
running suture of 2-0 Prolene. The limbs were taken down through tunnels, and
an end-to-side anastomosis was made between the graft and the femoral arteries with running suture of 4-0 Prolene. The inguinal incisions were closed with
running sutures of 2-0 Vicryl and steel staples in the skin. The subcutaneous tissue was closed with running suture of 3-0 Vicryl, and the skin was closed with steel
staples. A sterile dressing was applied. The patient tolerated the procedure well and
returned to the recovery room in adequate condition.

Code(s): _____

**3.11.**

**Preoperative Diagnosis:** Right trigeminal neuralgia

**Postoperative Diagnosis:** Same

**Operation:** Right percutaneous stereotactic radiofrequency destruction of trigeminal nerve

**Operative Procedure:** After the patient was positioned supine, intravenous sedation was administered. Lateral skull x-ray fluoroscopy was set. The right cheek was infiltrated dermally with Xylocaine, and a small nick in the skin, 2.5 cm lateral to the corner of the mouth, was performed with an 18-gauge needle. The radio-frequency needle with 2 mm exposed tip was then introduced using the known anatomical landmarks and under lateral fluoroscopy guidance into the foramen ovale. Confirmation of the placement of the needle was done by the patient grimacing to pain and by the lateral x-ray. The first treatment, 90 seconds in length, was administered with the tip of the needle 3 mm below the clival line at a temperature of 75 degrees Celsius. The needle was then advanced further to the mid clival line, and another treatment of similar strength and duration was also administered. Finally the third and last treatment was administered with the tip of the needle about 3 cm above the line. The needle was removed. The patient tolerated the procedure well. (Note: Do not code fluoroscopy.)

Code(s): _____

**3.12.**

**Preoperative Diagnosis:** Left inguinal hernia

**Postoperative Diagnosis:** Left inguinal hernia

**Operation:** Left initial inguinal hernia repair with mesh

**Procedure:** The patient is a 35-year-old male who presented with several weeks' history of pain in the left groin associated with a bulge. Examination revealed that the left groin did indeed have a bulge and the right groin was normal. We discussed the procedure as well as the choice of anesthesia.

After preoperative evaluation and clearance, the patient was brought into the operating suite and placed in the supine position on the OR table. General anesthesia was induced. The left groin was sterilely prepped and draped and an inguinal incision made. This was carried down through the subcutaneous tissues until the external oblique fascia was reached. This was split in a direction parallel with its fibers, and the medial aspect of the opening included the external ring. The cord structures were encircled and the cremasteric muscle fiber divided. At this point, the floor of the inguinal canal was examined and the patient did appear to have a weakness here. A piece of 3 × 5 mesh was obtained and trimmed to fit. It was placed down in the inguinal canal and tacked to the pubic tubercle. It was then run inferiorly along the pelvic shelving edge until lateral to the internal ring and tacked down superiorly using interrupted sutures of 0 Prolene. A single stitch was placed lateral to the cord to recreate the internal ring. Details of the mesh were tucked underneath the external oblique fascia. The cord and nerve were allowed to drop back into the wound, and the wound was infiltrated with 30 cc. of half percent Marcaine. The external oblique fascia was then closed with a running suture of 0 Vicryl. Subcutaneous tissues were approximated with interrupted sutures of 3-0 Vicryl. The skin was closed with a running subcuticular suture of 4-0 Vicryl. Benzoin and Steri-Strips and a dry sterile dressing were applied. All sponge, needle, and instrument counts were correct at the end of the procedure. The patient tolerated the procedure well and was taken to the recovery room in stable condition.

Code(s): _____

### 3.13.

**Preoperative Diagnosis:** Dysfunctional uterine bleeding

**Postoperative Diagnosis:** Same

**Operation:** Fractional D&C and Therma-Choice balloon endometrial ablation

**Procedure:** The patient was taken to the OR and under adequate general anesthesia she was prepped and draped in the dorsolithotomy position for a vaginal procedure. The uterus was sounded to approximately 9-10 cm. Using Pratt cervical dilators, the cervix was dilated to the point that a Sims sharp curette could be inserted. The Sims sharp curette was passed to obtain endometrial curetting. After the curetting was obtained, the Therma-Choice system was assembled and primed. The catheter with the balloon was placed inside the endometrial cavity and slowly filled with fluid until it stabilized at a pressure of approximately 175 to 180 mmHg. The system was then preheated and after preheating to 87 degrees Celsius, eight minutes of therapeutic heat was applied to the lining of the endometrium. The fluid was allowed to drain from the balloon and the system was removed. The procedure was then discontinued. All sponge, instrument, and needle counts were correct. The patient tolerated the procedure well and was taken to the recovery room.

Code(s): _____

### 3.14.

**Preoperative Diagnosis:** Right kidney stone

**Postoperative Diagnosis:** Right kidney stone

**Operation:** Extracorporeal shock wave lithotripsy of right kidney stone

**Procedure:** Under IV sedation, the patient was placed in the supine position. The stone in the upper right kidney was positioned at F2. The extracorporeal lithotripsy was started at 19 KV, which subsequently was increased to a maximum of 26 KV at 1,600 shocks. The stone was revisualized, and repositioning was done considering the transverse colon passing right anterior to the stone. Because the stone appeared to be in the same place after the repositioning, shocks were delivered. Apparent adequate fragmentation was obtained after a total of 2,400 shocks had been administered. The patient tolerated the procedure well.

Code(s): _____

> **Coding Guideline B3.11a. Inspection Procedures**
> Inspection of a body part(s) performed in order to achieve the objective of the procedure is not coded separately.

**3.15.**

**Preoperative Diagnosis:** Abdominal pain

**Postoperative Diagnosis:** Gastritis and duodenitis

**Procedure:** Esophagogastroduodenoscopy with biopsy

**Procedure:** The patient was premedicated and brought to the endoscopy suite where his throat was anesthetized with Cetacaine spray. He then was placed in the left lateral position and given 2 mg Versed, IV.

An Olympus gastroscope was advanced into the esophagus, which was well visualized with no significant segmental spasms. Subsequently, the scope was advanced into the distal esophagus which was essentially normal. Then the scope was advanced into the stomach, which showed evidence of erythema and gastritis. The pylorus was intubated and the duodenal bulb visualized. The duodenal bulb showed severe erythema, suggestive of duodenitis. Biopsies of both the duodenum and stomach were obtained. The scope was withdrawn. The patient tolerated the procedure well.

Code(s): _____

**3.16.**

**Preoperative Diagnosis:** Cataract, left eye

**Postoperative Diagnosis:** Cataract, left eye

**Operation:** Extracapsular cataract extraction with intraocular lens implantation, left eye

**Procedure:** The patient was given a retrobulbar injection of 2.5 to 3.0 cc of a mixture of equal parts of 2 percent lidocaine with epinephrine and 0.75 percent Marcaine with Wydase. The area above the left eye was infiltrated with an additional 6 to 7 cc of this mixture in a modified Van Lint technique. A self-maintaining pressure device was applied to the eye, and a short time later, the patient was taken to the OR.

The patient was properly positioned on the operating table, and the area around the left eye was prepped and draped in the usual fashion. A self-retaining eyelid speculum was positioned and 4-0 silk suture passed through the tendon of the superior rectus muscle, thereby deviating the eye inferiorly. A 160 degrees fornix-based conjunctival flap was created, followed by a 150 degrees corneoscleral groove with a #64 Beaver blade. Hemostasis was maintained throughout with gentle cautery. A 6-0 silk suture was introduced to cross this groove at the 12 o'clock position and looped out of the operative field. The anterior chamber was then entered superiorly temporally, and after injecting Occucoat, an anterior capsulotomy was performed. The nucleus was easily brought forward into the anterior chamber. The corneoscleral section was opened with scissors to the left and the nucleus delivered with irrigation and gentle lens loop manipulation. Interrupted 10-0 nylon sutures were placed at both the nasal and lateral extent of the incision.

At this point, a modified C-loop posterior chamber lens was removed from its package and irrigated and inspected. It was then positioned into the inferior capsular bag without difficulty and the superior haptic was placed behind the iris at the 12 o'clock location. Then the lens was rotated to a horizontal orientation in an attempt to better enhance capsular fixation. Miochol was then instilled into the anterior chamber. In addition, three or four interrupted 10-0 nylon sutures were used to close the corneal sclera section. The silk sutures were removed, and the conjunctiva advanced back into its normal location and was secured with cautery burns. Approximately 20 to 30 mg of both gentamicin and Kenalog were injected into the inferior cul-de-sac in a subconjunctival and sub-Tenon fashion. After instillation of 2 percent pilocarpine and Maxitrol ophthalmic solution, the eyelid speculum was removed and the eye dressed in a sterile fashion. The patient was released to the recovery room in satisfactory condition.

Code(s): _____

# Detailed and/or Complex Cases and Scenarios Using ICD-10-CM and ICD-10-PCS Codes

---

**ICD-10-PCS Coding Guideline B3.13. Release Procedures**
In the root operation Release, the body part value coded is the body part being freed and not the tissue being manipulated or cut to free the body part.

---

**3.17.**
**Preoperative Diagnosis:** Carpal tunnel syndrome, left

**Postoperative Diagnosis:** Carpal tunnel syndrome, left

**Operation:** Release, left carpal tunnel

**Procedure:** After successful axillary block was placed, the patient's left arm was prepared and draped in the usual sterile fashion. Tourniquet was inflated. A curvilinear hypothenar incision was made and the palmaris retracted radially. The carpal tunnel and the transverse carpal ligament were then opened and completely freed in the proximal directions. It was noted to be severely tight in the palm with flattening and swelling of the median nerve. The carpal tunnel was opened distally in the hand and noted to be clear. The wound was then closed with 4-0 Dexon in subcuticular tissues. Sterile bulky dressing was applied, and the patient was awakened and taken to the recovery room in satisfactory condition.

ICD-10-CM Code(s): _____

ICD-10-PCS Code(s): _____

---

**ICD-10-CM Coding Guideline I.15.b.5. Outcome of Delivery**
A code from category Z37, Outcome of Delivery, should be included on every maternal record when a delivery has occurred. These codes are not to be used on subsequent records or on the newborn record.

---

**ICD-10-PCS Coding Guideline C.1. Products of Conception**
Procedures performed on the products of conception are coded to the Obstetrics section. Procedures performed on the pregnant female other than the products of conception are coded to the appropriate root operation in the Medical and Surgical section.

---

**3.18.**
This is a 26-year-old patient who had a previous cesarean section for delivery due to fetal distress. During this pregnancy, she has had routine antepartum care with no complications. We are going to attempt a VBAC for this delivery. She is admitted in her 39th week in labor. The fetus is in cephalic position and no rotation is necessary. The labor continues to progress and five hours later she is taken to delivery. During the delivery she is fatigued, so mid forceps are required over a midline episiotomy which was subsequently repaired by an episiorrhaphy. A single liveborn infant is delivered.

ICD-10-CM Code(s): _____

ICD-10-PCS Code(s): _____

**3.19.**

**Discharge Summary**: The patient is a 45-year-old female who fell while walking her dog. She was walking on the sidewalk in her neighborhood and accidently tripped and subsequently fell. She sustained a comminuted fracture of the shaft of her right tibia confirmed by x-ray done in the emergency room. She also hit her head on a fire hydrant and suffered a slight concussion but no loss of consciousness. The patient was admitted and taken to surgery, where an open reduction with internal fixation was accomplished with good alignment of fracture fragments. Postop course was uneventful and the patient was discharged home with daily physical therapy.

ICD-10-CM Code(s): _____

ICD-10-PCS Code(s): _____

---

**ICD-10-CM Coding Guideline I.15.b.4. Selection of OB Principal Diagnosis When a Delivery Occurs**
When a delivery occurs, the principal diagnosis should correspond to the main circumstances or complication of the delivery. In cases of cesarean delivery, the selection of the principal diagnosis should be the condition established after study that was responsible for the patient's admission. If the patient was admitted with a condition that resulted in the performance of a cesarean procedure, that condition should be selected as the principal diagnosis. If the reason for the admission/ encounter was unrelated to the condition resulting in the cesarean delivery, the condition related to the reason for the admission/encounter should be selected as the principal diagnosis.

---

**Coding Note: Definition of Third Trimester**
The third trimester is defined as 28 weeks 0 days of gestation until delivery.

---

**3.20.**

**Inpatient Admission:** The patient, gravida II, para 1, was admitted at approximately 33 weeks gestation with mild contractions. She was contracting every 7–8 minutes. An ultrasound showed twins of approximately 4 pounds each. The patient was given magnesium sulfate to stop the contractions, but she contracted through the drug. After developing a fever with suspected chorioamnionitis, a low cervical cesarean section was performed. The umbilical cord was wrapped tightly around the neck of twin 1.

**Discharge Diagnoses:** Cesarean delivery of liveborn twins prematurely at 33 weeks gestation; chorioamnionitis; umbilical cord compression.

ICD-10-CM Code(s): _____

ICD-10-PCS Code(s): _____

> **ICD-10-CM Coding Guideline II.C. Selection of Principal Diagnosis—Two or More Diagnoses That Equally Meet the Definition of Principal Diagnosis**
> In the unusual instance when two or more diagnoses equally meet the criteria for principal diagnosis as determined by the admission, diagnostic workup, and/or therapy provided, and the Alphabetic Index, Tabular List, or another coding guideline does not provide sequencing direction, any one of these diagnoses may be sequenced first.

> **ICD-10-PCS Coding Guideline B3.4a Biopsy Procedures**
> Biopsy procedures are coded using the root operations: Excision, Extraction, or Drainage and the qualifier Diagnostic. The qualifier Diagnostic is used only for biopsies.

**3.21.**

This 19-year-old college student was brought to the ER and admitted with high fever, stiff neck, chest pain, cough, and nausea. A diagnostic lumbar puncture was performed, and results were positive for meningitis. Chest x-ray revealed pneumonia. Sputum cultures grew *pneumococcus*. Patient was treated with IV antibiotics and was discharged with the diagnosis of pneumococcal meningitis and pneumococcal pneumonia.

**Procedure Note:** The patient was placed in the left lateral decubitus position in a semi-fetal position. The area was cleansed and draped in usual sterile fashion. Anesthesia was achieved with 1 percent lidocaine. A 20-guage 3.5 inch spinal needle was placed in the L4-L5 interspace. On the first attempt cerebral spinal fluid was obtained. Four tubes were filled and these were sent for the usual tests. The patient had no immediate complications and tolerated the procedure well.

ICD-10-CM Code(s): _____

ICD-10-PCS Code(s): _____

**3.22.** The following documentation is from the health record of a 61-year-old female patient.

**Operative Report**

**Preoperative Diagnoses:** Acute gallstone pancreatitis with acute cholecystitis, evidence of bile duct obstruction

**Postoperative Diagnoses:** Acute cholecystitis with gallstone, acute gallstone pancreatitis, bile duct obstruction

**Operation:** Cholecystectomy; Exploration of common bile duct; Insertion of feed tube; Intraoperative cholangiogram performed under fluoroscopy.

**History:** The patient is a 61-year-old female admitted 48 hours ago with evidence of possible acute gallstone pancreatitis. The patient had some thickening of her gallbladder wall and pericholecystic fluid. The patient had marked elevation of amylase and was given 48 hours of medical therapy with chemical clearance of her pancreatitis. The patient was felt to be a candidate for open exploration of her biliary tract, with concomitant cholecystectomy and possible common duct exploration.

**Description of Procedure:** After discussion with the patient and her family and obtaining informed consent, she was taken to the operating room, where, after induction of general anesthesia, the abdomen was prepped and draped in a standard fashion. Following this, a right upper quadrant incision was used to gain access to the abdominal cavity. Manual exploration revealed no abnormalities of the uterus, ovaries, colon, or stomach. The pancreas was enlarged and edematous in the area of the head. Attention was then turned to the right upper quadrant, where the gallbladder was noted to be somewhat distended. This decompressed with a 2-0 Vicryl purse string stitch using the trocar. The cystic artery was dissected free and double clipped proximally, singly distally, and divided. The duct was then dissected free and subsequently clipped proximally.

Low osmolar cholangiogram with fluoroscopy was then obtained by opening the cystic duct and placing a cholangiogram catheter. The common bile duct measured roughly 1½ cm in size. The duct tapered out in the area of the intraduodenal portion of the common duct to near occlusion. The gallbladder was then removed by transecting the cystic duct and removing it in a retrograde fashion. The gallbladder contained several stones.

Following removal of the gallbladder, attention was turned to the common bile duct, which was opened. No stones were retrieved initially from the bile duct. A biliary Fogarty was passed distally and, with some difficulty, was negotiated into the duodenum. On return, no calculus material was obtained. Palpation of the distal duct revealed thickening due to the pancreatic inflammation, which was noted to improve somewhat over the inside portion of the C-loop to the duodenum. The patient was felt to have bile duct obstruction from some other primary duct process other than a stone or inflammation.

Following this, cholangiography revealed some mild emptying of the distal common bile duct into the duodenum. With the overall picture, it was felt the patient might benefit from a feeding jejunostomy, as she might well sustain postoperative or perioperative complications of respiratory insufficiency or perhaps other imponderables. As such, jejunum was identified roughly one foot beyond the ligament of Treitz, and 2-0 Vicryl pursestring stitches times two were placed. The jejunotomy was performed, and a 16 French T-tube was then placed and brought out through a stab wound in the left upper quadrant. The tube was anchored anteriorly with interrupted 2-0 silk stitches and externally with 2-0 stitches. Jackson-Pratt drain was placed through a lateral stab wound in the right upper quadrant and used to drain the duodenotomy and choledochotomy. This was anchored with several 3-0 silk stitches.

Following this, the wound was irrigated with Kantrex irrigation, 1 g per liter, and the wound was closed by closing the posterior rectus sheath with running #1 Vicryl suture. The sub-q was irrigated and the skin was closed with staples. The wound was then dressed, and the patient was taken to the recovery room postop in stable condition. Estimated blood loss was 400 cc. Sponge and needle counts were correct times two.

ICD-10-CM Code(s): _____

ICD-10-PCS Code(s): _____

**3.23.** The following documentation is from the health record of a 50-year-old female patient.

**Discharge Summary:** The patient is a 50-year-old female with known carcinoma of the right breast with widespread pulmonary and bone metastases. She recently completed the third of six outpatient chemotherapy treatments for the metastases. The patient also has a history of a right mastectomy for the breast carcinoma two years ago and is no longer receiving any treatment for this carcinoma. The patient was now admitted for treatment of lumps of the lower-outer quadrant of the left breast. This has been recommended as treatment for the lumps of the left breast due to the patient's history of right breast carcinoma with metastases. The patient has agreed to the recommended treatment.

The patient was taken to surgery, and a left simple mastectomy was performed via an Open approach to start the reconstruction process.

Pathology report revealed benign fibroadenoma.

The patient was discharged in satisfactory condition to see me in the office in 10 days.

ICD-10-CM Code(s): _____

ICD-10-PCS Code(s): _____

> **ICD-10-PCS Coding Guideline B3.15. Reposition for Fracture Treatment**
> Reduction of a displaced fracture is coded to the root operation Reposition, and the application of a cast or splint in conjunction with the Reposition procedure is not coded separately. Treatment of a nondisplaced fracture is coded to the procedure performed.

**3.24.** The following documentation is from the health record of an ORIF patient.

**Operative Report**

**Preoperative Diagnosis:** Displaced comminuted fracture of the shaft of the right humerus

**Postoperative Diagnosis:** Same

**Procedure:** Open reduction, internal fixation of fracture of shaft of right humerus

**History:** The patient is a fourth grader whose class was on a field trip at the local bowling alley. The patient tripped over an object on the alley and fell sustaining a fracture of the right humerus.

**Description:** The patient was anesthetized and prepped with Betadine, sterile drapes were applied, and the pneumatic tourniquet was inflated around the arm. An incision was made in the area of the lateral epicondyle through a Steri-drape, and this was carried through subcutaneous tissue, and the fracture site was easily exposed. Inspection revealed the fragment to be rotated in two planes about 90 degrees. It was possible to manually reduce this quite easily, and the judicious manipulation resulted in an almost anatomic reduction. This was fixed with two pins across the humerus. These pins were cut off below skin level. The wound was closed with some plain catgut subcutaneously and 5-0 nylon in the skin. Dressings were applied to the patient and tourniquet released.

ICD-10-CM Code(s): _____

ICD-10-PCS Code(s): _____

ICD-10-PCS Coding Guideline B3.2b. Multiple Procedures
During the same operative episode, multiple procedures are coded if the same root operation is repeated at different body sites that are included in the same body part value.

ICD-10-PCS Coding Guideline B3.11a. Inspection Procedures
Inspection of a body part(s) performed in order to achieve the objective of a procedure is not coded separately.

ICD-10-PCS Coding Guideline B3.4a. Biopsy Procedures
Biopsy procedures are coded using the root operations Excision, Extraction, or Drainage and the qualifier Diagnostic. The qualifier Diagnostic is used only for biopsies.

**3.25.**

| | |
|---|---|
| **Preoperative Diagnosis:** | Rectal mass |
| | Change in bowel habits |
| | |
| **Postoperative Diagnosis:** | Rectal prolapse |
| | Tubular adenoma of sigmoid colon, biopsies ×2 |
| | Sigmoid diverticulosis |
| | Nonspecific colitis |

**Procedure:** Colonoscopy performed to the level of the cecum (110 cm)

**Procedure:** The patient was prepped in the usual fashion, followed by placement in the left lateral decubitus position. I administered 3 mg of Versed. Monitoring of sedation was assisted by a trained registered nurse. Next, the Pentax Video Endoscope was passed through the rectal verge after a negative digital examination and advanced to the level of the cecum. The scope was then slowly retracted with a circular tip motion. There was mild nonspecific colitis noted. The patient also had significant sigmoid diverticulosis and several small polyps in the sigmoid colon area. Additionally, there was a large prolapsing mass of mucosa approximately 5 cm inside the rectum. This appears to have prolapsed previously. Two of the small polyps were biopsied using the cold biopsy forceps and sent to pathology for examination. The remainder of the exam was unremarkable. The patient tolerated the procedure well.

**Pathology Report**

**Diagnosis:** Tubular adenoma of sigmoid colon

ICD-10-CM Code(s): _____

ICD-10-PCS Code(s): _____

> **ICD-10-PCS Coding Guideline B3.1b. General Guidelines for Root Operation**
> Components of a procedure specified in the root operation definition and explanation are not coded separately. Procedural steps necessary to reach the operative site and close the operative site, including anastomosis of a tubular body part, are also not coded separately.

**3.26.** The following documentation is from the health record of a 79-year-old female patient.

**Operative Report**

**Preoperative Diagnosis:** Displaced right femoral neck hip fracture

**Postoperative Diagnosis:** Displaced right femoral neck hip fracture

**Operation:** Right hip hemiarthroplasty (metal Zimmer LDFX cemented monopolar)

**Indications:** This is a 79-year-old female that fractured the right femoral neck. The patient was doing some gardening in her back yard when she tripped and fell. The patient lives in a single family home. The patient also has the following chronic conditions: hypertensive heart disease, congestive heart failure, and emphysema.

**Procedure:** The patient was taken to the operating room and placed in the lateral position on the transfer bed where spinal anesthesia was administered. She was transferred to the left lateral decubitus position on a beanbag on the operative table. Padded all bony prominences. Peritoneum was sealed off with Steri-Drape. The right hip was prepped and draped in the usual sterile fashion. Longitudinal incision over the greater trochanter and proximal femur was performed curving posteriorly proximally along the gluteus maximus. Sharp dissection to the skin, Bovie dissection to the subcutaneous tissues down to tensor fascia lata, identifying the greater trochanter. Besides the tensor fascia lata and along with the incision splitting the fibrous gluteus maximus, controlling bleeders with Bovie cautery. Piriformis was identified and short external rotators were tagged with a #5 Tycron suture. These are moved from their insertion. T-capsulotomy was performed. Displaced hip fracture was identified, femoral head was removed and measured, copious irrigation was performed, and acetabulum was visible and palpable, appearing normal. Sagittal saw was used to make cut in the femoral neck. Box osteotome was used to gain lateral entrance to the canal. The canal finder was used, easily locating the femoral canal. Sequential broaching was performed up to a 14, which fit well. Had full range of motion without instability and grossly equal leg lengths. I could bring the hip and knee up to 90 degrees of flexion, neutral adduction, start to internally rotate to 30 degrees before it would become unstable. Hip was redislocated, trial components were removed. I then measured the central canal for a centralizer. I placed a distal cement restrictor 2 cm distal to the component. Copious lavage of the canal was performed and brushed. Acetabulum was irrigated clean, palpable and visibly free of loose fragments. It was packed off with lap sponge. Femoral canal was dried. Cement was placed in the femoral canal with retrograde manner using proximal pressurizer. The 14-mm Zimmer LDFX was placed with a distal centralizer in the appropriate anteversion and held in place with a cement set. Copious irrigation was performed. After the cement set, placed the final endo head, tapped into position with Morris taper, and reduced the head. I could then take the hip through the same range of motion without any instability. The short external rotator is in the drill holes in the greater trochanter. The tensor fascia lata was closed with interrupted 0-0 Vicryl sutures. We copiously irrigated each layer. Subcutaneous tissue was closed with interrupted 2-0 Vicryl sutures, skin was closed with staples. Patient tolerated the procedure well.

ICD-10-CM Code(s): _____

ICD-10-PCS Code(s): _____

**3.27.** The following documentation is from the health record of an 11-year-old boy.

**Preoperative Diagnoses:**   1. Ewing sarcoma, left scapula
                              2. Down syndrome

**Postoperative Diagnosis:** Same

**Procedure:** Biopsy of left scapula; Insertion of vascular access device

**Findings:** This is an 11-year-old boy with Down syndrome who presented four days ago with a large mass in the left scapular region. Outpatient x-ray and CT scan showed laminated new bone with a large expansile permeative lesion in the scapular body. It did not appear to involve the glenohumeral joint. Outpatient bone scan showed marked increased uptake and questionable area of uptake in the right seventh rib and left first vertebral body. At the time of biopsy there was obvious stretching of the posterior trapezius and deltoid musculature over the mass and a very soft calcific mass noted within the central area of the substance. Frozen pathology sections showed many small cells, but definitive diagnosis could not be made off the frozen section. Final pathologic diagnosis was malignant bone tumor consistent with Ewing's sarcoma. He will be started on a chemotherapy program, and definitive surgery will be planned.

**Procedure:** Following an adequate level of general endotracheal anesthesia, the patient was turned to the right lateral decubitus position with the left side up. The left shoulder region was prepped and draped in routine sterile fashion.

A 3 cm incision was then made over the spine of the scapula. Electrocautery was used for hemostasis and the incision deepened with electrocautery. When we were in the area of the soft tissue mass noted on the CT scan, biopsies were taken. The initial biopsies showed primarily muscle fibers, so we deepened the incision at this point and obtained a biopsy of the obvious calcific bone tissue. These cultures were more consistent with tumor, and, at this point, hemostasis was achieved with a combination of bone wax, packing, and electrocautery. Meticulous hemostasis was achieved prior to closure and then a two-layer interrupted closure was performed, closing the skin with a running subcuticular suture of 4-0 Vicryl. Bulky dry sterile dressing was applied, and the patient was awakened and returned to the recovery room in good condition.

ICD-10-CM Code(s): _____

ICD-10-PCS Code(s): _____

**3.28.** The following documentation is from the health record of a 32-year-old female patient.

**Delivery Record**

**Admit Note:** 7/20: Patient is a 32-year-old female with EDC 7/22 and EGA of 39 weeks. She has been having uterine contractions for 2 days, mild, more severe this a.m. with contractions every 2–4 minutes at admission. Cervix is 1 cm/20%/-1 station. EFW 3,500 g.

**Delivery Record Summary:** 7/21: Patient progressed to 5 cm and exhausted. No sleep for two nights. Patient is also in extreme pain of labor. A vacuum-assisted vaginal delivery of a live male was performed due to the prolonged first stage of labor. A first degree laceration of the perineum was repaired with 3-0 Vicryl. Estimated blood loss of 450 ml.

**Progress Note:** 7/22: Patient weak, slightly dizzy, sore perineum. Patient is afebrile and fundus firm. H/H 8.5/24.6. Assessment – s/p VD with first degree laceration; postpartum anemia. Slow Fe #30.

**Progress Note:** 7/23: PPD #2 – S – feeling better, ambulating without dizziness; O VSS, afebrile, fundus firm; A – s/p VD with first degree laceration; P – home today, FU 4 weeks, DC meds Vicodin #20, Colace #20, and Slow Fe #30.

ICD-10-CM Code(s): _____

ICD-10-PCS Code(s): _____

---

**ICD-10-CM Coding Guideline I.C.18.e. Coma Scale**

The coma scale codes (R40.2-) can be used in conjunction with traumatic brain injury codes, acute cerebrovascular disease or sequelae of cerebrovascular disease codes. These codes are primarily for use by trauma registries, but they may be used in any setting where this information is collected. The coma scale codes should be sequenced after the diagnosis code(s).

These codes, one from each subcategory, are needed to complete the scale. The seventh character indicates when the scale was recorded. The seventh character should match for all three codes.

At a minimum, report the initial score documented on presentation at your facility. This may be a score from the emergency medicine technician (EMT) or in the emergency department. If desired, a facility may choose to capture multiple coma scale score.

Assign code R40.24, Glasgow coma scale, total score, when only the total score is documented in the medical record and not the individual score(s).

---

**3.29.** The following documentation is from the health record of a 22-year-old male patient.

**Case Summary:** The patient is a 22-year-old male, admitted through the emergency department after the motorcycle he was driving collided with an elk while driving in the mountains. It was noted that when the accident occurred the patient was driving in the mountains and not on the road. The patient was not wearing a helmet and sustained a skull fracture over the left temporal and orbital roof areas with depressed zygomatic arch on the left side. The patient was unconscious at the scene and upon examination in the ED, with a Glasgow coma scale (GCS) score of 3: Eyes, never open; No verbal response; No motor response. Left pupil was blown (fixed and dilated), indicating intracranial injury. Hypoxemia, hypotension, and cerebral edema were noted. The patient was admitted to the ICU with continuous monitoring of intracranial pressure (percutaneous). The patient experienced increasing periods of apnea and was placed on a ventilator following endotracheal intubation. The patient's family (in another state) was notified and arrived two days later. There was no improvement in the patient's status over the following five days. The patient continued to be monitored and was unconscious. Attempts to wean from ventilation were unsuccessful. Brain wave measurement showed no brain wave electrical activity. The family made the decision to discontinue life support and the life-sustaining efforts were discontinued.

ICD-10-CM Code(s): _____

ICD-10-PCS Code(s): _____

**3.30.**

This 56-year-old female was admitted for resection of an adrenal mass. The patient has had hypertension of several years' duration. Ultrasound was done on an outpatient basis in consideration of the possibility of a mass, and catecholamine studies have been normal. A 4–5 cm right adrenal mass was identified. Dr. White had obtained a 24-hour urinary free cortisol, ACTH, and short suppression tests, all of which confirmed the presence of Cushing's syndrome. The patient was not diabetic. She did report weight gain, some shift in body configuration, and easy bruising of several years' duration.

**Surgery:** A 5 cm, well-circumscribed round, benign cortical tumor was resected from the adrenal gland via an open approach. Pathology diagnosis confirmed that the tumor was benign.

**Allergies:** No known drug allergies

**Medications on Discharge:** Hydrocortisone, rapidly tapering dose, currently on 40 mg daily; Toprol 50 mg q.a.m.; Prevacid 30 mg qd; Lipitor 10 mg q.a.m.; Prempro 0.625/2.5

**Physical Exam:** Vital signs stable. HEENT: Sclerae and conjunctivae clear. Neck: Supple. No palpable thyroid. Lungs: Somewhat decreased breath sounds currently. There is mild splinting with deep breathing. Abdomen: Tenderness in the incision area. She has active bowel sounds at this time. Extremities: No definite bruises currently. No edema noted.

**Discharge Diagnosis:** Right adrenal tumor with Cushing's syndrome secondary to tumor

**Plan:** The patient appears to have tolerated the surgery well. She will require steroid replacement. Excess cortisol output is presumed entirely due to her tumor, and her ACTH was suppressed previously. As with exogenous steroid therapy, there will be contralateral adrenal suppression. The patient will be tapered rapidly to replacement hydrocortisone levels. We will try the remaining hydrocortisone withdrawal over the next six months or so, depending on her ACTH and cortisol responses. She is discharged to home with follow-up in my office in 1 week.

ICD-10-CM Code(s): _____

ICD-10-PCS Code(s): _____

**3.31.** The following documentation is from the health record of a cardiac service patient.

**Discharge Summary**
Admit Date: 1/9/xx
Discharge Date: 1/12/xx

**Final Diagnoses:**   Coronary artery disease (CAD)
Sick sinus syndrome
Hypertensive heart disease
CHF

**Procedures:**   Percutaneous transluminal coronary angioplasty with stent insertion (1/10/xx)
Permanent dual chamber pacemaker insertion (1/9/xx)

**History of Present Illness:** The patient is a 62-year-old female who was admitted to another hospital on 1/8/xx after experiencing tachycardia. There she underwent a cardiac catheterization, showing the presence of severe two-vessel coronary artery disease. The patient does not have any history of a CABG in the past. The patient has a history of sick sinus syndrome, hypertensive heart disease, and CHF. She was transferred to our hospital to undergo a percutaneous transluminal angioplasty.

**Physical Examination:** No physical abnormalities were found on the cardiovascular examination. Pulse 50 and blood pressure 100/85. HEENT: PERRLA, faint carotid bruits. Lungs: Clear to percussion and auscultation. Heart: Normal sinus rhythm with a 2.6 systolic ejection murmur. Extremities and abdomen were negative.

**Hospital Course:** To manage the patient's sick sinus syndrome, a permanent dual chamber pacemaker with atrial and ventricular leads was implanted on 1/9/xx. An incision was made into the left chest wall with the dual chamber pacemaker being placed in the subcutaneous pocket. Next a small incision was made in the skin and the leads were percutaneously passed into the right ventricle and right atrium.

On 1/10 the patient underwent a PTCA of both the left anterior descending artery and the right coronary artery. A drug-eluting stent was placed in the right coronary artery without complications and good results were obtained.

Postoperatively, the patient was stable and was subsequently discharged. The patient's hypertensive heart disease and CHF were managed and monitored during the hospital stay and the patient continued taking her normal medications for these conditions.

ICD-10-CM Code(s): _____

ICD-10-PCS Code(s): _____

> **ICD-10-PCS Coding Guideline C2. Procedures Following Delivery or Abortion**
> Procedures performed following a delivery or abortion for curettage of the endometrium or evacuation of retained products of conception are all coded in the Obstetrics section, to the root operation Extraction and the body part Products of Conception, Retained. Diagnostic or therapeutic dilation and curettage performed during times other than the postpartum or post-abortion period are all coded in the Medical and Surgical section, to the root operation Extraction and the body part Endometrium.

### 3.32.

This 26-year-old gravid 1, para 1, female has been spotting and has been on bed rest. She awoke this morning with severe cramping and bleeding. Her husband brought her to the hospital. After examination, it was determined that she has had an incomplete early spontaneous abortion. She is in the 12th week of her pregnancy. She was taken to surgery, and a dilation and curettage was performed to remove the products of conception. The patient developed a urinary tract infection due to E. coli which was treated with intravenous antibiotics. The patient was subsequently discharged on oral antibiotics and she is to follow up with me in the office.

ICD-10-CM Code(s): _____

ICD-10-PCS Code(s): _____

**3.33.** The following documentation is from the health record of a 47-year-old female.

**Preoperative Diagnosis:** Menorrhagia

**Postoperative Diagnosis:** Menorrhagia

**Procedure:** Hysteroscopy with biopsy, dilatation and curettage

**Indications:** The patient is a 47-year-old female with increasing irregular vaginal bleeding. The uterus is very tender, and ultrasound reveals no specific adnexal masses. Pap smear shows some chronic inflammatory cells. Bleeding has not been controlled in the past month with conservation therapy; thus, the patient is admitted for dilatation and curettage, and a hysteroscopy and biopsy will be carried out.

**Technique:** Under general anesthesia, the patient was prepped and draped in the usual manner with Betadine, with her cervix retracted outward. The vaginal vault appeared to be clear, as did both adnexa. Sound was passed into the intrauterine cavity after the cervix was found to be 8 cm deep. The cervix was dilated with Hegar dilators up to #5. The 5 mm Wolff hysteroscope, with normal saline irrigation, was then inserted. An inspection of the endocervical canal showed no abnormalities.

Upon entering the uterine cavity, some irregular shedding of the endometrium was noted. Endometrial shedding was noted more to be the patient's left cornu area than the right. The contour of the cavity appeared to be normal; no bulging masses or septation was noted. An endometrial biopsy was then taken. The Wolff scope was removed. The cervix was further dilated with Hegar dilators up to #12. A medium-sharp curette was inserted into the uterine cavity and the endometrium was curettage in a clockwise manner, with a moderate amount of what appeared to be irregular proliferative endometrium being obtained. Again, the contour of the cavity appeared to be normal. The patient was transferred to the recovery room in good condition.

Pathology report reveals secretory proliferative endometrium without additional abnormalities noted.

ICD-10-CM Code(s): _____

ICD-10-PCS Code(s): _____

### 3.34.

**Preoperative Diagnosis:** Bucket-handle tear left medial meniscus

**Postoperative Diagnosis:** Bucket-handle tear left medial meniscus

**Procedure:** Arthroscopic partial medial meniscectomy

**Indications:** The patient is a 16-year-old male who torn his left medial meniscus while playing football at the local high school football field. The patient is a wide receiver for the high school football team and was tackled resulting in the torn medial meniscus. I saw and treated the patient initially in the emergency room three weeks ago for this injury.

**Technique:** After induction with general anesthesia, a standard three-portal approach of the knee was evaluated. Mild synovitic changes were noted in the suprapatellar pouch. No chondromalacia changes were noted. The anterior portion of the medial meniscus had a flap tear, which was removed.

After all instruments were withdrawn, 4-0 nylon horizontal mattress stitches were used to close the wound, and pressure dressings were applied. The patient was awakened and taken to the recovery room in good condition.

ICD-10-CM Code(s): _____

ICD-10-PCS Code(s): _____

**3.35.** The following documentation is from the health record of a 67-year-old male.

**Procedure:** Placement of a dual chamber implantable pacing cardioverter defibrillator

**Diagnoses:** Ischemic cardiomyopathy; history of myocardial infarction; status post PTCA

**Description of Procedure:** After informed consent was obtained, the patient was brought to the cardiac lab. The procedure was done under conscious sedation with fluoroscopic guidance. One percent Lidocaine was used to anesthetize the skin in the left abdominal area and a skin incision was made. A pocket was made in the subcutaneous tissue for the ICD generator, securing good hemostasis. The left subclavian vein was easily cannulated twice using a pediatric set, which was upsized to regular 037 wires, the position which was checked under fluoroscopy.

I then dilated the access volts with 9-French dilators and used 7-French access sheaths through which a 7-French right ventricular lead was advanced and placed under fluoroscopic guidance. It was an active fixation lead. The numbers looked good, and the lead was sutured down.

A 7-French lead was then advanced under fluoroscopic guidance and placed in the right atrial appendage. The numbers looked good. There was no diaphragmatic stimulation and the lead was sutured down. The leads were then attached to the generator, which was tested and sutured down in the pocket. The wound was irrigated several times with antibiotics at the end of the procedure. Wound was closed with layers. The patient tolerated the procedure well without any complications.

The ICD is Model Virtuoso DRD 154AWG. Atrial and ventricular leads are Medtronic. (Note: Do not code the fluoroscopy.)

ICD-10-CM Code(s): _____

ICD-10-PCS Code(s): _____

**3.36.**

**Preoperative Diagnosis:** Chronic right calf skin ulcer with necrosis of the bone and E. coli severe sepsis with acute respiratory failure

**Postoperative Diagnosis:** Same

**Procedure:** Right below-the-knee amputation

**Description of Procedure:** The patient was brought to the operating room and placed supine on the operating room table. The patient was placed under general endotracheal anesthesia. A tourniquet was placed on the right proximal thigh and the right lower extremity was prepped and draped in a standard sterile fashion.

A below-the-knee amputation was carried out directly below the tibial tubercle with a posteriorly based flap. The skin and soft tissue were cut sharply to bone along the line of the skin incision. Once the soft tissue was incised the tibia and fibula were provisionally cut with an oscillating saw and the remainder of the right lower extremity was removed and sent to pathology. Next, the tibia and fibula were dissected out subperiosteally proximal to the anterior portion of the skin incision and re-cut with the oscillating saw. The anterior portion of the tibia was beveled again with the oscillating saw and smoothed with a rasp. The fibular cut was beveled in a lateral to medial direction while extending posteriorly.

The nerves and blood vessels were then addressed. The anterior tibial and posterior tibial arteries, as well as the peroneal artery and attendant veins were suture ligated with #1 Vicryl suture. The anterior and posterior tibial nerves and peroneal nerve were also identified, pulled out of the wound, cut short, and allowed to retract back into the soft tissue. In addition, large veins were identified and ligated. The tourniquet was then released for a total tourniquet time of 32 minutes and minimal bleeding was encountered. Several smaller bleeders were ligated. There was some clotting observed, which was important as the blood clotting was of significant concern preceding this operation. The wound was closed over a medium Hemovac drain with 2 limbs, with the posterior flap brought anteriorly. The fascia was closed using interrupted 1 Vicryl suture, and the subcutaneous tissue was closed using interrupted 3-0 Monocryl suture in a simple buried fashion. Staples were placed at the level of the skin in the interest of time.

After a sterile compressive dressing was placed and Hemovac drain extension and reservoir were attached and activated, the patient was awoken from anesthesia and sent to the ICU in unchanged condition.

ICD-10-CM Code(s): _____

ICD-10-PCS Code(s): _____

> **ICD-10-PCS Coding Guideline B3.6a. Bypass Procedures**
> Bypass procedures are coded by identifying the body part bypassed "from" and the body part bypassed "to." The fourth character body part specifies the body part bypassed from, and the qualifier specifies the body part bypassed to.

> **ICD-10-PCS Coding Guideline B3.8. Excision vs. Resection**
> PCS contains specific body parts for anatomical subdivisions of a body part, such as lobes of the lungs or liver and regions of the intestine. Resection of the specific body part is coded whenever all of the body part is cut out or off, rather than coding Excision of a less specific body part.

**3.37.**

**Preoperative Diagnoses:** Extensive diverticulitis of sigmoid colon with perforation; Crohn's disease with obstruction of right colon and proximal transverse colon

**Postoperative Diagnoses:** Same

**Procedures:** Exploratory laparotomy; sigmoid colectomy; extended right hemicolectomy; colostomy

**Procedure Description:** After consent was obtained for the procedure, risks and benefits were described at length. The patient was taken to the operating room and placed supine on the operating room table. Preoperatively, the patient received 3 g of IV Unasyn. The patient was placed under general endotracheal anesthesia. PAS stockings were applied to both lower extremities. The patient's abdomen was then prepped and draped in the standard surgical fashion.

A midline laparotomy incision was made from just around the umbilicus to the pubic symphysis. The midline of the fascia was divided, and the abdomen was entered. With exploration of the abdomen, extensive diverticular disease of the distal sigmoid colon was noted.

First order of business was to mobilize the sigmoid colon for a sigmoid colectomy. The left ureter was identified and was far from the area of the sigmoid colon. The sigmoid colon was mobilized laterally to include the area of the diverticulitis. The sigmoid colon was mobilized down to the peritoneal reflection. The medial aspect of the sigmoid colon was also mobilized. The colon was then completely mobilized. A point of transaction was chosen at the proximal sigmoid colon. The mesentery was then taken down across the sacrum. The vessels were tied with 2-0 silk sutures. The sigmoid colon was mobilized down to the proximal rectum. Once the proximal rectum was identified, the sigmoid colon was again transected this time using a contour Ethicon stapler with a blue load. Both the right and left ureters were identified prior to any transection of the sigmoid colon. A 3-0 Prolene suture was then tagged to either edge of the rectal staple line. The specimen was then passed off the field.

The right colon was then inspected. Multiple perforations with sites of deserosalization with exposed mucosa were identified in the right colon. The right colon was mobilized by taking down the white line of Toldt all the way up to and including the hepatic flexure. The omentum was taken off the transverse colon with electrocautery.

Once the colon was completely mobilized and became a medial structure, the terminal ileum was transected this time also using a 45-mm GIA stapler with a blue load. A point of transection was chosen in the mid transverse colon just proximal to the middle colic artery where the last site of deserosalization was identified. The mid transverse colon was divided with a GIA 45-mm stapler with a blue load. The mesentery to the right colon and transverse colon were then taken down with Pean clamps and tied with 2-0 silk sutures. The specimen was then passed off the field.

The abdomen was then irrigated. Hemostasis was assured. The ileocolic anastomosis was then created between the terminal ileum and the mid transverse colon. The bowel were positioned to lie along side each other, and a side-to-side functional end-to-end anastomosis was created using a 45-mm GIA stapler with a blue load. The enterostomies were then closed together with a running 3-0 PDS suture followed by interrupted 3-0 GI silks in a Lembert fashion. A stitch was placed at the crotch of each of the bowel connections. A finger was palpated at the anastomosis, and it was widely patent. Mesenteric defect was then closed using 3-0 Vicryl suture in a running fashion.

Attention then turned toward formation of the end-descending colostomy. The descending colon had already been mobilized enough to make it to the anterior abdominal wall without any difficulty. A point on the anterior abdominal wall on the left-hand side just below the umbilicus was chosen for the colostomy. A small 1.5 to 2-cm circular incision was made on the anterior abdominal wall midway through the rectus muscle. The anterior fascia was divided in a cruciate fashion. The rectus muscles were split, and two fingers were palpated through the defect into the abdominal cavity. The descending colon was then grasped with an Allis clamp and passed through the defect and exteriorized. There was no tension on the colon. On the undersurface of the peritoneum, the colon was tagged with 3-0 GI silk sutures ×2.

The midline fascial incision was then closed with a running #1 looped PDS ×2. The surgical incision was then irrigated with copious saline. The skin was then closed with surgical staples. The ostomy was then matured by removing the staple line and sewing the ostomy in place with 3-0 Vicryl sutures. The sutures were sewn in circumferentially. An ostomy appliance was applied.

Sterile dressings were applied, and the patient was awakened from general anesthesia and transported to the recovery room in stable condition.

     ICD-10-CM Code(s): _____

     ICD-10-PCS Code(s): _____

**3.38.**

**Preoperative Diagnosis:** Primary osteoarthritis of right knee

**Postoperative Diagnosis:** Primary osteoarthritis of right knee

**Procedure:** Right posterior stabilized total knee arthroplasty

**Implants:** DePuy Sigma System size 4 right posterior stabilized femoral component, size 3 modular tibial tray with 8 mm. noncrosslinked polyethylene spacer and 35 mm × 8.5 mm thick patella. Antibiotic cement was used.

**Procedure Description:** After obtaining informed consent, the patient was brought to the operating room whereupon the smooth induction of right femoral block and general anesthesia was performed. The patient was positioned in supine fashion on the operating room table, and all bony prominences were well-padded. A bump was placed under the right hip, and a tourniquet was placed on the right proximal thigh. A gram of Kefzol was given intravenously. The right lower extremity was prepped and draped in standard sterile fashion for arthroplasty including an alcohol pre-prep.

After exsanguinations of the extremity with an Ace wrap, the tourniquet was inflated to 300 mg Hg. An approximately 6-inch longitudinal incision was made about the anterior aspect of the knee centered on the inferior pole of the patella. The skin and subcutaneous tissue were dissected sharply down to the level of the fascia, and a medial parapatellar incision was made in the fascia with the medial most split proximally. The patella was everted, and the knee was flexed. Care was taken to protect the patellar tendon insertion. The osteophytes about the femoral notch were removed and a partial resection of the posterior patellar fat pad was carried out. The femoral canal was entered with a drill, and the sword with distal femoral cutting guide were attached set for a resection of 10 mm. The lateral femoral condyle was noted to be eroded distally and posteriorly; however, a 10 mm cut was sufficient for the distal cut.

Using anterior-referenced system, the femur was sized to a size 4. Rotation was set at 3 degrees external rotation. This was checked using the epicondylar axis. The four-in-one cutting guide was then applied, and the distal femoral anterior and posterior cuts as well as the chamfer cuts were completed. Care was taken to protect the collateral ligaments during these cuts. The femoral notch was then completed using the notch-cutting guide supplied with the system. Once that was done, attention was turned to the tibia. Using an external referenced guide, a tibial cut was made with a zero degree posterior slope with 2 mm off the low (lateral) side. This resection resulted in a similar amount of resection medially and laterally. The tibia was exposed using a Homan placed posteriorly and laterally. The osteophytes were removed laterally and posteriorly.

At this point the osteophytes about the posterior femoral condyles were removed using a curved osteotome under direct visualization. The tibia was then sized to a size 3. A thin cut was then made for the modular tibial tray system. An 8-mm posterior stabilized trial spacer, size 3 tibia tray, and size 4 femur were then applied. The knee was taken through a range of motion. Following this, stability was symmetric medially and laterally. The patella was then prepared. The osteophytes were removed with a rongeur, and the thickness was measured to be 25 mm. An 8.5 mm resection was made down to 16.5 mm and a 16.5 × 35 mm patellar trial was applied after the cut was completed. Stability of this component was then trialed, and it was found to be excellent.

The trial components were removed, and the knee was copiously irrigated with normal saline. The final components were then cemented into place in the sizes mentioned above. Order of cement was patella, tibia, femur. The tibial tray was placed and the knee brought out into full extension to compress the tibial and femoral components. Again, antibiotic gentamicin-containing cement was used. The wound was then cleared of excess cement and bony debris and irrigated one final time. It was then closed in layers over a ConstaVac drain. Number 1 Vicryl was used for the extensor fascia and Scarpa fascia in a simple interrupted fashion, 3-0 Monocryl was used for the subcutaneous tissue in a simple buried fashion, and staples were placed at the level of the skin.

A sterile dressing was placed. The ConstaVac drain extension and reservoir were attached and activated, and a compressive wrap was placed from the toes to the thigh. The tourniquet was released for a total tourniquet time of 112 minutes. EBL was minimal. Postoperatively the patient was taken to the recovery room in stable condition.

ICD-10-CM Code(s): _____

ICD-10-PCS Code(s): _____

---

**ICD-10-PCS Coding Guideline B3.10a. Fusion Procedures of the Spine**
The body part coded for a spinal vertebral joint(s) rendered immobile by a spinal fusion procedure is classified by the level of the spine (e.g., thoracic). There are distinct body part values for a single vertebral joint and for multiple vertebral joints at each spinal level.

---

**ICD-10-PCS Coding Guideline B3.10c. Fusion Procedures of the Spine**
Combinations of devices and materials are often used on a vertebral joint to render the joint immobile. When combinations of devices are used on the same vertebral joint, the device value coded for the procedure is as follows:
- If an interbody fusion device is used to render the joint immobile (alone or containing other material like bone graft), the procedure is coded with the device value Interbody Fusion Device.
- If bone graft is the *only* device used to render the joint immobile, the procedure is coded with the device value Nonautologous Tissue Substitute or Autologous Tissue Substitute.
- If a mixture of autologous and nonautologous bone graft (with or without biological or synthetic extenders or binders) is used to render the joint immobile, code the procedure with the device value Autologous Tissue Substitute.

---

**ICD-10-PCS Coding Guideline B3.9. Excision for Graft**
If an autograft is obtained from a different body part in order to complete the objective of the procedure, a separate procedure is coded.

---

**3.39.**
**Preoperative Diagnosis:** Degenerative disk disease, L3-4, L4-5

**Postoperative Diagnosis:** Degenerative disk disease, L3-4, L4-5

**Operation:** Posterior lumbar interbody fusion, anterior column, L3-4 and L4-5, using BAK threaded fusion cages and Danek pedicle screws with autogenous bone graft

**Procedure Description:** The patient was brought to the operating room, and after induction of satisfactory general endotracheal anesthesia, he was placed in the prone position on the spinal frame. The back was prepped and draped in the usual sterile fashion.

A #18 gauge needle was used to identify the posterior spinous process of L3-4, L4-5, marked with Indigo Carmine stain and substantiated by x-ray. Just to the left of the midline an incision was made and the incision was carried down through the skin and subcutaneous tissue and fascia. The tissues just under the skin were separated and the left and right lower back muscles were moved aside, exposing the back of the spinal column.

Using the same lumbar incision, dissection of a suprafascial plane was made to identify the posterior superior iliac spine (PSIS). Using an osteotome, the cortical bone of the PSIS was chipped off to expose the cancellous undersurface. A large bone gouge was utilized to harvest the cancellous bone from left iliac crest. The bone is then morselized and stored for use later in the procedure. The graft site was then irrigated with antibiotic irrigation and packed with Gelfoam. The fascial opening was then closed. Laminectomy was then performed.

Next, the fusion was completed using the posterior lumbar interbody technique utilizing BAK instrumentation. The L3-L4 level was addressed first. An alignment guide was placed over the L3-L4 disk space and the disk was incised with a knife. A drill was used to make a hole into the disk space and then spacers were put in sequentially up to a size #11. Cross-table lateral x-rays were then taken of the lumbar spine. A C-ring retractor was placed over the spacer on the left side and the locking tube sleeve was inserted into the body of L3 and L4. The hole was then drilled and loose fragments were moved with the straight pituitary. The BAK was then selected and packed with bone graft obtained earlier from the iliac crest. The bone graft was packed into the cage at the distal end and then the cage was inserted on the left side. The proximal end of the cage was then packed with bone. The same technique was then completed on the right hand side. After completion of the procedure at the L3-L4 level the same technique was done at the L4-L5 level. Because this was a two-level cage procedure, the pedicle screw instrumentation was used to augment the stabilization. The pedicle screw was put into the L3 vertebral body by making a burr hole at the junction of the facet joint and transverse process on the left. The curette was used to make an entry hole into the pedicle and the screw was inserted. The same technique was done on the contralateral side and at the L5 level bilaterally. The screw from L3-L5 was connected to the other L5 screw with a rod on both sides and then the rods were locked into place with the locking nuts, and the rods were then connected with a transverse connector piece. Final x-rays were taken. The wound was then closed in anatomic layers using interrupted Vicryl suture for the deep layer and staples for the skin. Sterile dressing was applied and the patient was taken to the recovery room in satisfactory condition.

ICD-10-CM Code(s): _____

ICD-10-PCS Code(s): _____

# Procedures in the Medical and Surgical-related Sections

ICD-10-PCS contains a total of nine Medical and Surgical-related sections:

| Section Value | Description |
|---|---|
| Section 1 | Obstetrics |
| Section 2 | Placement |
| Section 3 | Administration |
| Section 4 | Measurement and Monitoring |
| Section 5 | Extracorporeal Assistance and Performance |
| Section 6 | Extracorporeal Therapies |
| Section 7 | Osteopathic |
| Section 8 | Other Procedures |
| Section 9 | Chiropractic |

## Coding Procedures in the Obstetrics Section – Section 1

## Obstetrics Guidelines

**C.1.** *Products of Conception*
Procedures performed on the Products of Conception are coded to the Obstetrics section. Procedures performed on the pregnant female other than the products of conception are coded to the appropriate root operation in the Medical and Surgical section.

**C.2.** *Procedures Following Delivery or Abortion*
Procedures performed following a delivery or abortion for curettage of the endometrium or evacuation of retained products of conception are all coded in the Obstetrics section, to the root operation Extraction and the body part Products of Conception, Retained. Diagnostic or therapeutic dilation and curettage performed during times other than the postpartum or post-abortion period are all coded in the Medical and Surgical section, to the root operation Extraction and the body part Endometrium.

---

**Coding Note: Products of Conception**
- Products of conception refer to all components of pregnancy, including fetus, embryo, amnion, umbilical cord, and placenta.
- There is no differentiation of the products of conception based on gestational age.

---

## Characters of Obstetrics Section

The seven characters in the Obstetrics section are

| Character 1 | Character 2 | Character 3 | Character 4 | Character 5 | Character 6 | Character 7 |
|---|---|---|---|---|---|---|
| Section | Body System | Root Operation | Body Part | Approach | Device | Qualifier |

The **Obstetrics** section follows the same conventions established in the Medical and Surgical section, with all seven characters retaining the same meaning.

Character 2 (Body System) – one single body system, **Pregnancy**
Character 4 (Body Part) – three body part values:
- Products of conception
- Products of conception, retained
- Products of conception, ectopic

## Root Operations in Obstetrics Section

Refer to Root Operation Definitions in the *ICD-10-PCS 2016 Code Book*.

There are a total of 12 root operations in the Obstetrics section; 10 of the root operations are found in other sections of ICD-10-PCS and two are unique to the Obstetrics section. The two unique root operations to the Obstetrics section are **Abortion** and **Delivery**.

| Obstetrics Section Root Operations | | | |
|---|---|---|---|
| ***Abortion*** | Change | ***Delivery*** | Drainage |
| Extraction | Insertion | Inspection | Removal |
| Repair | Reposition | Resection | Transplantation |

## Obstetrics Section Qualifier

The qualifier values are dependent on the root operation, approach, or body system.

*Examples*
- Methods of extraction – low forceps, vacuum, low cervical
- Methods of terminating pregnancy – laminaria, abortifacient
- Substances drained – amniotic fluid, fetal cerebrospinal fluid

## *Abortion – Root Operation A*

| Abortion A | Definition | Artificially terminating a pregnancy |
|---|---|---|
| | Explanation | Subdivided according to whether an additional device such as a laminaria or abortifacient is used, or whether the abortion was performed by mechanical means |
| | Examples | Transvaginal abortion using vacuum aspiration technique |

**Abortion** is subdivided according to whether an additional device such as a laminaria or abortifacient is used, or whether the abortion was performed by mechanical means. If either a laminaria or abortifacient is used, the approach is Via Natural or Artificial Opening. All other abortion procedures are those done by mechanical means (the products of conception are physically removed using instrumentation) and the device value is Z, No Device.

**3.41.** Transvaginal abortion using vacuum aspiration technique

Code(s): _____

## *Delivery – Root Operation E*

| Delivery E | Definition | Assisting the passage of the products of conception from the genital canal |
|---|---|---|
| | Explanation | Applies only to manually assisted, vaginal delivery |
| | Example | Manually assisted delivery |

**Delivery** applies only to manually assisted, vaginal delivery and is defined as assisting the passage of products of conception from the genital canal. Cesarean deliveries are coded in this section to the root operation Extraction.

**3.42.**   Manually assisted delivery

Code(s): _____

## Drainage – Root Operation 9

| Drainage 9 | Definition | Taking or letting out fluids and/or gases from a body part |
|---|---|---|
| | Explanation | The qualifier identifies the substance that is drained from the products of conception (fetal blood, fetal spinal fluid, amniotic fluid) |
| | Examples | Amniocentesis, percutaneous fetal spinal tap |

The root operation **Drainage** is coded for both diagnostic and therapeutic drainage procedures. For the Obstetrics section the qualifier values identify the substance that is drained from the products of conception (e.g., fetal blood, amniotic fluid).

**3.43.** Fetal spinal tap, percutaneous

Code(s): _____

# Coding Procedures in the Placement Section – Section 2

## Characters of Placement Section

The seven characters in the Placement section are

| Character 1 | Character 2 | Character 3 | Character 4 | Character 5 | Character 6 | Character 7 |
|---|---|---|---|---|---|---|
| Section | Body System | Root Operation | Body Region | Approach | Device | Qualifier |

The **Placement** section follows the same conventions established in the Medical and Surgical section, with all seven characters retaining the same meaning.

Character 2 (Body System) – two body system values:
- Anatomical Regions
- Anatomical Orifices

Character 4 (Body Region) – two body region types:
- External body regions (e.g., chest wall)
- Natural orifices (e.g., mouth and pharynx)

## Root Operations in Placement Section

Refer to Root Operation Definitions in the *ICD-10-PCS 2016 Code Book*.

The root operations in the **Placement** section include only those procedures performed without making an incision or puncture. There are a total of seven root operations in the **Placement** section of which two are common to other sections—**Change** and **Removal**. The five additional root operations unique to the **Placement** section are **Compression, Dressing, Immobilization, Packing**, and **Traction**.

| Placement Section Root Operations | | | |
|---|---|---|---|
| Change | *Compression* | *Dressing* | *Immobilization* |
| *Packing* | Removal | *Traction* | |

## Devices in Placement Section

- Specifies the material or device in placement procedure (e.g., splint, traction apparatus, pressure dressing, bandage)
- Includes casts for fractures and dislocations
- Devices in the Placement section are off the shelf and do not require any extensive design, fabrication, or fitting
- The placement of devices that require extensive design, fabrication, or fitting are coded in the Rehabilitation section of ICD-10-PCS

## *Packing – Root Operation 4*

| Packing 4 | Definition | Putting material in a body region |
|---|---|---|
| | Explanation | Procedures performed without making an incision or puncture |
| | Example | Placement of nasal packing |

**3.44.** Placement of nasal packing

Code(s): _____

## *Immobilization – Root Operation 3*

| Immobilization 3 | Definition | Limiting or preventing motion of a body region |
|---|---|---|
| | Explanation | Procedures to fit a device, such as splints or braces, apply only to the rehabilitation setting |
| | Example | Placement of splint on left finger |

**Coding Note: Immobilization**
The procedures to fit a device, such as splints and braces as described in F0DZ6EZ and F0DZ7EZ, apply only to the rehabilitation setting. Splints and braces placed in other inpatient settings are coded to **Immobilization**, Table 2W3 in the **Placement** section.

**3.45.** Placement of splint, left hand

Code(s): _____

## *Compression – Root Operation 1*

| Compression 1 | Definition | Putting pressure on a body region |
|---|---|---|
| | Explanation | Procedures performed without making an incision or puncture |
| | Example | Placement of pressure dressing on abdominal wall |

**3.46.** Placement of intermittent pneumatic compression device, covering left lower leg

Code(s): _____

## Dressing – Root Operation 2

| Dressing 2 | Definition | Putting material on a body region for protection |
|---|---|---|
| | Explanation | Procedures performed without making an incision or puncture |
| | Example | Application of sterile dressing to head wound |

**3.47.** Sterile dressing placement to wound of the chest wall

Code(s): _____

## Traction – Root Operation 6

| Traction 6 | Definition | Exerting a pulling force on a body region in a distal direction |
|---|---|---|
| | Explanation | Traction in this section includes only the task performed using a mechanical traction apparatus |
| | Example | Lumbar traction using motorized split-traction table |

**Traction** in this section includes only the task performed using a mechanical traction apparatus. Manual traction performed by a physical therapist is coded to Manual Therapy Techniques in section F, Physical Rehabilitation and Diagnostic Audiology.

**3.48.** Mechanical traction of entire right leg

Code(s): _____

# Coding Procedures in the Administration Section – Section 3

## Characters of Administration Section
The seven characters in the Administration section are

| Character 1 | Character 2 | Character 3 | Character 4 | Character 5 | Character 6 | Character 7 |
|---|---|---|---|---|---|---|
| Section | Body System | Root Operation | Body System/ Region | Approach | Substance | Qualifier |

Character 2 (Body System) – three body system values:
- Physiological Systems and Anatomical Regions
- Circulatory
- Indwelling Device

Character 5 (Approach)
- Uses values defined in the Medical and Surgical section
- The approach value for intradermal, subcutaneous, and intramuscular introduction (i.e., injections) is percutaneous
- If a catheter is used to introduce a substance into a site within the circulatory system, the approach value is percutaneous

Character 6 (Substance)
- Substances are specified in broad categories
- Substance values depend on body part

## Root Operations in Administration Section
Refer to Root Operation Definitions in the *ICD-10-PCS 2016 Code Book.*

The root operations in this section are classified according to the broad category of substance administered. If the substance given is a blood product or a cleansing substance, then the procedure is coded to **Transfusion** and **Irrigation** respectively. All other substances administered, such as antineoplastic substances, are coded to the root operation **Introduction**.

| Administration Section Root Operations | | |
|---|---|---|
| *Introduction* | *Irrigation* | *Transfusion* |

## Substances in Administrative Section

Character 6 in the Administrative section specifies the substances given and broad categories are specified with the substance values dependent on the body part.

| Administrative Section Substances Physiological Systems and Anatomical Regions | | | |
|---|---|---|---|
| Anti-inflammatory | Anti-infective | Antineoplastic | Antiarrhythmic |
| Dialysate | Electrolytic and Water Balance Substance | Gas | Intracirculatory Anesthetic |
| Local Anesthetic | Nutritional Substance | Pancreatic Islet Cells | Pigment |
| Platelet Inhibitor | Radioactive Substance | Regional Anesthetic | Serum, Toxoid, and Vaccine |
| Sperm | Stem Cells, Embryonic | Stem Cells, Somatic | Thrombolytic |

| Administrative Section Substances Circulatory | | | |
|---|---|---|---|
| Antihemolytic factor | Bone Marrow | Factor IX | Fibrinogen |
| Fresh Plasma | Frozen Plasma | Globulin | Platelets |
| Red Blood Cells | Frozen Red Cells | Serum Albumin | Whole Blood |

**Coding Note: Administration Section**

The **Administration** section includes infusions, injections, and transfusions, as well as other related procedures, such as irrigation and tattooing. All codes in this section define procedures where a diagnostic or therapeutic substance is given to the patient.

## Transfusion – Root Operation 2

| Transfusion 2 | Definition | Putting in blood or blood products |
|---|---|---|
| | Explanation | Substance given is a blood product or a stem cell substance |
| | Example | Transfusion of cell saver red cells into central venous line |

**3.49.** Bone marrow transplant using donor marrow from identical twin, central vein infusion

Code(s): _____

**3.50.** Transfusion of cell saver red cells via central venous catheter

Code(s): _____

## *Irrigation – Root Operation 1*

| Irrigation 1 | Definition | Putting in or on a cleansing substance |
|---|---|---|
| | Explanation | Substance given is a cleansing substance or dialysate |
| | Example | Flushing of eye |

**Coding Note: Body Part Value**
For the root operation Irrigation, the body part value specifies the site of the irrigation.

**3.51.** Peritoneal dialysis via indwelling catheter

Code(s): _____

**3.52.** Percutaneous irrigation of knee joint

Code(s): _____

## *Introduction – Root Operation 0*

| Introduction 0 | Definition | Putting in or on a therapeutic, diagnostic, nutritional, physiological, or prophylactic substance except' blood or blood products |
|---|---|---|
| | Explanation | All other substances administered, such as antineoplastic substance |
| | Example | Nerve block injection to median nerve |

**Coding Note: Substance for Mixed Steroid and Local Anesthetic**
When a substance of mixed steroid and local anesthetic is given for pain control it is coded to the substance value **Anti-inflammatory**. The anesthetic is only added to lessen the pain of the injection.

**Coding Note: Body Part Value**
For the root operation Introduction, the body part value specifies where the procedure occurs and not necessarily the site where the substance introduced has an effect.

**3.53.** Lumbar epidural injection of mixed steroid and local anesthetic for pain control

Code(s): _____

# Coding Procedures in the Measurement and Monitoring Section – Section 4

## Characters of Measurement and Monitoring Section

The seven characters in the Measurement and Monitoring section are

| Character 1 | Character 2 | Character 3 | Character 4 | Character 5 | Character 6 | Character 7 |
|---|---|---|---|---|---|---|
| Section | Body System | Root Operation | Body System | Approach | Function/ Device | Qualifier |

Character 2 (Body System) – two body system values
- Physiological Systems
- Physiological Devices (Note: Physiological Devices is a body system value for Measurement only.)

Character 6 (Function/Device) – specifies physiological or physical function being tested (e.g., nerve conductivity, respiratory capacity)

## Root Operations in Measurement and Monitoring Section

Refer to Root Operation Definitions in the *ICD-10-PCS 2016 Code Book.*

There are only two root operations in the **Measurement and Monitoring** section. **Measurement** is the first root operation and is used when the procedure determines the level of a physiological or physical function at a point in time. **Monitoring** is the second root operation and is used when the procedure determines the level of a physiological or physical function repetitively over a period of time. These two root operations differ in only one respect: Measurement defines one procedure, and Monitoring defines a series of procedures.

| Measurement and Monitoring Section Root Operations ||
|---|---|
| *Measurement* | *Monitoring* |

## Measurement – Root Operation 0

| Measurement 0 | Definition | Determining the level of a physiological or physical function at a point in time |
|---|---|---|
| | Explanation | A single temperature reading is considered a measurement |
| | Example | EGD with biliary flow measurement, Cardiac catheterization |

**3.54.** Left heart catheterization with sampling and pressure measurements

Code(s): _____

## *Monitoring – Root Operation 1*

| Monitoring 1 | Definition | Determining the level of a physiological or physical function repetitively over a period of time |
| --- | --- | --- |
| | Explanation | Temperature taken every half hour for 8 hours is considered monitoring |
| | Example | Urinary pressure monitoring |

**3.55.** Ambulatory Holter monitoring

Code(s): _____

**3.56.** Transvaginal fetal heart rate monitoring over a period of 16 hours

Code(s): _____

# Coding Procedures in the Extracorporeal Assistance and Performance Section – Section 5

## Characters of Extracorporeal Assistance and Performance Section

The seven characters in the Extracorporeal Assistance and Performance section are

| Character 1 | Character 2 | Character 3 | Character 4 | Character 5 | Character 6 | Character 7 |
|---|---|---|---|---|---|---|
| Section | Body System | Root Operation | Body System | Duration | Function | Qualifier |

Character 2 (Body System) – single body system value: **Physiological Systems**

Character 5 (Duration) – describes the duration of the procedure

Character 6 (Function) – describes the body function being acted upon

---

**Coding Note: Character 5 – Duration**

For respiratory ventilation assistance or performance, the range of consecutive hours is specified (<24 hours, 24–96 hours, or >96 hours).

---

## Root Operation in Extracorporeal Assistance and Performance Section

Refer to Root Operation Definitions in the *ICD-10-PCS 2016 Coding Book.*

There are three unique root operations in the **Extracorporeal Assistance and Performance** section: **Assistance, Performance**, and **Restoration. Assistance** and **Performance** are two variations of the same kinds of procedures, varying only in the degree of control exercised over the physiological function. **Assistance** is taking over partial control of the physiological function and **Performance** is taking complete control of the physiological function. **Restoration** is returning a physiological function to its original state.

| Extracorporeal Assistance and Performance Section Root Operations | | |
|---|---|---|
| *Assistance* | *Performance* | *Restoration* |

### Assistance – Root Operation 0

| Assistance 0 | Definition | Taking over a portion of a physiological function by extracorporeal means |
|---|---|---|
| | Explanation | Procedures that support a physiological function but do not take complete control of it, such as intra-aortic balloon pump to support cardiac output and hyperbaric oxygen treatment |
| | Example | Hyperbaric oxygenation of wound |

3.57.  Intra-aortic balloon pump (IABP), continuous

Code(s): _____

## *Performance – Root Operation 1*

| Performance 1 | Definition | Completely taking over a physiological function by extracorporeal means |
|---|---|---|
| | Explanation | Procedures in which complete control is exercised over a physiological function, such as total mechanical ventilation, cardiac pacing, and cardiopulmonary bypass |
| | Example | Cardiopulmonary bypass in conjunction with CABG |

**3.58.** Hemodialysis, single encounter

Code(s): _____

**3.59.** Cardiopulmonary bypass with CABG, 8 hours

Code(s): _____

---

**ICD-10-PCS Coding Guideline B3.6b. Bypass Procedures**
Coronary arteries are classified by number of distinct sites treated, rather than number of coronary arteries or anatomic name of coronary artery (e.g., left anterior descending). Coronary artery bypass procedures are coded differently than other bypass procedures as described in the previous guideline. Rather than identifying the body part bypassed "from," the body part identifies the number of coronary artery sites bypassed "to," and the qualifier specifies the vessel bypassed "from."

---

**ICD-10-PCS Coding Guideline B3.6c. Bypass Procedures**
If multiple coronary artery sites are bypassed, a separate procedure is coded for each coronary artery site that uses a different device and/or qualifier.

---

**3.60.**
**History:** The patient is a 67-year-old male who was transferred from a local community hospital where he was admitted six days ago with chest pain, shortness of breath, elevated cardiac enzymes, and EKG changes indicating an anterolateral ST elevation myocardial infarction. The patient subsequently underwent a cardiac catheterization, which revealed significant four-vessel disease. He was transferred here for a coronary artery bypass procedure.

**Past History:** Type 2 diabetes (on insulin), hypercholesterolemia and history of carcinoma of the sigmoid colon which was treated with resection of the sigmoid colon and chemotherapy five years ago (the patient has had no recurrence and is currently not being treated). Patient has no past history of a CABG.

**Impression and Plan:** Anterolateral myocardial infarction, coronary artery disease, diabetes mellitus, and hypercholesterolemia

**Operative Report**

**Preoperative Diagnosis:** CAD

**Postoperative Diagnosis:** CAD

**Procedure:** CABG ×4; saphenous vein graft to the obtuse marginal, diagonal artery and posterior descending artery; left internal mammary artery to the left anterior descending artery; cardiopulmonary bypass.

**Description of Procedure:** After obtaining adequate anesthesia, the patient was prepped and draped in the usual fashion. A primary median sternotomy incision was made, and the pericardium was opened. The left internal mammary artery was dissected as a pedicle using electrocautery and small hemoclips at the same time that the greater saphenous vein was harvested endoscopically from the left lower extremity. Cardiopulmonary bypass was instituted and the patient was taken to a mild degree of hypothermia.

The aorta was cross-clamped and electrical arrest effect was administered via cold blood cardioplegia. The saphenous vein graft was placed end-to-side with the posterior descending artery, then a separate graft was placed to the obtuse marginal and finally a separate graft was placed to the diagonal artery. Each anastomosis was done with running 7-0 Prolene suture and verified no bleeders were present. The left internal mammary artery was subsequently brought through a subthalamic tunnel and placed end-to-side with the left anterior descending coronary artery.

Following completion of the grafts, warm blood cardioplegia was administered. During this time, two atrial and ventricular pacing wires were attached to the heart's surface; in addition, mediastinal tubes were also placed. The cross clamps were released following this, and sinus rhythm returned spontaneously. The patient was weaned from cardiopulmonary bypass without incident.

After all grafts were checked for diastolic flow, which revealed no problems, the incisions were closed. The patient was taken to the recovery room in good condition and will be monitored in the intensive care unit. The procedure took approximately 5 hours.

ICD-10-CM Code(s): _____

ICD-10-PCS Code(s): _____

## *Restoration – Root Operation 2*

| Restoration 2 | Definition | Returning, or attempting to return, a physiological function to its original state by extracorporeal means |
|---|---|---|
| | Explanation | Restoration defines only external cardioversion and defibrillation procedures. Failed cardioversion procedures are also included in the definition of Restoration and are coded the same as successful procedures. |
| | Example | Attempted cardiac defibrillation, unsuccessful |

**3.61.** External cardioversion

Code(s): _____

## Coding Procedures in the Extracorporeal Therapies Section – Section 6

### Characters of Extracorporeal Therapies Section

The seven characters in the Extracorporeal Therapies section are

| Character 1 | Character 2 | Character 3 | Character 4 | Character 5 | Character 6 | Character 7 |
|---|---|---|---|---|---|---|
| Section | Body System | Root Operation | Body System | Duration | Qualifier | Qualifier |

Character 2 (Body System) – single body system value: **Physiological Systems**

Character 5 (Duration) – specifies whether the procedure was single occurrence, multiple occurrence, or intermittent

Character 6 (Qualifier) – no specific qualifier values (Z, No Qualifier)

Character 7 (Qualifier) – identifies various blood components separated out in pheresis procedures

### Root Operation in Extracorporeal Therapies Section

Refer to Root Operation Definitions in the *ICD-10-PCS 2016 Code Book*.

There are 10 root operations within the **Extracorporeal Therapies** section and the meaning of each root operation is consistent with the term as used in the medical community.

- Atmospheric Control (value 0) – extracorporeal control of atmospheric pressure and composition
- Decompression (value 1) – extracorporeal elimination of undissolved gas from body fluids
- Electromagnetic Therapy (value 2) – extracorporeal treatment by electromagnetic rays
- Hyperthermia (value 3) – extracorporeal raising of the body temperature
- Hypothermia (value 4) – extracorporeal lowering of the body temperature
- Pheresis (value 5) – extracorporeal separation of blood products
- Phototherapy (value 6) – extracorporeal treatment by light rays
- Ultrasound Therapy (value 7) – extracorporeal treatment by ultrasound
- Ultraviolet Light Therapy (value 8) – extracorporeal treatment by ultraviolet lights
- Shock Wave Therapy (value 9) – extracorporeal treatment by shock waves

| Extracorporeal Therapies Section Root Operations | | | |
|---|---|---|---|
| *Atmospheric Control* | *Decompression* | *Electromagnetic Therapy* | *Hyperthermia* |
| *Hypothermia* | *Pheresis* | *Phototherapy* | *Ultrasound Therapy* |
| *Ultraviolet Light Therapy* | *Shock Wave Therapy* | | |

---

**Coding Note: Decompression**
Decompression describes a single type of procedure—treatment for decompression sickness (the bends) in a hyperbaric chamber.

---

**Coding Note: Hyperthermia**
Hyperthermia is used both to treat temperature imbalance, and as an adjunct radiation treatment for cancer. When performed to treat temperature imbalance, the procedure is coded to this section.

When performed for cancer treatment, whole-body hyperthermia is classified as a modality qualifier in section D, Radiation Therapy.

---

**Coding Note: Pheresis**
Pheresis is used in medical practice for two main purposes: to treat diseases where too much of a blood component is produced, such as leukemia, or to remove a blood product such as platelets from a donor, for transfusion into a patient who needs them.

---

**Coding Note: Phototherapy**
Phototherapy to the circulatory system means exposing the blood to light rays outside the body, using a machine that recirculates the blood and returns it to the body after phototherapy.

---

**3.62.** Whole body hypothermia, single treatment (for treatment of temperature imbalance)

Code(s): _____

**3.63.** Ultraviolet light phototherapy, single treatment

Code(s): _____

# Coding Procedures in the Osteopathic Section – Section 7

## Characters of Osteopathic Section

The seven characters in the Osteopathic section are

| Character 1 | Character 2 | Character 3 | Character 4 | Character 5 | Character 6 | Character 7 |
|---|---|---|---|---|---|---|
| Section | Body System | Root Operation | Body Region | Approach | Method | Qualifier |

Character 2 (Body System) – single body system value: **Anatomical Regions**

Character 6 (Method) – method of the osteopathic treatment; these methods are not explicitly defined in ICD-10-PCS and rely on the standard definitions as used in this specialty

## Root Operation in Osteopathic Section

Refer to Root Operation Definitions in the *ICD-10-PCS 2016 Code Book*.

The Osteopathic section contains a single root operation: **Treatment**.

## Osteopathic Methods

Character 6 in the Osteopathic section defines the osteopathic method of the procedure.

| Osteopathic Methods | | | |
|---|---|---|---|
| Articulatory – Raising | Fascial Release | General Mobilization | High Velocity – Low Amplitude |
| Indirect | Low Velocity – High Amplitude | Lymphatic Pump | Muscle Energy – Isometric |
| Muscle Energy – Isotonic | Other Method | | |

> **Coding Note: Osteopathic Section**
> Section 7, Osteopathic, is one of the smallest sections in ICD-10-PCS. There is a single body system, **Anatomic Regions**, and a single root operation, **Treatment**.

## *Treatment – Root Operation 0*

| Treatment 0 | Definition | Manual treatment to eliminate or alleviate somatic dysfunction and related disorder |
|---|---|---|
| | Explanation | None |
| | Example | Fascial release of abdomen, osteopathic treatment |

**3.64.** Indirect osteopathic treatment of sacrum

Code(s): _____

# Coding Procedures in the Other Procedures Section – Section 8

## Characters of Other Procedures Section

The seven characters in the Other Procedures section are

| Character 1 | Character 2 | Character 3 | Character 4 | Character 5 | Character 6 | Character 7 |
|---|---|---|---|---|---|---|
| Section | Body System | Root Operation | Body Region | Approach | Method | Qualifier |

Character 2 (Body System) – two body system values:
- Indwelling Device
- Physiological Systems and Anatomical Regions

Character 6 (Method) – defines the method of the procedure, such as robotic-assisted procedure, computer-assisted procedure, or acupuncture

## Root Operation in Other Procedures Section

Refer to Root Operation Definitions in the *ICD-10-PCS 2016 Code Book*.

The Other Procedures section contains a single root operation, **Other Procedures**.

---

**Coding Note: Other Procedures Section**

The Other Procedures section contains codes for procedures not included in the other Medical and Surgical-related sections. There are relatively few procedures coded in this section. Whole-body therapies including acupuncture and meditation are included in this section along with a code for the fertilization portion of an in-vitro fertilization procedure. This section also contains codes for robotic-assisted and computer-assisted procedures.

---

## *Other Procedures – Root Operation 0*

| Other Procedures 0 | Definition | Methodologies that attempt to remediate or cure a disorder or disease |
|---|---|---|
| | Explanation | For nontraditional, whole-body therapies including acupuncture and meditation |
| | Example | Acupuncture |

**3.65.** Robotic-assisted transurethral prostatectomy via endoscopy

Code(s): _____

**3.66.** Suture removal, right leg

Code(s): _____

# Coding Procedures in the Chiropractic Section – Section 9

## Characters of Chiropractic Section

The seven characters in the Chiropractic section are

| Character 1 | Character 2 | Character 3 | Character 4 | Character 5 | Character 6 | Character 7 |
|---|---|---|---|---|---|---|
| Section | Body System | Root Operation | Body Region | Approach | Method | Qualifier |

Character 2 (Body System) – single body system value: **Anatomical Regions**

## Root Operation in Chiropractic Section

Refer to Root Operation Definitions in the *ICD-10-PCS 2016 Code Book*.

The Chiropractic Section contains a single root operation, **Manipulation**.

---

**Coding Note: Chiropractic Section**
Section 9, Chiropractic section, consists of a single body system, **Anatomical Regions**, and a single root operation, **Manipulation**.

---

## *Manipulation – Root Operation B*

| Manipulation B | Definition | Manual procedures that involves a direct thrust to move a joint past the physiological range of motion, without exceeding the anatomical limit |
|---|---|---|
| | Explanation | None |
| | Example | Chiropractic treatment of cervical spine, short lever specific contact |

3.67. Chiropractic treatment of lumbar spine using long and short lever specific contact

Code(s): _____

218

## *Procedures in the Ancillary Sections*

ICD-10-PCS contains a total of seven ancillary sections as follows:

| Section Value | Description |
|---|---|
| Section B | Imaging |
| Section C | Nuclear Medicine |
| Section D | Radiation Therapy |
| Section F | Physical Rehabilitation and Diagnostic Audiology |
| Section G | Mental Health |
| Section H | Substance Abuse Treatment |
| Section X | New Technology |

**Note:** Ancillary sections (sections B–D, F–H, and X) do not include root operations.

Character 3 represents root type of the procedure for these sections.

## *Coding Procedures in the Imaging Section – Section B*

### Characters of Imaging Section

The seven characters in the Imaging section are

| Character 1 | Character 2 | Character 3 | Character 4 | Character 5 | Character 6 | Character 7 |
|---|---|---|---|---|---|---|
| Section | Body System | Root Type | Body Part | Contrast | Qualifier | Qualifier |

Character 3 (Root Type) – defines procedure by root type, instead of root operation

Character 5 (Contrast) – defines contrast if used; contrast is differentiated by the concentration of the contrast material (e.g., high or low osmolar)

Character 6 (Qualifier) – for majority of imaging codes is a qualifier that specifies an image is taken without contrast followed by one with contrast (unenhanced and enhanced (0)); occasionally also specifies laser (1) or intravascular optical coherence (2)

Character 7 (Qualifier) – for majority of imaging codes is a qualifier that is not specified in this section; occasionally specifies intraoperative (0), densitometry (1), intravascular (3), transesophageal (4), or guidance (A)

## Root Types in Imaging Section

The Imaging section has a total of five root types:

- Plain Radiography (value 0) – Planar display of an image developed from the capture of external ionizing radiation on photographic or photoconductive plate.
- Fluoroscopy (value 1) – Single plane or bi-plane real time display of an image developed from the capture of external ionizing radiation on a fluorescent screen. The image may also be stored by either digital or analog means.
- Computerized Tomography (CT scan) (value 2) – Computer reformatted digital display of multiplanar images developed from the capture of multiple exposures of external ionizing radiation.
- Magnetic Resonance Imaging (MRI) (value 3) – Computer reformatted digital display of multiplanar images developed from the capture of radio-frequency signals emitted by nuclei in a body site excited within a magnetic field.
- Ultrasonography (value 4) – Real time display of images of anatomy or flow information developed from the capture of reflected and attenuated high-frequency sound waves.

**3.68.** MRI of thyroid gland, without contrast material followed by with other contrast material

Code(s): _____

**3.69.** Chest x-ray, anteroposterior (AP) and posteroanterior (PA)

Code(s): _____

**3.70.** The following documentation is from the health record of a 42-year-old male.

**Procedure:** Left heart catheterization, coronary angiography and left ventriculography

**Indications:** This is a 42-year-old male who presented to the emergency room with unstable angina and was subsequently admitted. Serial EKGs and cardiac enzymes ruled out a myocardial infarction. The patient has no history of any previous cardiac interventions including angioplasty or CABG. The patient also is being treated for hypertension.

**Procedure:** The patient was premedicated with 2 mg of Versed in the catheterization laboratory. The right groin was prepped and draped using aseptic technique. The skin and subcutaneous tissues were locally anesthetized with 1 percent Xylocaine. The right femoral artery was entered with 18 gauge needle and 0.035 J guide wire was introduced into the descending aorta. A #6 French left coronary artery catheter was introduced over the guide wire. Selective injections using low osmolar dye were made in the left coronary artery. The right coronary artery catheter was then exchanged with #6 French pigtail catheter and left heart catheterization was performed at rest with pressures being measured. The left ventriculogram was then performed using low osmolar dye. At the end of the procedure, the catheter was removed and pressure held over the right groin until adequate hemostasis was achieved. The patient had good right posterior tibial and dorsalis pedis arterial pulsations following the catheterization. The patient was stabilized and then transferred to his room.

**Findings**

**Hemodynamics:** Pressures: Aortic and left ventricular pressures were normal

**Left ventriculography:** The overall left ventricular systolic function is mildly reduced. Left ventricular ejection fraction is 40 percent by left ventriculogram. Mild hypokinesis of the anterior wall of the left ventricle. Mitral valve regurgitation is not seen.

**Coronary angiography:** Left main coronary artery: There were no obstructing lesions in the left main coronary artery. Blood flow appeared to be normal.

**Left anterior descending artery:** There was a 45 percent stenosis in the mid left anterior descending artery.

**Left circumflex:** There was a 40 percent stenosis in the left circumflex artery.

**Right coronary artery:** Right coronary artery is dominant to the posterior circulation. There were no obstructing lesions in the right coronary artery. Blood flow appeared normal.

**Impression**
1. Atherosclerotic heart disease with unstable angina
2. Family history of heart disease
3. Tobacco use

ICD-10-CM Code(s): _____

ICD-10-PCS Code(s): _____

# Coding Procedures in the Nuclear Medicine Section – Section C

## Characters of Nuclear Medicine Section

The seven characters in the Nuclear Medicine section are

| Character 1 | Character 2 | Character 3 | Character 4 | Character 5 | Character 6 | Character 7 |
|---|---|---|---|---|---|---|
| Section | Body System | Root Type | Body Part | Radionuclide | Qualifier | Qualifier |

Character 3 (Root Type) – defines procedure by root type, instead of root operation

Character 5 (Radionuclide) – defines the source of the radiation used in the procedure; an Other Radionuclide option is included for new FDA radiopharmaceuticals

Characters 6 and 7 (Qualifiers) – are not specified in this section (Z)

## Root Types in Nuclear Medicine Section

The Nuclear Medicine section has a total of seven root types:
- Planar Nuclear Medicine Imaging (value 1) – Introduction of radioactive materials into the body for single plane display of images developed from the capture of radioactive emissions
- Tomographic (Tomo) Nuclear Medicine Imaging (value 2) – Introduction of radioactive materials into the body for three-dimensional display of images developed from the capture of radioactive emissions
- Positron Emission Tomography (PET) (value 3) – Introduction of radioactive materials into the body for three-dimensional display of images developed from the simultaneous capture, 180 degrees apart, of radioactive emissions
- Nonimaging Nuclear Medicine Uptake (value 4) – Introduction of radioactive materials into the body for measurements of organ function, from the detection of radioactive emissions
- Nonimaging Nuclear Medicine Probe (value 5) – Introduction of radioactive materials into the body for the study of distribution and fate of certain substances by the detection of radioactive emissions from an external source
- Nonimaging Nuclear Medicine Assay (value 6) – Introduction of radioactive materials into the body for the study of body fluids and blood elements, by the detection of radioactive emissions
- Systemic Nuclear Medicine Therapy (value 7) – Introduction of unsealed radioactive materials into the body for treatment

3.71.   PET scan of myocardium using Fluorine 18 (F-18)

   Code(s): _____

3.72.   Technetium tomo scan of the spleen

   Code(s): _____

# Coding Procedures in the Radiation Therapy Section – Section D

## Characters of Radiation Therapy Section

The seven characters in the Radiation Therapy section are

| Character 1 | Character 2 | Character 3 | Character 4 | Character 5 | Character 6 | Character 7 |
|---|---|---|---|---|---|---|
| Section | Body System | Root Type | Treatment Site | Modality Qualifier | Isotope | Qualifier |

Character 3 (Root Type) – specifies the basic modality (beam radiation, brachytherapy, stereotactic radiosurgery, and other radiation)

Character 4 (Treatment Site) – specifies the treatment site that is the target of the radiation therapy

Character 5 (Modality Qualifier) – further specifies treatment modality (photons, electrons, heavy particles, contact radiation)

Character 6 (Isotope) – specifies the radioactive isotope administered in the oncology treatment

**3.73.** Brachytherapy of prostate, HDR using Cesium 137

Code(s): _____

**3.74.** Contact radiation of esophagus

Code(s): _____

## Coding Procedures in the Physical Rehabilitation and Diagnostic Audiology Section – Section F

### Characters of Physical Rehabilitation and Diagnostic Audiology Section

The seven characters in the Physical Rehabilitation and Diagnostic Audiology section are

| Character 1 | Character 2 | Character 3 | Character 4 | Character 5 | Character 6 | Character 7 |
|---|---|---|---|---|---|---|
| Section | Section Qualifier | Root Type | Body System/ Region | Type Qualifier | Equipment | Qualifier |

Character 2 (Section Qualifier) – specifies whether the procedure is a rehabilitation or diagnostic audiology procedure

Character 3 (Root Type) – specifies general procedure root type

Character 4 (Body System/Region) – specifies the body system and body region combined, where applicable

Character 5 (Type Qualifier) – specifies the precise test or method employed. The *ICD-10-PCS 2016 Code Book* provides Type and Qualifier Definitions.

Character 6 (Equipment) – specifies the general categories of equipment used, if any (Note: Specific types of equipment are not listed.)

### Root Types in Physical Rehabilitation and Diagnostic Audiology Section

The Physical Rehabilitation and Diagnostic Audiology section classifies procedures into 14 root types:
- Speech Assessment (value 0) – Measurement of speech and related functions
- Motor and/or Nerve Function Assessment (value 1) – Measurement of motor, nerve, and related functions
- Activities of Daily Living Assessment (value 2) – Measurement of functional level for activities of daily living
- Hearing Assessment (value 3) – Measurement of hearing and related functions
- Hearing Aid Assessment (value 4) – Measurement of the appropriateness and/or effectiveness of a hearing device
- Vestibular Assessment (value 5) – Measurement of the vestibular system and related functions
- Speech Treatment (value 6) – Application of techniques to improve, augment, or compensate for speech and related functional impairment
- Motor Treatment (value 7) – Exercise or activities to increase or facilitate motor function
- Activities of Daily Living Treatment (value 8) – Exercise or activities to facilitate functional competence for activities of daily living
- Hearing Treatment (value 9) – Application of techniques to improve, augment, or compensate for hearing and related functional impairment

- Hearing Aid Treatment (value B) – Application of techniques to improve the communication abilities of individuals with cochlear implant
- Vestibular Treatment (value C) – Application of techniques to improve, augment, or compensate for vestibular and related functional impairment
- Device Fitting (value D) – Fitting of a device designed to facilitate or support achievement of a higher level of function
- Caregiver Training (value F) – Training in activities to support patient's optimal level of function

---

**Coding Note: Treatment**

Use of specific activities or methods to develop, improve, and/or restore the performance of necessary functions; compensate for dysfunction; and/or minimize debilitation.

Treatment procedures include swallowing dysfunction exercises, bathing and showering techniques, wound management, gait training, and a host of activities typically associated with rehabilitation.

---

**Coding Note: Assessment**

Assessment includes a determination of the patient's diagnosis when appropriate, need for treatment, planning for treatment, periodic assessment, and documentation related to these activities.

Assessments are further classified into more than 100 different tests or methods. The majority of these focus on the faculties of hearing and speech, but others focus on various aspects of body function, and on the patient's quality of life, such as muscle performance, neuromotor development, and reintegration skills.

---

**Coding Note: Device Fitting**

The fifth character used in Device Fitting procedures describes the device being fitted rather than the method used to fit the device. Where definitions of devices are provided, they are located in the definitions portion of the ICD-10-PCS Tables and Index, under section F, character 5

---

**Coding Note: Caregiver Training**

Educating caregiver with the skills and knowledge used to interact with and assist the patient. Caregiver Training is divided into 18 different broad subjects taught to help a caregiver provide proper patient care.

---

**3.75.** Wound care treatment of right lower leg ulcer (staged to muscle) using pulsatile lavage

Code(s): _____

**3.76.** Bekesy assessment using audiometer

Code(s): _____

## *Coding Procedures in the Mental Health Section – Section G*

### Characters of Mental Health Section

The seven characters in the Mental Health section are

| Character 1 | Character 2 | Character 3 | Character 4 | Character 5 | Character 6 | Character 7 |
|---|---|---|---|---|---|---|
| Section | Body System | Root Type | Type Qualifier | Qualifier | Qualifier | Qualifier |

Character 2 (Body System) – does not convey specific information about the procedure; the value Z functions as a placeholder for this character

Character 3 (Root Type) – specifies the mental health procedure root type

Character 4 (Type Qualifier) – further specifies the procedure type as needed

Characters 5, 6, and 7 (Qualifier) – do not convey specific information about the procedure; the value Z functions as a placeholder for these characters

### Root Types in Mental Health Section

There are 12 root type values in the Mental Health section:
- Psychological Tests – value 1
- Crisis Intervention – value 2
- Medication Management – value 3
- Individual Psychotherapy – value 5
- Counseling – value 6
- Family Psychotherapy – value 7
- Electroconvulsive Therapy – value B
- Biofeedback – value C
- Hypnosis – value F
- Narcosynthesis – value G
- Group Therapy – value H
- Light Therapy – value J

**3.77.**   Electroconvulsive therapy (ECT), bilateral, multiple seizures

Code(s): _____

**3.78.**   Personality and behavioral testing

Code(s): _____

# Coding Procedures in the Substance Abuse Treatment Section – Section H

## Characters of Substance Abuse Treatment Section

The seven characters in the Substance Abuse Treatment section are

| Character 1 | Character 2 | Character 3 | Character 4 | Character 5 | Character 6 | Character 7 |
|---|---|---|---|---|---|---|
| Section | Body System | Root Type | Type Qualifier | Qualifier | Qualifier | Qualifier |

Character 2 (Body System) – does not convey specific information about the procedure; the value Z functions as a placeholder for this character

Character 3 (Root Type) – specifies the root type

Character 4 (Type Qualifier) – further classifies the root type

Characters 5, 6, and 7 (Qualifier) – do not convey specific information about the procedure; the value Z functions as a placeholder for these characters

## Root Types in Substance Abuse Treatment Section

There are seven different root type values in the Substance Abuse Treatment section:
- Detoxification Services – value 2
- Individual Counseling – value 3
- Group Counseling – value 4
- Individual Psychotherapy – value 5
- Family Counseling – value 6
- Medication Management – value 8
- Pharmacotherapy – value 9

**3.79.** Alcohol detoxification treatment

Code(s): _____

**3.80.** Individual 12-step psychotherapy for substance abuse

Code(s): _____

# References

American Hospital Association. 1991. *Coding Clinic,* 1st Quarter. Chicago: AHA.

American Hospital Association. 2014. *Coding Clinic,* 4th Quarter. Chicago: AHA.

Centers for Medicare and Medicaid Services. 2016a. 2016 Development of the ICD-10 Procedure Coding System (ICD-10-PCS). http://www.cms.gov/ICD10/.

Centers for Medicare and Medicaid Services. 2016b. *2016 ICD-10-PCS Reference Manual* and Slides. http://www.cms.gov/ICD10/.

Centers for Medicare and Medicaid Services. 2016c. *2016 Official ICD-10-PCS Coding Guidelines.* http://www.cms.gov/ICD10/.

Dorland. 2007. *Dorland's Illustrated Medical Dictionary.* Philadelphia: W.B. Saunders.

Kuehn, L. and T. Jorwic. 2011. *ICD-10-PCS: An Applied Approach.* Chicago: AHIMA.

Kuehn, L. and T. Jorwic. 2013. *ICD-10-PCS: An Applied Approach,* Second Edition. Chicago: AHIMA.

Kuehn, L. and T. Jorwic. 2014. *ICD-10-PCS: An Applied Approach,* 2015 Edition. Chicago: AHIMA.

Merriam-Webster. 2010. *Merriam-Webster's Medical Dictionary.* Springfield, MA: Merriam-Webster, Inc.

Stedman's. 2006. *Stedman's Electronic Medical Dictionary.* Philadelphia: Lippincott Williams & Wilkins.

# ICD-10-PCS Coder Training Manual Answer Key

# Introduction: ICD-10-PCS Overview

**Activity 1: Matching Procedures with Sections**

1. Medical and Surgical

2. Other Procedures

3. Physical Rehabilitation and Diagnostic Audiology

4. Administration

5. Measurement and Monitoring

6. Imaging

## Section 1 Review Questions

1.   d. 5A2204Z

2.   a . True

3.   a. Root Operation

4.   c. CMS

5.   d. October 1, 2015

6.   d. 7

7.   b. False

8.   c. 34

9.   d. Uniaxial

10.   c. D

**Activity 2: Identifying Problems with ICD-9-CM Procedure Codes**

1. c. Standardized terminology

2. c. Standardized terminology

3. d. Standardized level of specificity

4. b. Diagnosis information excluded

5. a. NOS code options excluded

**Activity 3: ICD-10-PCS Key Attribute – Completeness**

1. Character 1: Section is the same for both codes

0 = Medical and Surgical section

Character 2: Body system is different

In 0C9P00Z, C = Mouth and Throat; In 0B0100Z, B = Respiratory System

Character 3: Root operation is the same for both codes

9 = Drainage

Character 4: Body part is different

In 0C9P00Z, P = Tonsils; In 0B9100Z, 1 = Trachea

Character 5: Approach is the same for both codes

0 = Open

Character 6: Device is the same for both codes

0 = Drainage device

Character 7: Qualifier is the same for both codes

Z = No qualifier

2. Character 1: Sections is the same for both codes

0 = Medical and Surgical section

Character 2: Body system is the same for both codes

B = Respiratory system

Character 3: Root operation is the same for both codes

9 = Drainage

Character 4: Body part is the same for both codes

3 = Right main bronchus

Character 5: Approach is different

In 0B9300Z, 0 = Open; In 0B933ZX, 3 = Percutaneous

Character 6: Device is different

In 0B9300Z, 0 = Drainage device; In 0B933ZX, Z = No device

Character 7: Qualifier is different

In 0B9300Z, Z = No qualifier; In 0B933ZX, X = Diagnostic

3. Character 1: Section is the same for both codes

0 = Medical and Surgical section

Character 2: Body system is the same for both codes

H – Skin and Breast

Character 3: Root operation is the same for both codes

9 = Drainage

Character 4: Body part is the same for both codes

0 = Skin, scalp

Character 5: Approach is the same for both codes

X = External

Character 6: Device is different

In 0H90X0Z, 0 = Drainage device; In 0H90XZZ, Z = No device

Character 7: Qualifier is the same for both codes

Z = No qualifier

## Section 2 Review Questions

1.    a. Multiaxial structure

2.    a. True

3.    d. Limited NEC code options

4.    d. Repair

5.    a. True

6.    b. False

7.    c. Partial lobectomy of lung

8.    d. Character 4

9.    b. False

10.   a. True

## Activity 4: Root Operations

1.  Detachment
2.  Excision
3.  Removal
4.  Revision
5.  Extraction

## Activity 5: Medical and Surgical Approaches

1.  Method
2.  Skin
3.  3
4.  7

## Activity 6: Approach Definiitions

1.  Percutaneous
2.  Via Natural or Artificial Opening with Percutaneous Endoscopic Assistance
3.  Percutaneous Endoscopic
4.  Via Natural or Artificial Opening Endoscopic
5.  Via Natural or Artificial Opening

## Activity 7: Coding Exercise

1.  0DB68ZX
2.  0FT44ZZ
3.  0HBU0ZZ

# Section 3 Review Questions

1.  c. Musculoskeletal system

2.  a. Removal

3.  b. False

4.  c. Peripheral Nervous System

5.  a. True

6.  a. True

7.  b. Insertion

8.  b. False

9.  c. Repair

10. b. Open

---

**Activity 8: Coding Exercise**

1.  3E1U38Z - Index Irrigation, Joint, Irrigation Substance (3E1U38Z)

2.  10T24ZZ - Index Resection, Products of conception, ectopic (10T2)

3.  3E1M39Z - Index: Dialysis, Peritoneal (3E1M39Z)
4.  5A09 - Index: Intermittent positive pressure breathing, see Assistance, Respiratory 5A09
    Assistance, Respiratory, 24-96 Consecutive Hours, Intermittent Positive Airway Pressure 5A09458

---

**Activity 9: Root Operations in the Medical and Surgical-related Sections**

1.  Dressing

2.  Measurement

3.  Performance

4.  Hypothermia

5.  Irrigation

# Section 4 Review Questions

1.    b. Holter monitoring

2.    a. Function

3.    a. True

4.    b. Function/Device

5.    b. False

6.    b. False

7.    c. 3

8.    b. False

9.    c. Extraction

10.    a. True

# Section 5 Review Questions

1.    c. Routine fetal ultrasound, second trimester, twin gestation

2.    d. Isotope

3.    a. True

4.    b. False

5.    a. Administration

6.    a. True

7.    d. Modality Qualifier

8.    b. False

9.    c. Pharmacotherapy

10.    a. True

**Activity 10: ICD-10-PCS Coding Guidelines**

   1.  e. Multiple procedures

   2.  c. Biopsy followed by more definitive treatment

   3.  d. Excision vs. Resection

   4.  b. Approach

   5.  c. Excision for graft

## Section 6 Review Questions

1.     b. False

2.     b. Guideline B3.11a Inspection of a body part(s) performed in order to achieve the objective of a procedure is not coded separately.

3.     b. The site, left hand

4.     a. True

5.     a. External

6.     a. True

7.     c. Proximal

8.     b. False

9.     b. It is required to consult the Index first before proceeding to the Tables to complete the code.

10.    a. True


## Final Review Questions

1.     c. Single axis

2.     d. Seven characters long

3.     b. Characters

4.     b. Section value D

5.     d. Four columns and a varying number of rows

6.     a. True

7.     a. True

8.     a. True

9.     b. Standardized terminology

10.    a. Total mastectomy

11.    c. Entry, by puncture or minor incision, of instrumentation through the skin or mucous membrane and/or any other body layers necessary to reach and visualize the site of the procedure.

12.  c. Diagnostic

13.  b. 10E0XZZ

14.  b. Revision

15.  b. False

16.  d. Epidural injection of mixed steroid and local anesthetic for pain control

17.  a. True

18.  d. Obstetrics

19.  a. True

20.  b. False

# Part I: ICD-10-PCS Coding

# ICD-10-PCS Training—Day 1

## *ICD-10-PCS Guidelines and Root Operations Review*

### ICD-10-PCS Guidelines

1.  a. True

2.  b. False

3.  b. False

4.  b. False

5.  a. True

6.  b. False

7.  a. True

8.  b. False

9.  a. True

10. a. True

### Root Operations

11. a. True

12. a. True

13. a. True

14. b. False

15. a. True

16. b. False

17. a. True

18. a. True

19. a. True

20. b. False

# Coding Procedures in the Medical and Surgical Section – Section 0

**2.1.**    0HTT0ZZ     Root Operation, Resection
                                   Resection, Breast, Right (0HTT0ZZ)
                                   Mastectomy, *see* Resection, Skin and Breast (0HT)

          0HBT3ZX     Root Operation, Excision
                                   Excision, Breast, Right (0HBT)
                                   Biopsy, *see* Excision with qualifier Diagnostic

**Rationale:**

In this case Resection is selected because this was a total mastectomy. While the Table is required for most code selections in ICD-10-PCS, there are some codes that can be obtained directly from the Index. This is one example in which the entire code was listed in the Alphabetic Index. ICD-10-PCS Coding Guideline A7 states that the PCS Tables should always be consulted to find the most appropriate valid code. Therefore, the Table should be consulted.

**2.2.**    0X690Z2     Root Operation: Detachment
                                   Detachment, Arm, Upper, Left (0X690Z)
                                   Amputation, *see* Detachment

**Rationale:**

Amputation, *see* Detachment

**2.3.**    0U5C7ZZ     Root Operation: Destruction
                                   Destruction, Cervix (0U5C)

          0U5G7ZZ     Root Operation: Destruction
                                   Destruction, Vagina (0U5G)

          0U5MXZZ     Root Operation: Destruction
                                   Destruction, Vulva (0U5M)

**Rationale:**

Three codes are required for this procedure since condylomas were removed from three separate and distinct body parts, cervix, vagina and vulva. The root operation Destruction is the correct root operation for all three procedures, as a laser was utilized to obliterate the condylomas. The approach for the cervix and vagina is 7, Via Natural or Artificial Opening, and the approach for the vulva is X, External.

**2.4.**    0GTG4ZZ     Root Operation: Resection
                                   Resection, Thyroid Gland, Left Lobe (0GTG)

          07B24ZX     Root Operation: Excision
                                   Excision, Lymphatic, Neck, Left (07B2)

**Rationale:**

The lobes of the thyroid have their own distinct body part values in ICD-10-PCS. Therefore, this is a Resection of the left thyroid lobe rather than an Excision of the thyroid gland.

**2.5.**    015H3ZZ     Root Operation: Destruction
                                   Destruction, Nerve, Peroneal (015H)
                                   Denervation, Peripheral nerve, *see* Destruction, Peripheral Nervous System (015H)

**Rationale:**
The common fibular nerve does not have its own distinct body part value. ICD-10-PCS Coding Guideline B4.2 states: "Where a specific branch of a body part does not have its own body part value in PCS, the body part is coded to the closest proximal branch that has a specific body part value." The Alphabetic Index has the following entry: Common fibular nerve, *use* Nerve, Peroneal.

**2.6.**　0DB64Z3　Root Operation: Excision
　　　　　　　　　　Excision, Stomach (0DB6)

**Rationale:**
The seventh character, qualifier, captures that the procedure is a vertical sleeve gastrectomy.

**2.7.**　0UDB7ZX　Root Operation: Extraction
　　　　　　　　　　Extraction, Endometrium (0UDB)

**Rationale:**
The approach for this procedure was via a natural opening (vagina). This case should be coded as diagnostic due to the *curettage for tissue sampling*.

**2.8.**　0BBF8ZX　Root Operation: Excision
　　　　　　　　　　Excision, Lung, Lower Lobe, Right (0BBF)
　　　　　　　　　　Biopsy, *see* Excision with qualifier Diagnostic

**Rationale:**
ICD-10-PCS Coding Guideline B3.2b states to code multiple procedure codes if the same root operation is repeated at different body sites that have the same body part value, but *Coding Clinic* Q4 2014 clarifies Guideline B3.2b as referring to distinct body parts, not different locations within the same body part, so the code is only assigned once.

**2.9.**　0B538ZZ　Root Operation: Destruction
　　　　　　　　　　Destruction, Bronchus, Main, Right (0B53)

**Rationale:**
During this procedure, the Nd:YAG laser is used to obliterate the lesion in the right main bronchus so that the lesion is no longer present.

**2.10.**　0SB20ZZ　Root Operation: Excision
　　　　　　　　　　Excision, Disc, Lumbar Vertebral (0SB2)

**Rationale:**
The correct root operation is Excision, since only a partial discectomy of L4 was performed. The correct body part is 2, Lumbar Vertebral Disc.

**2.11.**　0HDRXZZ　Root Operation: Extraction
　　　　　　　　　　Extraction, Toe Nail (0HDRXZZ)
　　　　　　0H5RXZZ　Root Operation: Destruction
　　　　　　　　　　Destruction, Toe Nail (0H5RXZZ)

**Rationale:**
ICD-10-PCS Coding Guideline B3.2c states that multiple procedures are coded if multiple root operations with distinct objectives are performed on the same body part. Two codes are assigned to this case since two distinct root operations were performed. The root operation Extraction is coded due to the fact that the nail plate is pulled out. The body part value R, Toe Nail is assigned for the fourth character. The nail matrix, still part of the body part R, Toenail, is destroyed by electrocautery.

**2.12.**   0BTJ0ZZ        Root Operation: Resection
                          Resection, Lung, Lower Lobe, Left (0BTJ)

**Rationale:**
ICD-10-PCS Coding Guideline B3.8 states that PCS contains specific body parts for anatomical subdivisions of a body part, such as lobes of the lungs or liver and regions of the intestine. Resection of the specific body part is coded whenever all of the body part is cut out or off, rather than coding Excision of a less specific body part.

**2.13.**   0UBC7ZZ        Root Operation: Excision
                          Excision, Cervix (0UBC)

**Rationale:**
The root operation Excision is used for the procedure on the cervix. Destruction is not appropriate in this case because the loop electrode excised a cone-shaped piece of tissue, as stated in the documentation. If the documentation stated that the electrocautery was used to completely destroy the tissue, the root operation Destruction would be appropriate.

**2.14.**   0FT40ZZ        Root Operation: Resection
                          Resection, Gallbladder (0FT4)
            0FJ44ZZ        Root Operation: Inspection
                          Inspection, Gallbladder (0FJ4)

**Rationale:**
In this case, a laparoscopic procedure was attempted, but converted to an open procedure. See Coding Guideline B3.2d. Multiple procedures are coded if the intended root operation is attempted using one approach, but is converted to a different approach.

**2.15.**   0Y6D0Z3        Root Operation: Detachment
                          Detachment, Leg, Upper Left (0Y6D0Z)
                          Amputation *see* Detachment

**Rationale:**
The upper leg (body part value C) is detached at the distal end of the femur, qualifier value 3 or Low amputation.

**2.16.**   0DBM8ZX        Root Operation: Excision
                          Excision, Colon, Descending (0DBM)
                          Biopsy *see* Excision
            0DBN8ZX        Root Operation, Excision
                          Excision, Colon, Sigmoid (0DBN)
            0DBP8ZZ        Root Operation: Excision
                          Excision, Rectum (0DBP)

**Rationale:**
Two biopsies were performed during this procedure, one in the descending colon and one in the sigmoid colon. ICD-10-PCS Coding Guideline B3.2a states that if the same root operation is performed on different body parts that have their own distinct body part value, a code should be assigned for each of the different body parts, but *Coding Clinic* Q4 2014 clarifies Guideline B3.2b as referring to distinct body parts, not different locations within the same body part. Additionally, polypectomies were performed at two different body sites within the rectum.

**2.17.**   0S9C3ZX        Root Operation: Drainage
                          Drainage, Joint, Knee, Right (0S9C)
                          Arthrocentesis, *see* Drainage, Lower Joints (0S9)

**Rationale:**

The knee joint is a lower joint since it is located below the diaphragm

**2.18.** OTC33ZZ     Root Operation: Extirpation
                              Extirpation, Kidney Pelvis, Right (OTC3)

**Rationale:**

The explanation for the root operation Extirpation states that the solid matter may or may not have been previously broken into pieces.

**2.19.** OTF4XZZ     Root Operation: Fragmentation
                              Fragmentation, Kidney Pelvis, Left (OTF4)

**Rationale:**

The root operation Fragmentation is coded to describe the breaking up of the calculus. The approach for extracorporeal shock wave lithotripsy is always X, External.

**2.20.** OW9B30Z     Root Operation: Drainage
                              Drainage, Pleural Cavity, Left (OW9B)

**Rationale:**

The approach for this procedure is percutaneous (3) as the instrumentation was introduced to the operative site via the skin. The sixth character (device) is drainage device (0) since the drainage device was left at the operative site at the end of the procedure.

**2.21.** OFF98ZZ     Root Operation: Fragmentation
                              Fragmentation, Duct, Common Bile (OFF9)

**Rationale:**

There is an entry in the Alphabetic Index for ERCP *see* Fluoroscopy, Hepatobiliary System and Pancreas BF1. This would identify the imaging component of this procedure and would be added to the surgical code if one codes to this degree of specificity with ICD-10-PCS codes. The Charge Description Master would most likely assign the component of the procedure.

ERCP is performed with a scope entering through the mouth to the biliary system via the duodenum, so the approach value is Via Natural or Artificial Opening Endoscopic. This would be considered integral to performing the procedure, and would not be separately coded to Inspection.

**2.22.** OTC78ZZ     Root Operation: Fragmentation
                              Extirpation, Ureter, Left (OTC7)
                              Lithotripsy, with removal of fragments – see Extirpation

**Rationale:**

For this case only one code is assigned, OTC78ZZ, for the extirpation of the fragmented calculi. In the ICD-10-PCS Alphabetic Index, the main term is Lithotripsy, with removal of fragments – *see* Extirpation. *AHA Coding Clinic, 4*[th] *Q 2013* states that the fragmentation would not be coded separately since it is inherent to the extirpation.

**2.23.** OY910ZZ     Root Operation: Drainage
                              Drainage, Buttock, Left (OY91)

**Rationale:**
This procedure was performed via an open approach as an incision was made in order to drain the abscess.

**2.24.** 03C93ZZ    Root Operation: Extirpation
                          Extirpation, Artery, Ulnar, Right (03C9)
                          Thrombectomy, see Extirpation

**Rationale:**
In order to select the body system and body part, one must know where the common interosseous artery is located. The Alphabetic Index can be utilized to find the correct body part value for the right common interosseous artery. Index: Common interosseous artery – *use* Artery, Ulnar, Right.

**2.25.** 08943ZZ    Root Operation: Drainage
                          Drainage, Vitreous, Right (0894)

**Rationale:**
Sclerotomy *see* Drainage, Eye 089

**2.26.** 0DC38ZZ    Root Operation: Extirpation
                          Extirpation, Esophagus, Lower (0DC3)
      0DB68ZX    Root Operation: Excision
                          Excision, Stomach (0DB6)

**Rationale:**
The root operation Extirpation is used to code the removal of the foreign body. Even though the foreign body was not removed through the mouth, it was removed from the distal esophagus by sending it through the normal digestive route. The body part value of 3, Esophagus, Lower is assigned. There is no device or qualifier value. The root operation Excision is used to code the stomach biopsy. The body part value 6, Stomach is assigned and the qualifier value of X, Diagnostic is assigned because this was a biopsy. Both procedures are performed using an endoscopic approach through a natural opening, approach value 8.

**2.27.** 0RNK4ZZ    Root Operation: Release
                          Release, Joint, Shoulder, Left (0RNK)

**Rationale:**
The sole objective of the manipulation is to free the frozen left shoulder; therefore, Release is the correct root operation. The procedure was performed arthroscopically, which codes to a percutaneous endoscopic approach.

**2.28.** 0SND0ZZ    Root Operation: Release
                          Release, Joint, Knee, Left (0SND)
      0SNC0ZZ    Root Operation: Release
                          Release, Joint, Knee, Right (0SNC)

**Rationale:**
ICD-10-PCS Coding Guideline B4.3 states that if no bilateral body part value exists, each procedure is coded separately using the appropriate body part value. The table 0SN does not contain a bilateral body part value for the knee joints, so two codes are required, one for the left knee and one for the right knee.

**2.29.** 0W8NXZZ    Root Operation: Division
                          Division, Perineum, Female (0W8N)
                          Episiotomy, *see* Division, Perineum, Female (0W8N)

**Rationale:**
The body part on which the episiotomy was performed is the perineum.

**2.30.** 0SNCXZZ    Root Operation: Release
Release, Joint, Knee, Right (0SNC)
Manipulation, Adhesions, *see* Release

**Rationale:**
The root operation is release. The right knee is manipulated under anesthesia to release the joint from an abnormal constraint. The approach is external.

**2.31.** 0P8M3ZZ    Root Operation: Division
Division, Carpal, Right (0P8M)
0P8M3ZZ    Root Operation: Division
Division, Carpal, Right (0P8M)

**Rationale:**
*See* Division, Head and Facial Bones (0N8), *see* Division, Lower Bones (0Q8), and *see* Division, Upper Bones (0P8) are all choices. It is necessary to know the location of the capitates to assign the body system. In this case, Upper Bones is selected as the body system. Next, to assign the body part, it is necessary to review Coding Guideline B4.1a. Since the capitate is not a choice in the Table, the body part would be the value corresponding to the whole body part. The capitate is one of the carpal bones of the wrist in the hand. The Alphabetic Index has the following entry: Capitate bone, *use* Carpal, Right.

Since the lunate is not a choice in the Table, the body part would be the value corresponding to the whole body part. The lunate is also one of the carpal bones of the wrist in the hand. The Alphabetic Index has the following entry: Lunate bone, *use* Carpal, Right.

**2.32.** 0BYM0Z0    Root Operation: Transplantation
Transplantation, Lung, Bilateral (0BYM0Z)

**Rationale:**
ICD-10-PCS provides a body part value for bilateral lungs, therefore only one code is assigned for this procedure. Coding Guideline B 4,3. states that if the identical procedure is performed on contralateral body parts, and a bilateral body part value exists for that body part, a single procedure is coded using the bilateral body part value. The seventh character of transplantation procedures defines genetic compatibility of the body part being transplanted. The seventh character for this procedure is 0, Allogenic, since the organs can from a cadaver donor. Allogenic is defined as being taken from different individuals of the same species.

**2.33.** 01X50Z4    Root Operation: Transfer
Transfer, Nerve, Median (01X5)

**Rationale:**
The anterior interosseous nerve does not have its own distinct body part value. ICD-10-PCS Coding Guideline B4.1b. states that when a specific branch of a body part does not have its own body part value in PCS, the body part is coded to the closest proximal branch that has a specific body part value. Utilization of the Alphabetic Index indicates that the median nerve is the closest proximal branch for the anterior interosseous nerve.

**2.34.** 0XMF0ZZ    Root Operation: Reattachment
Reattachment, Arm, Lower, Left

**Rationale:**
The root operation Reattachment involves putting back on all or a portion of a separated body part. For the case the separated body part was the left lower arm.

**2.35.**  0QS906Z    Root Operation: Reposition
Reposition, Femoral Shaft, Left (0QS9)
Reduction, Fracture, *see* Reposition
0QSJ0CZ    Root Operation: Reposition
Reposition, Fibula, Right
0QSG0CZ    Root Operation: Reposition
Reposition, Tibia, Right

**Rationale:**
The patient sustained fractures of three different bones, and since each of the three bones have their own distinct body part value, three procedure codes are required. The first fracture is of the shaft of the left femur which was repaired by an open reduction with intramedullary fixation. The device value for this first fracture is 6. Both the second and third fractures of the tibia and fibula were repaired with an open reduction with an external ring fixation device. The device value for these fractures is C.

**2.36.**  0TY00Z0    Root Operation: Transplantation
Transplantation, Kidney, Right (0TY00Z)

**2.37.**  0KXL0Z6    Root Operation, Transfer
Transfer, Muscle, Abdomen, Left (0KXL)
TRAM (transverse rectus abdominis myocutaneous) flap, Pedicle, *see* Transfer, Muscles (0KX)

**Rationale:**
The root operation for a pedicle flap transfer is Transfer. During a pedicle flap transfer the body part transferred remains connected to its vascular and nervous supply. The qualifier identifies that this is a TRAM pedicle graft.

**2.38.**  0PSH34Z    Root Operation: Reposition
Reposition, Radius, Right (0PSH)
Reduction, Fracture, *see* Reposition
0PSKXZZ    Root Operation: Reposition
Reposition, Ulna, Right (0PSK)

**Rationale:**
Two procedure codes are required for this case with Reposition being the root operation for both fracture reductions. The definition for Reposition is moving to its normal location, or other suitable location, all or a portion of a body part. The right radius fracture was first reduced and then K wire pins (internal fixation) were placed percutaneously The fracture of the right ulna was only reduced externally.

**2.39.**  01X64Z5    Root Operation: Transfer
Transfer, Nerve, Radial (01X6)

**Rationale:**
During this procedure the radial nerve was transferred to the median nerve. In the Alphabetic Index, the body part selected is Radial because that is the nerve being transferred. The qualifier for this procedure describes the site receiving the transfer (median).

**2.40.**  0VSC0ZZ    Root Operation: Reposition
Reposition, Testis, Bilateral (0VSC)

**Rationale:**
During this procedure, the testes are moved into the Inner thigh to protect them because the scrotum has been damaged in some way.

**2.41.** 0LXW0ZZ    Root Operation: Transfer
                     Transfer, Tendon, Foot, Left (0LXW)

**Rationale:**
Utilizing the Alphabetic Index, the flexor digitorum brevis tendon is in the foot. There is no specific index entry for Flexor digitorum brevis tendon, but there is an Alphabetic Index entry for Flexor digitorum brevis muscle (*use* Muscle, Foot). Knowing that tendons are named for their muscles will also help in the selection of the correct body part values.

**2.42.** 08SL0ZZ    Root Operation: Reposition
                     Reposition, Muscle, Extraocular, Right (08SL)

**Rationale:**
The root operation Reposition is used because the eye muscle is moved to a more posterior position to repair the hypertropia. Utilizing the Alphabetic Index, the body value assigned for the right superior rectus muscle is an extraocular eye muscle, right. Since the body part (the eye) was removed from the socket, the approach would be Open.

**2.43.** 0LMM0ZZ    Root Operation: Reattachment
                     Reattachment, Tendon, Upper Leg, Left (0LMM)

**Rationale:**
The root operation Reattachment is used to code the repair (reattachment) of the tendon rupture. Utilizing the Alphabetic Index, the body part value assigned for the left quadriceps tendon is the body part value for upper leg tendon, left.

**2.44.** 0PSR04Z    Root Operation: Reposition
                     Reposition, Phalanx, Thumb, Right (0PSR)
                     Reduction, Fracture, *see* Reposition

**Rationale:**
The root operation Reposition is used to code the reduction of the fracture. The body part value, R, Thumb Phalanx, Right, is assigned.

**2.45.** 087X0DZ    Root Operation: Dilation
                     Dilation, Duct, Lacrimal, Right (087X)

**Rationale:**
This procedure is coded to the root operation Dilation since the right lacrimal duct was dilated. The osteotomy is the approach which is open. The sixth character for the device (silicone tube) is D, Intraluminal device.

**2.46.** 0B110F4    Root Operation: Bypass
                     Bypass, Trachea (0B11)
                     Tracheostomy, *see*, Bypass, Respiratory System (0B1)

**Rationale:**
This procedure is coded to the root operation Bypass. A tracheostomy is a bypass between the trachea and skin. The body part value 1, Trachea, is the source of the bypass (or where the bypass is coming from) and the skin (Cutaneous, 4) is the body part bypassed to. A Shiley trach was left at the operative site, therefore the device value of F, Tracheostomy, is assigned for the sixth character.

**2.47.** 0TL70ZZ    Root Operation: Occlusion
                     Occlusion, Ureter, Left (0TL7)
                     Ligation *see* Occlusion

**Rationale:**
Ligation *see* Occlusion

**2.48.** 0UVC0CZ    Root Operation: Restriction
Restriction,Cervix (0UVC)
Cerclage, *see* Restriction

**Rationale:**
The root operation for the cervical cerclage is Restriction. The objective of this procedure is to partially close the cervix. The device value is C, Extraluminal Device, to capture the band that was placed around or on the outside of the cervix.

**2.49.** 0DV64CZ    Root Operation: Restriction
Restriction, Stomach (0DV6)
Banding, *see* Restriction

**2.50.** 03VG3DZ    Root Operation: Restriction
Restriction, Artery, Intracranial (03VG)

**Rationale:**
The anterior cerebral artery does not have its own body part value in ICD-10-PCS. Utilizing the Alphabetic Index, the anterior cerebral artery maps to the intracranial artery body part in ICD-10-PCS. A cerebral aneurysm is also known as an intracranial or intracerebral aneurysm and is a weak area on a blood vessel in the brain that balloons out and fills with blood.

The device value for the coated platinum coils is D, Intraluminal Device. Utilizing the Device Table or the Alphabetic Index the term Embolization coils maps to an Intraluminal Device.

**2.51.**   021109W    Root Operation: Bypass
Bypass, Artery, Coronary, Two Sites (0211)
02100Z9    Root Operation: Bypass
Bypass, Artery, Coronary, One Site (0210)
06BQ4ZZ    Root Operation: Excision
Excision, Vein, Greater Saphenous, Left (06BQ)

**Rationale:**
The diagonal and obtuse margin arteries were bypassed using the aortocoronary bypass grafting technique. This technique involves graft material which for this case was autologous venous tissue. The graft material came from the patient's own left greater saphenous vein.

The coronary artery bypass graft of the left anterior descending artery was done using the left internal mammary artery. Review Coding Guideline B3.6b for coronary arteries. The body part value identifies the number of coronary artery sites bypassed to and the qualifier identifies the vessel bypassed from. The sixth character, No Device, was selected because internal mammary coronary artery bypass procedures do not involve the use of free graft material, but rather a pedicled graft. The internal mammary is loosened from one side and brought around to the occluded coronary artery, restoring blood flow (AHA 1991).

If cardiopulmonary bypass was performed with the CABG, an additional code would be assigned from the procedures in the Medical and Surgical-related sections (Extracorporeal Assistance and Performance – Section 5). This section will be studied later in the training.

**2.52.**   027034Z    Root Operation: Dilation
Dilation, Artery, Coronary, One Site (0270)
02703ZZ    Root Operation: Dilation
Dilation, Artery, Coronary, One Site (0270)

**Rationale:**
Two codes are required for this procedure with a separate code required for each artery dilated, because the device value differs for each artery. For the body part value, select Coronary Artery, One Site (0), because a drug-eluting stent was used in one artery, but not the other. The device character 4 was assigned for the procedure with the drug-eluting stent (Coding Guideline B4.4).

If the same example had a stent inserted in both arteries, the code would be 027134Z.

**2.53.**  0UL74CZ    Root Operation: Occlusion
                          Occlusion, Fallopian Tubes, Bilateral (0UL7)

**Rationale:**
Ligation *see* Occlusion

**2.54.**  0D738ZZ    Root Operation: Dilation
                          Dilation, Esophagus, Lower (0D73)

**Rationale:**
The dilation was performed in the distal, or lower, part of the esophagus.

**2.55.**  0D1M0Z4    Root Operation: Bypass
                          Bypass, Colon, Descending (0D1M)

**Rationale:**
The fourth character of this procedure code specifies the body part bypassed from (descending colon) and the seventh character specifies the body part bypassed to (skin).

**2.56.**  04LE3DT    Root Operation: Occlusion
                          Occlusion, Artery, Internal Iliac, Right Uterine Artery (04LE)
           04LF3DU    Root Operation: Occlusion
                          Occlusion, Artery, Internal Iliac, Left Uterine Artery (04LF)

**Rationale:**
Two codes are required for this procedure – one for the embolization of the right uterine artery and one for the embolization of the left uterine artery. The uterine arteries do not have their own body part values in ICD-10-PCS. Utilizing the Alphabetic Index, the closest proximal branch to the uterine arteries are the left and right internal iliac arteries.

**2.57.**  0F798ZZ    Root Operation: Dilation
                          Dilation, Duct, Common Bile (0F79)

**Rationale:**
The ERCP is the approach; therefore, it is not separately coded.

**2.58.**  041K09N    Root Operation: Bypass
                          Bypass, Artery, Femoral, Right (041K)
           06BP0ZZ    Root Operation: Excision
                          Excision, Vein, Greater Saphenous, Right (06BP)

**2.59.**  0D160ZA    Root Operation: Bypass
                          Bypass, Stomach (0D16)

**Rationale:**
Bypass procedure are coded by identifying the body part bypassed "from" and the body part bypass "to". In this case, the body part bypassed from is the Stomach and the body part bypassed to is the Jejunum.

A Roux-en-Y anastomosis is defined as an anastomosis of the distal end of the divided jejunum to the stomach, bile duct, or another structure, with implantation of the proximal end into the side of the jejunum at a suitable distance (usually greater than 40 cm) below the first anastomosis, the bowel then forming a Y-shaped pattern (Stedman's 2010).

**2.60.** 0C7S8ZZ    Root Operation: Dilation
                            Dilation, Larynx (0C7S)

**2.61.** 0JHN0NZ    Root Operation: Insertion
                            Insertion of device in, Subcutaneous Tissue and Fascia, Lower Leg, Right (0JHN)

**2.62.** 0YU60JZ    Root Operation: Supplement
                            Supplement, Inguinal Region, Left (0YU6)

**Rationale:**
The body system is one of the General Anatomic Regions and Lower Extremities would be selected because the inguinal region is below the diaphragm. See Coding Guideline B2.1b. The device is a Synthetic Substitute (J).

**2.63.** 0W29X0Z    Root Operation: Change
                            Change device in, Pleural Cavity, Right (0W29X)

**Rationale:**
A chest tube is a flexible plastic tube that is inserted through the side of the chest into the pleural space. The body part would be the pleural cavity, which is part of the Anatomical Regions, General (0W2).

**2.64.** 08R93KZ    Root Operation: Replacement
                            Replacement, Cornea, Left (08R9)
       08R83KZ    Root Operation: Replacement
                            Replacement, Cornea, Right (08R8)

**Rationale:**
Keratoplasty, *see* Repair, Eye; *see* Replacement, Eye; *see* Supplement, Eye. In this case, Replacement meets the intent of the procedure.

There is not a body part value for bilateral cornea, so therefore the right and left cornea are coded separately. The device is Nonautologous Tissue Substitute (K) because the tissue came from a donor.

**2.65.** 02PA3MZ    Root Operation: Removal
                            Removal of device from, Heart (02PA)
       02PA3MZ    Root Operation: Removal
                            Removal of device from, Heart (02PA)
       02H63JZ    Root Operation: Insertion
                            Insertion of device in, Atrium, Right (02H6)
       02HK3JZ    Root Operation: Insertion
                            Insertion of device in, Ventricle, Right (02HK)

**Rationale:**
Based on the ICD-10-PCS definitions, this procedure is not a Replacement. This procedure is coded to the root operation Removal to remove the old leads and the root operation Insertion to insert the new leads. Based on Coding Guideline B3.2b, two codes are required for the removal of the leads because the same root operation is repeated on different body sites (atrium and ventricle) that are included in the same body part value (heart).

The insertion also requires two codes because the right atrium and right ventricle are identified with individual body part values.

**2.66.** 02U50JZ      Root Operation: Supplement
Supplement, Septum, Atrial (02U5)

**Rationale:**
Since the septal defect is repaired with mesh, the root operation is Supplement.

**2.67.** 0JH606Z      Root Operation: Insertion
Insertion of device in, Subcutaneous Tissue and Fascia, Chest (0JH6)
02H63JZ      Root Operation: Insertion
Insertion of device in, Atrium, Right (02H6)
02HK3JZ      Root Operation: Insertion
Insertion of device in, Ventricle, Right (02HK)

**Rationale:**
The root operation Insertion is used to code all three procedures. Three codes are required since three different devices were inserted: the generator, the right ventricle lead, and the right atrium lead.

**2.68.** 02RF08Z      Root Operation: Replacement
Replacement, Valve, Aortic (02RF)

**Rationale:**
The device used is Zooplastic Tissue (8) because a porcine valve is from a pig heart.

**2.69.** 02WA3MZ      Root Operation: Revision
Revision of device in, Heart (02WA)

**2.70.** 0HR8X73      Root Operation: Replacement
Replacement, Skin, Buttock (0HR8)
0HRJX73      Root Operation: Replacement
Replacement, Skin, Upper Leg, Left (0HRJ)

**Rationale:**
The root operation Replacement is used to code free skin grafts. Replacement procedures can use tissue-cultured epidermal autograft. This type of graft is from the patient's own skin that was previously harvested and grown in a laboratory to a larger size to be used as a skin replacement approximately 14 days later. This type of tissue is coded with the device value of 7, Autologous Tissue Substitute, because the origin is the patient's own skin. Character 4, partial thickness is used for the qualifier character to reflect the epidermal graft which is a partial thickness graft.

**2.71.** 0TP98DZ      Root Operation: Removal
Removal of device from, Ureter (0TP9)

**Rationale:**
There is no distinction for right versus left in the body part of Ureter for this code assignment.

The device is an Intraluminal Device because the stent is placed into the lumen of the ureter.

**2.72.** 0B21XFZ      Root Operation: Change
Change device in, Trachea (0B21)

**Rationale:**
Exchange, *see* Change device in. Tracheostomy Device, Change device in, Trachea (0B21XFZ)

**2.73.** 0RRK00Z      Root Operation: Replacement
Replacement, Joint, Shoulder, Left (0RRK)

**Rationale:**
During this procedure the left shoulder joint is replaced with a reverse prosthesis (ball on glenoid and socket on humerus). The removal of the native shoulder joint is included in the replacement procedure and is not coded separately.

**2.74.** 02HV33Z  Root Operation: Insertion
Insertion of device in, Vena Cava, Superior (02HV)

**Rationale:**
The ICD-10-PCS Device Table indicates to use Infusion Device as the device character for a peripherally inserted central catheter (PICC). Additionally the following entry appears in the ICD-10-PCS Alphabetic Index: Peripherally inserted central catheter (PICC) *use* Infusion Device.

**2.75.** 0PPF04Z  Root Operation: Removal
Removal of device from, Humeral Shaft, Right (0PPF)

**Rationale:**
Utilizing the Alphabetic Index, the body part value for the distal humerus is the humeral shaft.

**2.76.** 0SH03BZ  Root Operation: Insertion
Insertion of device in, Joint, Lumbar Vertebral (0SH0)

**2.77.** 0QHG08Z  Root Operation: Insertion
Insertion of device in, Tibia, Right (0QHG)

0QHJ08Z  Root Operation, Insertion
Insertion of device in, Fibula, Right (0QHJ)

**2.78.** 0JH608Z  Root Operation: Insertion
Insertion of device in, Subcutaneous Tissue and Fascia, Chest (0JH6)

02H63KZ  Root Operation: Insertion
Insertion of device in, Atrium, Right (02H6)

02HK3KZ  Root Operation, Insertion
Insertion of device in, Ventricle, Right (02HK)

**Rationale:**
Three codes are required for this procedure with the root operation being Insertion for all three procedures. Three devices were inserted: Generator, Right Ventricle Lead and Right Atrium Lead.

**2.79.** 0SRR019  Root Operation: Replacement
Replacement, Joint, Hip, Right, Femoral Surface (0SRR)

**Rationale:**
During this procedure only, the femoral surface of the right hip was replaced. The prosthesis is a metal synthetic substitute and the qualifier indicates that the device was cemented. The removal of the native femoral head is included in the replacement procedure and not coded separately.

**2.80.** 0QHY3MZ  Root Operation: Insertion
Insertion of device in, Bone, Lower (0QHY)

**Rationale:**
When indexing Insertion of device in, there is a subterm for Femoral Shaft, Left (0QH9). When reviewing the Table, Femoral Shaft, Left (9) is not an option for the bone growth stimulator. In the row for Bone Growth Stimulator (M), the only body part available is Lower Bone (Y).

**Coding Note:** Several electrical bone growth stimulators are available:

The noninvasive type of stimulator is comprised of coils or electrodes, which are placed on the skin near the fracture site.

The invasive type includes percutaneous and implanted devices. The percutaneous type involves electrode wires inserted through the skin into the bone while implanted devices include a generator placed under the skin or in the muscles near the gap between the ends of the bones, which have not fused. The implanted devices are surgically placed and later surgically removed.

**2.81.** 0WJP0ZZ     Root Operation: Inspection
                       Inspection, Gastrointestinal Tract (0WJP)

**Rationale:**
During this procedure, the gastrointestinal tract was explored with no disease being found. Therefore, Inspection is the root operation. Inspection is defined as visually exploring a body part.

**2.82.** 00K73ZZ     Root Operation: Map
                       Map, Cerebral Hemisphere (00K7)

**2.83.** 0BTD0ZZ     Root Operation: Resection
                       Resection, Lung, Middle Lobe, Right (0BTD)
        0WJ94ZZ     Root Operation: Inspection
                       Inspection, Pleural Cavity, Right (0WJ9)

**Rationale:**
Two codes are required to completely code this procedure. ICD-10-PCS Coding Guideline B3.2d states that during the same operative episode, multiple procedures are coded if the intended root operation is attempted using one approach, but is converted to a different approach. Because the procedure was discontinued due to the pleural effusion, the root operation Inspection is coded for the initial endoscopic evaluation, with a percutaneous endoscopic approach. The root operation Resection is coded for the completed procedure of the open lobectomy of the right middle lobe, because the right middle lobe is an entire body part in ICD-10-PCS.

**2.84.** 0BJ08ZZ     Root Operation: Inspection
                       Inspection, Tracheobronchial Tree (0BJ0)

**Rationale:**
ICD-10-PCS Coding Guideline B3.11b states if multiple tubular body parts are inspected, the most distal body part inspected is coded. If multiple non-tubular body parts in a region are inspected, the body part that specifies the entire area inspected is coded.

**2.85.** 0DJD8ZZ     Root Operation: Inspection
                       Inspection, Intestinal Tract, Lower (0DJD)

**Rationale:**
ICD-10-PCS Coding Guideline B4.8 states in the gastrointestinal body system, the general body part values Upper Intestinal Tract and Lower Intestinal Tract are provided as an option for the root operations Change, Inspection, Removal and Revision. Upper Intestinal Tract includes the portion of the gastrointestinal tract from the esophagus down to and including the duodenum, and Lower Intestinal Tract includes the portion of the gastrointestinal tract from the jejunum down to and including the rectum and anus.

**2.86.** 02K83ZZ     Root Operation: Map
                       Map, Conduction Mechanism (02K8)

**2.87.** 0TJB8ZZ      Root Operation: Inspection
Inspection, Bladder (0TJB)

**2.88.** 0MQ24ZZ      Root Operation: Repair
Repair, Bursa and Ligament, Shoulder, Left (0MQ2)

**Rationale:**
The glenoid labrum ligament does not have its own distinct body part value in ICD-10-PCS. Utilizing the Alphabetic Index, the body part value assigned is for the Shoulder Bursa and Ligament, Right.

**2.89.** 0W3D0ZZ      Root Operation: Control
Control, postoperative bleeding in, Pericardial Cavity (0W3D)

**Rationale:**
The site of the bleeding for a control procedure is coded as an anatomical region and not a specific body part.

**2.90.** 0X334ZZ      Root Operation: Control
Control postprocedural bleeding in, Shoulder Region, Left (0X33)

**Rationale:**
The site of the bleeding for a control procedure is coded as an anatomical region and not a specific body part.

**2.91.** 0WQF0ZZ      Root Operation: Repair
Repair, Abdominal Wall (0WQF)

**Rationale:**
The root operation repair is coded to restore the abdominal wall to the normal anatomic structure. During the procedure, the hernia was repaired with sutures, which are not considered to be a device

**2.92.** 0JQR0ZZ      Root Operation: Repair
Repair, Subcutaneous Tissue and Fascia, Foot, Left (0JQR)

**Rationale:**
The approach is considered to be Open even though the surgical exposure may have been created by the wound itself.

**2.93.** 0W33XZZ      Root Operation: Control
Control postprocedural bleeding in, Oral Cavity and Throat (0W33)

**Rationale:**
The root operation Control is coded because the bleeder is the result of a previous procedure. When cautery is used to stop postprocedural bleeding, Control is the appropriate root operation. The tonsillar area is coded to the body part value of 3, Oral cavity and Throat

**2.94.** 0LQ80ZZ      Root Operation: Repair
Repair, Tendon, Hand, Left (0LQ8)

**Rationale:**
ICD-10-PCS Coding Guideline B4.7 states that if a body system does not contain a separate body part value for fingers, procedures performed on the fingers are coded to the body part value for the hand. In this case, the body system Tendons does not have a separate body part value for left fingers, therefore the body part value is 8, Hand Tendon, Left.

**2.95.** 0SG10AJ      Root Operation: Fusion
Fusion, Lumbar Vertebral, 2 or more (0SG1)

**Rationale:**

Two joints were fused, so the body part for the fusion is 1, Lumbar Vertebral Joints, 2 or more. The insertion of the pedicle screws is not coded separately. A code is not assigned for the nonautologous bone graft per ICD-10-PCS Coding Guideline B3.10c which states that if an interbody fusion device is used to render the joint immobile (alone or containing other material like bone graft), the procedure is coded with the device value Interbody Fusion Device.

**2.96.** 090K0JZ    Root Operation: Alteration
                            Alteration: Nose (090K)

**Rationale:**

Rhinoplasty, *see* Alteration, Nose

**2.97.** 0RGS34Z    Root Operation: Fusion
                            Fusion, Metacarpocarpal, Right (0RGS)

**Rationale:**

There are only two choices of body systems for Fusion procedures: Lower Joints (0SG) and Upper Joints (0RG). The thumb is located above the diaphragm, therefore is considered to be an upper joint.

**2.98.** 0W4M070    Root Operation: Creation
                            Creation, Male (0W4M0)

**Rationale:**

There is only one body system: Anatomical Regions, General (0W4) and only two body part values: Perineum, Female (0W4N) and Perineum, Male (0W4M) for the root operation Creation. The body part value pertains to the current sex of the patient and the qualifier identifies the body part being created.

**2.99.** 0W4N0J1    Root Operation: Creation
                            Creation, Female (0W4N0)

**Rationale:**

There is only one body system: Anatomical Regions, General (0W4) and only two body part values: Perineum, Female (0W4N) and Perineum, Male (0W4M) for the root operation Creation. The body part value pertains to the current sex of the patient and the qualifier identifies the body part being created.

**2.100.** 0SG107J    Root Operation: Fusion
                            Fusion, Lumbar Vertebral, 2 or more (0SG1)
          0PB10ZZ    Root Operation: Excision
                            Excision, Rib, Right (0PB1)

**Rationale:**

Two joints were fused, so the body part for the fusion is 1, Lumbar Vertebral Joints, 2 or more. A code is not assigned for the nonautologous bone graft per ICD-10-PCS Coding Guideline B3.10c which states that if an interbody fusion device is used to render the joint immobile (alone or containing other material like bone graft), the procedure is coded with the device value Interbody Fusion Device. A second code is assigned for the harvesting of bone graft material from the patient's right rib. Coding Guideline B3.9 states that if an autograft is obtained from a different body part in order to complete the objective of the procedure, a separate procedure is coded. The insertion of the pedicle screws are coded separately.

**2.101.** 0H0V0JZ    Root Operation: Alteration
                            Alteration, Breast Bilateral (0H0V)

**Rationale:**
There is no Alphabetic Index term for Augmentation. It is necessary to understand that the root operation for this procedure is Alteration because it is done for cosmetic purposes.

**2.102.** 0W0F0ZZ          Root Operation: Alteration
                                        Alteration, Abdominal Wall (0W0F)

**Rationale:**
Abdominoplasty – *see* Alteration, Abdominal Wall (0W0F); *see* Repair, Abdominal Wall (0WQF); *see* Supplement, Abdominal Wall (0WUF). There is no documentation this was done for medical reasons; in fact, it is called a "tummy tuck" so Alteration is selected

# Part II: ICD-10-PCS Coding

# ICD-10-PCS Training—Day 2

## Case Studies from Inpatient Health Records

### Detailed and/or Complex Cases and Scenarios Using ICD-10-PCS Procedure Codes

**3.1.**      0UT90ZZ          Resection, Uterus (0UT9)
                                        Hysterectomy, *see* Resection, Uterus (0UT9)
              0UTC0ZZ          Resection, Cervix (0UTC)
              0UT20ZZ          Resection, Ovary, Bilateral (0UT2)
              0UT70ZZ          Resection, Fallopian Tubes, Bilateral (0UT7)
              0FB20ZX          Excision, Liver, Left Lobe (0FB2)
                                        Biopsy, *see* Excision with qualifier Diagnostic

**Rationale:**
The ICD-10-PCS Root Operation Guidelines for coding multiple procedures state that if the same root operation is performed on different body parts as defined by distinct values of the body part character, each should be coded separately (B3.2.a). During this procedure, four distinct body parts were removed: uterus, cervix, both ovaries, and both fallopian tubes, and therefore should be coded separately. By definition, a total hysterectomy includes resection or removal of both the uterus and cervix. Two codes are needed for this procedure: resection of the uterus and resection of the cervix. The resection of the uterus is coded to 0UT90ZZ and resection of the cervix is coded to 0UTC0ZZ. The root operation Resection is selected since the entire uterus and cervix is removed during a total abdominal hysterectomy. Removal of bilateral ovaries is coded to 0UT20ZZ with the body part value of 2 indicating bilateral ovaries. Removal of bilateral fallopian tubes is coded to 0UT70ZZ with the body part value of 7 indicating bilateral fallopian tubes. ICD-10-PCS Coding Guideline B.4.3 states that bilateral body part values are available for a limited number of body parts. If the identical procedure is performed on contralateral body parts, and a bilateral body part value exists for that body part, a single procedure is coded using the bilateral body part value. For all four of these codes, the approach is 0 for open. The liver biopsy is coded to 0FB20ZX. The root operation for the biopsy is Excision (B) since only a portion of the liver is removed. The approach for the liver biopsy is Open. In ICD-10-PCS, the approach is the technique used to reach the site of the procedure. In this case, the laparotomy was the technique used to reach the liver. The needle was simply the instrument used to obtain the sample. The qualifier for the liver biopsy is Diagnostic (X), which is used to identify excision procedures that are biopsies. Additionally, *Coding Clinic*, Third Quarter 2013 states a total hysterectomy includes the removal of the uterus and cervix. Therefore, code both the resection of the uterus and cervix.

| | | |
|---|---|---|
| **3.2.** | 0PSV04Z | Reposition, Phalanx, Finger, Left (0PSV) |
| | | Reduction, Fracture, *see* Reposition |
| | 0JQK0ZZ | Repair, Subcutaneous Tissue and Fascia, Hand, Left (0JQK) |
| | | Suture, Laceration repair, *see* Repair |

**Rationale:**
Two separate procedures were performed during this operation: open reduction internal fixation of the left index finger and repair of a laceration of the left middle finger. The code for the open reduction internal fixation of the distal left index finger is 0PSV04Z. ICD-10-PCS Root Operation Guideline for fracture treatment (B3.15) states that reduction of a fracture is coded to the root operation Reposition. The body system is Upper Bones, since it was the bone that was repositioned. The code for the suture repair of left middle finger is 0JQK0ZZ. The code for the nonexcisional debridement of the subcutaneous tissue is 0JDK0ZZ. The body part value for this procedure is the Left Hand (K) because there is not a body part value for finger.

| | | |
|---|---|---|
| **3.3.** | 08QPXZZ | Repair, Eyelid, Upper, Left (08QP) |
| | | Suture, Laceration repair, *see* Repair |
| | 0HQ1XZZ | Repair, Skin, Face (0HQ1XZZ) |

**Rationale:**
The root operation Repair represents a broad range of procedures for restoring the anatomic structure of a body part such as suture of lacerations. The code for suturing the left upper eyelid is 08QPXZZ. The code for suturing the chin laceration is 0HQ1XZZ. Review of the body part values reveals that there is not a separate body part value for the chin. ICD-10-PCS Body Part Guidelines indicate that if a procedure is performed on a portion of a body part that does not have a separate body part value, code the body part value corresponding to the whole body part (B4.1a). In this case, the whole body part value is the Face, body part value of 1. Procedures performed directly on the skin or mucous membranes have an External (X) approach.

| | | |
|---|---|---|
| **3.4.** | 0VB08ZZ | Excision, Prostate (0VB0) |
| | | Prostatectomy, *see* Excision, Prostate (0VB0) |

**Rationale:**
The code for TURP is 0VB08ZZ. The root operation Excision is used for the TURP since only a portion of the prostate, the posterior lobe, was removed. Excision is defined as cutting out or off, without replacement, a portion of a body part. The correct approach for this procedure is Via Natural or Artificial Opening Endoscopic (8). During this surgical approach, instrumentation is entered through a natural or artificial external opening to reach and visualize the site of the procedure. For this procedure, a resectoscope (instrumentation) was entered through the urethra (natural opening) to reach and visualize the site of the procedure. A resectoscope is an instrument with a wide-angle telescope and an electronically activated wide loop for transurethral removal or biopsy of lesions of bladder, prostate, or urethra. ICD-10-PCS Coding Guideline B3.1b states that components of a procedure necessary to complete the objective of the procedure specified in the root operation are considered integral to the procedure and are not coded separately. The Foley catheter with continuous bladder irrigation is considered a component of the main procedure and is not coded separately.

**3.5.**      0BTL0ZZ      Resection, Lung, Left (0BTL)
                               Pneumonectomy, *see* Resection, Respiratory System (0BT)

**Rationale:**
The code for the left total pneumonectomy is 0BTL0ZZ. The root operation is Resection because the entire left lung was excised. ICD-10-PCS Root Operation Guideline B3.8 states "PCS contains specific body parts for anatomical subdivisions of a body part, such as lobes of the lungs or liver and regions of the intestine. Resection of the specific body part is coded whenever all of the body part is cut out or off, rather than coding Excision of a less specific body part." The left lung has its own body part value in ICD-10-PCS. The exploratory left thoracotomy is not coded because it is the approach to the procedure and is considered to be integral to the pneumonectomy. ICD-10-PCS Root Operations Guideline B3.1b states "Components of a procedure specified in the root operation definition and explanation are not coded separately. Procedural steps necessary to reach the operative site and close the operative site, including anastomosis of a tubular body part, are also not coded separately.

**3.6.**      0HBT0ZZ      Excision, Breast, Right (0HBT)
                               Mastectomy, *see*, Excision, Skin and Breast (0HB)
                               Quadrant resection of breast, *see* Excision, Skin and Breast (0HB)

**Rationale:**
The code for a quadrectomy of the right breast is 0HBT0ZZ. The correct root operation for this procedure is Excision, which is cutting out or off, without replacement, a portion of a body part. During this procedure, only a quadrant of the right breast was removed. The approach is open as an incision was made to get to the operative site. The body part value T specifies the procedure was performed on the right breast.

**3.7.**      10D17ZZ      Extraction, Products of Conception, Retained (10D1)

**Rationale:**
The code for the manual extraction of the retained placenta is 10D17ZZ. This procedure is coded to the Obstetrics section, which includes only the procedures performed on the products of conception. Coding Guideline C2 states "Procedures performed following a delivery or abortion for curettage of the endometrium or evacuation of retained products of conception are all coded in the Obstetrics section, to the root operation Extraction and the body part Products of Conception, Retained." The approach to perform the manual extraction was Via a Natural Opening (7).

**3.8.**       0DB60ZZ        Excision, Stomach (0DB6)
                                    Gastrectomy, Partial, *see* Excision, Stomach (0DB6)
               0D160ZA        Bypass, Stomach (0D16)
               0DHA0UZ        Insertion of device in, Jejunum (0DHA)

**Rationale:**
During this procedure, a subtotal excision of the stomach is performed followed by a gastrojejunostomy (closure of the proximal end of the duodenum and side-to-side anastomosis of the jejunum to the remaining portion of the stomach). A jejunostomy feeding tube was then placed. ICD-10-PCS Root Operation Guideline for multiple procedures states that if during the same operative episode, multiple procedures are coded if multiple root operations with distinct objectives are performed on the same body part (B3.2c). The first procedure performed was a subtotal gastrectomy, which codes to 0DB60ZZ. The root operation Excision is used since only a portion of the stomach (subtotal) was removed. The second procedure performed is the gastrojejunostomy which codes to 0D160ZA. The root operation Bypass is used because the objective of the gastrojejunostomy is to reroute the content. The ICD-10-PCS Root Operation Guideline for Bypass states that bypass procedures are coded by identifying the body part bypass from and the body part bypassed to. The fourth character body part specifies the body part bypassed from, (Stomach, value 6) and the qualifier specifies the body part bypassed to (Jejunum, value A) (B3.6a). The third procedure performed was the insertion of the feeding tube into the jejunum, which codes to 0DHA0UZ.

**3.9.**       0HRMX74        Replacement, Skin, Foot, Right (0HRM)
                                    Graft, *see* Replacement
               0HBHXZZ        Excision, Skin, Upper Leg, Right (0HBHXZ)

**Rationale:**
Two separate procedures were performed during this operative episode. The first procedure was the harvesting of the skin graft from the upper aspect of the right anterior thigh, which codes to 0HBHXZZ. ICD-10-PCS Root Operation Guideline B3.9 states that if, as part of a procedure, an autograft is obtained from a different body part a separate procedure is coded. The second procedure is the split thickness skin graft of the right foot, which codes to 0HRMX74. In order to code this procedure, you need to be familiar with and apply the

definition of the root operation, Replacement. *Replacement* is defined as putting in or on biological or synthetic material that physically takes the place and/or function of all or a portion of a body part. The sixth character value for the device is 7 for autologous tissue substitute. The seventh character value is 4 for partial thickness because a split thickness skin graft consists of only the superficial layers of the dermis. When coding this case, consideration may have been given to using the root operation Transfer. This would have been incorrect because during a Transfer procedure the body part transferred remains connected to its vascular and nervous supply. The debridement is not coded as it is integral to the skin graft. The explanation for Replacement states that the body part may have been previously taken out, previously replaced, or may be taken out concomitantly with the Replacement procedure.

**3.10.**      04100JK        Bypass, Aorta, Abdominal (0410)

**Rationale:**
The code for the aorto-bifemoral bypass graft is 04100JK. ICD-10-PCS Root Operation Guideline B3.6a states that for bypass procedures the fourth character body part specifies the body part bypassed from and the qualifier specifies the body part bypassed to. For this procedure, the body part bypassed from is the Aorta (0) and the body part bypassed to is the Femoral Arteries, Bilateral (K). The device character value is J for Synthetic Substitute (bifurcated microvelour graft).

**3.11.**   005K3ZZ   Destruction, Nerve, Trigeminal (005K)

**Rationale:**

The code for radiofrequency destruction of the trigeminal nerve is 005K3ZZ. *Destruction* is defined as the physical eradication of all or a portion of a body part by the direct use of energy, force, or a destructive agent. The approach for this procedure was percutaneous. The small nick in the skin does not constitute an open approach. The small nick was made so that the radiofrequency needle could be advanced to the operative site. Although three treatments were done, only code the procedure code once due to the fact that the needle was not reintroduced each time and the ablation was all on the same branch of the trigeminal nerve. In this case, the procedure does not meet the full intent of ICD-10-PCS Coding Guideline B3.2b. Only codes from the Medical and Surgical section were used for this question.

**3.12.**   0YU60JZ   Supplement, Inguinal Region, Left (0YU6)
Herniorrhaphy, with synthetic substitute, *see* Supplement Anatomical Regions, Lower Extremities (0YU)

**Rationale:**

The correct root operation is Supplement for a herniorrhaphy with mesh. *Supplement* is defined as putting in or on biological or synthetic material (such as mesh) that physically reinforces and/or augments the function of a portion of a body part. A herniorrhaphy without mesh is coded with the root operation Repair.

**3.13.**   0U5B7ZZ   Destruction, Endometrium (0U5B)
Ablation, *see* Destruction

**Rationale:**

The procedure code is 0U5B7ZZ for the ablation of the endometrium. The dilatation and curettage would not be coded as it is integral to the endometrial ablation. The operative approach for was Via a Natural Opening (vagina).

**3.14.**   0TF3XZZ   Fragmentation, Kidney Pelvis, Right (0TF3)
ESWL (extracorporeal shock wave lithotripsy), *see* Fragmentation

**Rationale:**

The extracorporeal shock wave lithotripsy is coded to the root operation Fragmentation. ESWL is an externally applied, focused, high-intensity acoustic pulse using shockwaves to break up stones into small pieces.

**3.15.**   0DB98ZX   Excision, Duodenum (0DB9)
0DB68ZX   Excision, Stomach (0DB6)
Biopsy, *see* Excision with qualifier Diagnostic

**Rationale:**

Root Operation Guideline B3.2.a states multiple procedures are coded if the same root operation is performed on different body parts as defined by distinct values of the body part character. Two biopsies were obtained during the EGD and both the duodenum and stomach have their own distinct value; therefore, two codes are necessary. The EGD is not coded because the inspection is integral to the performance of the duodenal biopsy. Coding Guideline B3.11a states that inspection of a body part(s) performed in order to achieve the objective of a procedure is not coded separately.

**3.16.**    08RK3JZ        Replacement, Lens, Left (08RK)

**Rationale:**

The extracapsular cataract extraction with insertion of intraocular lens code is 08RK3JZ with the root operation of Replacement because the patient's left lens is replaced with a prosthetic lens. The removal of the patient's lens is not coded because Replacement includes taking out the body part.

### *Detailed and/or Complex Cases and Scenarios Using ICD-10-CM and ICD-10-PCS Codes*

**3.17.**    G56.02         Syndrome, carpal tunnel
             01N50ZZ        Release, Nerve, Median Nerve (01N5)

**Rationale:**

Diagnosis: The patient is being seen for carpal tunnel syndrome of the left wrist, which codes to G56.02. When referencing the code in the Alphabetic Index, one obtains G56.0-. Referencing the Tabular reveals that the code requires a fifth digit of 2 for the left side

Procedure: The correct root operation for the carpal tunnel release is Release. Release is defined as freeing a body part from an abnormal constraint and is coded to the body part being freed, not the structure cut to obtain the release. During a carpal tunnel release, the median nerve is the body part being freed.

**3.18.**    O75.81         Pregnancy, complicated by, fatigue, during labor and delivery
             O34.21         Delivery, vaginal, following previous cesarean delivery
             Z37.0          Outcome of delivery, single, liveborn
             Z3A.39         Pregnancy, weeks of gestation, 39 weeks
             10D07Z4        Extraction, Products of Conception, Mid Forceps (10D07Z4)
                            Delivery, Forceps, *see* Extraction, Products of Conception (10D0)
             0W8NXZZ        Division, Perineum, Female (0W8NXZZ)
                            Episiotomy, *see* Division, Perineum, Female (0W8N)

**Rationale:**

Diagnoses: The principal diagnosis for this case is O75.81. ICD-10-CM Coding Guideline I.C.15.b.4 states that when a delivery occurs, the principal diagnosis should correspond to the main circumstances or complication of the delivery. The code for a VBAC after previous cesarean delivery is O34.21. The secondary diagnosis code of Z37.0 indicates that the outcome of the delivery was a single liveborn infant. ICD-10-CM Coding Guideline I.15.b.5 states that a code from category Z37, Outcome of Delivery, should be included on every maternal record when a delivery has occurred. These codes are not to be used on subsequent records or on the newborn record. In the Tabular at the beginning of Chapter 15, the following note appears: "Use additional code from category Z3A, Weeks of gestation, to identify specific week of pregnancy."

Procedures: ICD-10-PCS Coding Guideline C.1 states that the Obstetrics section includes only the procedures performed on the products of conception. Procedures performed on the pregnant female other than the products of conception are coded to a root operation in the Medical and Surgical section. *Products of conception* refer to all components of pregnancy, including fetus, embryo, amnion, umbilical cord, and placenta. There is no differentiation of the products of conception based on gestational age. Therefore, since the mid forceps delivery is performed on the fetus, it is coded to the Obstetrics section of ICD-10-PCS. The use of the mid forceps to deliver the fetus is coded to the root operation Extraction. *Extraction* is defined as the pulling or stripping out of all or a portion of a body part. In this case, the mid forceps are used to pull out the body part (products of conception). The episiotomy is coded to the Medical and Surgical section because it is performed on the pregnant female. The code for episiotomy is 0W8NXZZ. The main term Episiotomy in the Alphabetic Index refers the coding professional to "*see* Division, Perineum, Female (0W8N)." The root operation Division is coded when the objective of the procedure is to cut into, transect, or otherwise separate all or a portion of a body part. The episiorrhaphy is not coded separately, per ICD-10-PCS Guideline B3.1b which states that procedural steps necessary to reach the operative site and close the operative site are not coded separately.

**3.19.**

| | |
|---|---|
| S82.251A | Fracture, traumatic, tibia (shaft), comminuted (displaced) |
| S06.0X0A | Concussion (brain) (cerebral) (current) |
| W01.198A | Index to External Causes, Fall, due to, slipping, with subsequent striking against object, specified NEC |
| Y92.480 | Index to External Causes, Place of occurrence, sidewalk |
| Y93.K1 | Index to External Causes, Activity, walking an animal |
| Y99.8 | Index to External Causes, Status of external cause, leisure activity |
| 0QSG04Z | Reposition, Tibia, Right (0QSG) |
| | Reduction, Fracture *see* Reposition |

**Rationale:**

Diagnoses: The reason for the visit was a fracture of the shaft of the right tibia which codes to S82.251 with the sixth digit indicating the right side. The fracture code requires a seventh character (code extension). The code extension A is used on the fracture code to indicate that this is the initial encounter for a closed fracture. The notes under S82 instruct the coder to code the fracture as closed if the documentation does not designate whether open or closed. An additional note indicates that a fracture not identified as displaced or nondisplaced should be coded to displaced. W01.198A is the external cause of injury code for tripping, falling, and subsequently hitting her head on the fire hydrant. Code Y92.480 indicates the place of occurrence for the injury. A note under Y92 indicates that a place of occurrence code should be recorded only at the initial encounter for treatment. An additional note under Y92 states to use in conjunction with an activity code. Activity code Y93.K1 is coded because the patient was walking her dog when the injury occurred. A note under Y93 states that activity codes should be used in conjunction with codes for external cause status (Y99) and place of occurrence (Y92). The external cause status code is Y99.8.

Procedure: The open reduction with internal fixation of the tibial fracture is coded to 0QSG04Z. The correct root operation is Reposition, which is defined as moving to its normal location or other suitable location all or a portion of a body part.

**3.20.**

| | |
|---|---|
| O60.14X0 | Delivery, preterm (*see also* Pregnancy, complicated by, preterm labor) Pregnancy, complicated by, preterm labor, third trimester, with third trimester preterm delivery |
| O30.003 | Pregnancy, twin – *see* Tabular for required extensions |
| O41.1230 | Chorioamnionitis; or Pregnancy, complicated by, chorioamnionitis |
| O69.1XX1 | Compression, umbilical cord, complicating delivery, cord around neck; or Delivery, complicated by, cord, around neck, tightly or with compression |
| Z37.2 | Outcome of delivery, twins, both liveborn |
| Z3A.33 | Pregnancy, weeks of gestation, 33 weeks |
| 10D00Z1 | Extraction, Products of Conception, Low Cervical (10D00Z1) Cesarean Section, see Extraction, Products of Conception (10D0) |

**Rationale:**
Diagnoses: Code O60.14X0, preterm delivery at 33 weeks, is sequenced as the principal diagnosis. ICD-10-CM Coding Guideline I.15.b.4 states that if the reason for the admission/encounter was unrelated to the condition resulting in the cesarean delivery, the condition related to the reason for the admission/encounter should be selected as the principal diagnosis. In this case, the reason for the admission was the preterm labor that could not be stopped. The third trimester of pregnancy is defined as 28 weeks 0 days until delivery. A note appears prior to O60.1 stating that a seventh character is to be assigned to each code under subcategory O60.1. The seventh character 0 is for single gestations and multiple gestations where the fetus is unspecified. Code O30.003 indicates the twin gestation with the sixth character indicating the third trimester. The code for the chorioamnionitis complication is O41.1230 with the sixth digit indicating the third trimester and the seventh character indicating an unspecified fetus. A note appears under O41 stating that a seventh character is to be assigned to each code under category O41. Seventh character 0 is for single gestations and multiple gestations where the fetus is unspecified. The code for the complication of cord around the neck of twin 1 is O69.1xx1 with the seventh character indicating that it is fetus 1 that is affected by the complication. A note appears under O69 stating that a seventh character is to be assigned to each code under category O69. The characters 1 through 9 are for cases of multiple gestations to identify the fetus for which the code applies. This code also requires the use of a character X in the fifth and sixth character positions in order for the code to be a valid code. ICD-10-CM Coding Guideline I.A.5 states that if a code that requires a seventh character is not six characters, a placeholder X must be used to fill in the empty characters. The correct outcome of delivery code is Z37.2 indicating that both twins were liveborn. In the Tabular at the beginning of Chapter 15, the following note appears: "Use additional code from category Z3A, Weeks of gestation, to identify specific week of pregnancy."

Procedure: The cesarean section is coded to 10D00Z1 with the seventh character indicating a low cervical cesarean section.

Note: Although most hospitals do not code the magnesium sulfate tocolysis, it would not be incorrect to also assign a code for this procedure. If coded, the code would be assigned from the Administration section, root operation Introduction.

| 3.21. | G00.1 | Meningitis, pneumococcal |
| | J13 | Pneumonia, pneumococcal |
| | 009U3ZX | Drainage, Spinal Canal, (009U) |

**Rationale:**
Diagnoses: The correct code for the meningitis is G00.1 and the code for the pneumonia is J13. Per Coding Guideline II.C, either the meningitis or the pneumonia can be sequenced as the principal diagnosis because both equally meet the criteria for principal diagnosis.

Procedure: A lumbar puncture is a technique of using a needle to withdraw cerebrospinal fluid from the spinal canal. The lumbar puncture codes to 009U3ZX. Although the documentation states that the lumbar puncture is diagnostic, a seventh character of Z, No Qualifier, is assigned. Coding Guideline B3.4 states that the qualifier Diagnostic is used only for biopsies.

**3.22.**  K80.01  Calculus, calculi, calculous, gallbladder, with, cholecystitis, acute, with,obstruction

Cholecystitis, with calculus, stones, in, gallbladder, *see*, Calculus, gallbladder, with cholecystitis

K85.1  Pancreatitis, acute, gallstone

0FT40ZZ  Resection, Gallbladder (0FT4)

Cholecystectomy, *see* Resection, Gallbladder (0FT4)

0FJB0ZZ  Inspection, Duct, Hepatobiliary (0FJB)

Exploration, *see* Inspection

0DHA0UZ  Insertion of device in, Jejunum (0DHA)

Feeding device, Insertion of device in, Jejunum (0DHA)

BF101ZZ  Fluoroscopy, bile duct (BF10)

Cholangiogram, *see* Fluoroscopy, Hepatobiliary System and Pancreas (BF1)

**Rationale:**

Diagnoses: The acute cholecystitis with gallbladder calculus codes to K80.01. Though the physician suspected a stone in the bile duct, none was found and the diagnosis after study was "evidence of bile duct obstruction." The code for the acute gallstone pancreatitis is K85.1. Code K83.1, Obstruction of bile duct, is not coded for the bile duct obstruction due to the Excludes1 note: obstruction of bile duct with cholelithiasis (K80.-).

Procedures; The procedure for the cholecystectomy is 0FT40ZZ with the approach (fifth character) being open since the procedure was performed via an abdominal incision. The root operation is Resection since the entire gallbladder was removed. The definition of Resection is to cut out or off, without replacement, all of a body part. The code for exploration of the common bile duct is 0FJB0ZZ. A feeding device was also inserted into the jejunum which codes to 0DHA0UZ. The operative cholangiogram code is BF101ZZ with the fifth character indicating that low osmolar contrast was used. ICD-10-PCS draft Device Guideline B6.1b states that materials such as sutures, ligatures, radiological markers, and temporary postoperative wound drains are considered integral to the performance of a procedure and are not coded as devices. Therefore, the placement of the Jackson-Pratt drain is not coded.

**3.23.**  D24.2  Fibroadenoma, specified site NEC – *see* Neoplasm, benign

Neoplasm Table, Breast, lower-outer quadrant, benign

C79.51  Neoplasm Table, Bone, malignant, secondary

C78.00  Neoplasm Table, Lung, lobe NEC, malignant, secondary

Z85.3  History, personal (of), malignant neoplasm (of), breast

Z90.11  Absence, breast(s) (and nipple(s)) (acquired)

0HTU0ZZ  Resection, Breast, Left (0HTU0ZZ)

Mastectomy, *see* Resection, Skin and Breast (0HT)

**Rationale:**

Diagnoses: The patient was admitted for a left mastectomy due to a fibroadenoma of the left breast which is the principal diagnosis and codes to D24.2. The patient is currently still under treatment for both the bone and lung metastases, and therefore both should be coded as an active condition. The bone metastases' code is C79.51 and the lung metastases' code is C78.00 for unspecified lung. The patient also has a history of right breast carcinoma, Z85.3 and an acquired absence of the right breast due to a previous mastectomy, Z90.11.

Procedures: The left mastectomy code is 0HTU0ZZ with the root operation of Resection since the entire left breast was removed.

**3.24.**

| | | |
|---|---|---|
| | S42.351A | Fracture, traumatic, humerus, shaft, comminuted (displaced), right |
| | W01.0XXA | Fall, same level, from, slipping, stumbling, tripping |
| | Y92.39 | Place of occurrence, bowling alley |
| | Y93.54 | Activity, bowling |
| | Y99.8 | Status of External Cause, student activity |
| | 0PSF04Z | Reposition, Humeral Shaft, Right (0PSF) |
| | | Reduction, Fracture *see* Reposition |

**Rationale:**

Diagnoses: The code for the fracture of the shaft of the humerus is S42.351A. The sixth digit of the fracture code specifies that it is the right humerus and the seventh character (code extension) specifies that this is the initial encounter for a closed fracture. A note appears under category S42 that states that a fracture that is not designated as open or closed should be coded to closed. ICD-10-CM Coding Guideline I.C.20.a.2 states to assign the external cause code, with the appropriate seventh character, for each encounter for which the injury or condition is being treated.

Procedure: 0PSF04Z is the code for the ORIF of the right humeral shaft. ICD-10-PCS Coding Guideline B3.15 states that reduction of a displaced fracture is coded to the root operation Reposition. Treatment of a nondisplaced fracture is coded to the procedure performed. The fourth character of the code, body part, is F for the Right Humeral Shaft and the sixth character, device, is 4 for Internal Fixation Device.

**3.25.**

| | | |
|---|---|---|
| | D12.5 | Adenoma – *see also* Neoplasm, benign, by site |
| | | Neoplasm Table: intestines, large, colon, sigmoid |
| | K62.3 | Prolapse, prolapsed, rectum (mucosa) (sphincter) |
| | K57.30 | Diverticulosis, large intestine |
| | K52.9 | Colitis (acute) (catarrhal) (chronic) (noninfectious) (hemorrhagic) |
| | 0DBN8ZX | Excision, Colon, Sigmoid (0DBN) |
| | | Biopsy, see Excision with qualifier Diagnostic |

**Rationale:**

Diagnoses: The code for the tubular adenoma of the sigmoid colon is D12.5. The code for the prolapsed rectum is K62.3; the code for the diverticulosis is K57.30; and the colitis code is K52.9.

Procedures: The code for a colonoscopy with sigmoid colon biopsies is 0DBN8ZX. The body part value is N for the Sigmoid Colon, which is the location of the biopsy. The approach is 8 Via Natural Opening Endoscopic and the qualifier is X for Diagnostic. The qualifier Diagnostic is used to identify excision procedures that are biopsies. *Coding Clinic* Q4 2014 clarifies Guideline B3.2b as referring to distinct body parts, not different locations within the same body part..

**3.26.**

| | | |
|---|---|---|
| | S72.001A | Fracture, traumatic, femur, upper end, neck |
| | I11.0 | Hypertension, hypertensive, heart, with heart failure |
| | I50.9 | Failure, heart, congestive |
| | J43.9 | Emphysema (atrophic) (bullous) (chronic) (interlobular) (lung) (obstructive) (pulmonary) (senile) (vesicular) |
| | W01.0XXA | Index to External Causes, Fall, same level, from, slipping, stumbling, tripping |
| | Y92.017 | Index to External Causes, Place of occurrence, residence, house, single-family, yard |
| | Y93.H2 | Index to External Causes, Activity, gardening |
| | Y99.8 | Index to External Causes, External cause status, leisure activity |
| | 0SRR019 | Replacement, Joint, Hip, Right, Femoral Surface (0SRR) |

**Rationale:**

Diagnoses: The code for the fracture of the neck of the right femur is S72.001A. The sixth character of the fracture code specifies that it is the right femur and the seventh character specifies that this is the initial encounter for a closed fracture. A note appears under category S72 that states that a fracture that is not designated as open or closed should be coded to closed. Hypertensive heart disease with CHF codes to I11.0 with a note appearing in the Tabular under I11.0 to use an additional code to identify the type of heart failure, I50.9. W01.0xx.A is the external cause of injury code for tripping and falling. A note in the Tabular under category W01 indicates that a seventh character is required. Code Y92.017 is the place of occurrence for the injury. A note under Y92 indicates that a place of occurrence code should be recorded only at the initial encounter for treatment. An additional note under Y92 states to use in conjunction with an activity code. Activity code Y93.H2 is coded since the patient was gardening when the injury occurred. A note under Y93 states that activity codes should be used in conjunction with codes for external cause status (Y99) and place of occurrence (Y92). The external cause status code is Y99.8.

Procedure: The right hip hemiarthroplasty is coded to 0SRR019. The definition of the root operation Replacement is putting in or on biological or synthetic material that physically takes the place and/or function of all or a portion of a body part. During this procedure, the patient's right femoral head was removed and replaced with a synthetic substitute, metal Zimmer LDFX cemented monopolar. Replacement includes taking out the body part; therefore, the removal of the femoral head is not coded separately.

| 3.27. | C40.02 | Neoplasm Table, bone, scapula, left side, malignant, primary |
| | | Sarcoma, Ewings, *see* Neoplasm, bone, malignant |
| | Q90.9 | Down syndrome |
| | | Syndrome, Down, *see also* Down Syndrome |
| | 0PB60ZX | Excision, Scapula, Left (0PB6) |
| | | Biopsy – *see* Excision with qualifier Diagnostic |

**Rationale:**

Diagnoses: The reason for this encounter, after study, was the Ewing's sarcoma of the scapula which codes to C40.02. The bone scan also revealed questionable areas of the ribs and vertebra but the physician does not document a diagnosis of sarcoma of these areas. Down syndrome codes to Q90.9.

Procedures: The procedure code for biopsy of the left scapula is 0PB60ZX. The body part value, character 4, is the left scapula (6). The qualifier Diagnostic is used to identify excision procedures that are biopsies; therefore, the seventh character is X.

| 3.28. | O63.0 | Delivery (childbirth) (labor), complicated, by, prolonged labor, first stage |
| | O70.0 | Delivery (childbirth) (labor) (complicated by), complicated, by, laceration (perineal), perineum, first degree |
| | O75.81 | Exhaustion, exhaustive, maternal, complicating delivery |
| | O90.81 | Puerperal, puerperium (complicated by, complications), anemia |
| | | Anemia, postpartum |
| | Z37.0 | Outcome of delivery, single, liveborn |
| | Z3A.39 | Pregnancy, weeks of gestation, 39 weeks |
| | 10D07Z6 | Extraction, Products of Conception, Vacuum (10D07Z6) |
| | | Delivery, Vacuum-assisted, *see* Extraction, Products of Conception (10D0) |
| | 0WQNXZZ | Repair, Perineum, Female (0WQNXZZ) |
| | | Episiorrhaphy – *see* Repair, Perineum, Female |

**Rationale:**

Diagnoses: The delivery was complicated by a prolonged first stage of labor which codes to O63.0. The patient also experienced a first degree perineal laceration during delivery which codes to O70.0. Code O75.81 is used to classify that the patient's exhaustion further complicated the delivery. The patient also developed anemia following delivery and was given Slow Fe #3 during the stay in addition to being discharged with the medication. The code for postpartum anemia is O90.81. The outcome of delivery is a single liveborn, Z37.0.

Procedures: ICD-10-PCS Coding Guideline C.1 states that the Obstetrics section includes only the procedures performed on the products of conception. Procedures performed on the pregnant female other than the products of conception are coded to a root operation in the Medical and Surgical section. Products of conception refer to all components of pregnancy, including fetus, embryo, amnion, umbilical cord, and placenta. There is no differentiation of the products of conception based on gestational age. Therefore, since the vacuum-assisted delivery is performed on the fetus, it is coded to the Obstetrics section of ICD-10-PCS. The vacuum-assisted delivery codes to 10D07Z6 with the qualifier indicating the use of a vacuum. The repair of the first degree laceration is coded to the Medical and Surgical section because it is performed on the pregnant female. The code for the repair is 0WQNXZZ.

| | | |
|---|---|---|
| **3.29.** | S02.19XA | Fracture, traumatic, skull, temporal bone |
| | S02.402A | Fracture, traumatic, zygoma |
| | S06.1X7A | Injury, intracranial, cerebral edema, traumatic |
| | R40.2312 | Coma, with, motor response (none) |
| | R40.2112 | Coma, with, opening of eyes (never) |
| | R40.2212 | Coma, with, verbal response (none) |
| | V20.0XXA | Index to External Causes, Accident, transport, motorcyclist, driver, collision (with), animal, nontraffic |
| | | Accident, motorcycle NOS, *see* Accident, transport, motorcyclist |
| | Y92.828 | Index to External Causes, Place of occurrence, mountain |
| | 5A1955Z | Performance, Respiratory, Greater than 96 Consecutive Hours, Ventilation (5A1955Z) |
| | 0BH17EZ | Insertion of Endotracheal Airway into Trachea, via Natural or Artificial Opening |
| | 4A103BD | Monitoring, Central Nervous, Pressure, Intracranial (4A10) |
| | 4A00X4Z | Measurement, Central Nervous, Electrical Activity (4A00) |

**Rationale:**

Diagnoses: The code for the fracture over the left temporal and orbital roof areas of the skull is S02.19XA. Review of the Includes notes for this code indicates that the code includes the fracture of both the temporal bone and the orbital roof. Review of the notes under S02 indicates that the appropriate seventh character is to be added to each code from category S02. This is the initial encounter for this closed fracture; therefore, the seventh character is A. A note under S02 indicates that if a fracture is not indicated as open or closed it should be coded as closed. There is an additional note that states to code also any associated intra-cranial injury (S06.-). This code is only five characters in length; therefore, a placeholder character of X must be utilized for the sixth character to make this a valid ICD-10-CM code. ICD-10-CM Coding Guideline I.A.5 states that if a code that requires a seventh character is not six characters, a placeholder X must be used to fill in the empty characters. The code for the fracture of the zygomatic arch is S02.402A, again with the seventh character indicating this is the initial encounter for a closed fracture.

Because the patient was comatose and the elements of the coma scale were documented (eyes never open, no verbal response, and no motor response) each of these can be identified and the seventh character of 2 is used to indicate that the coma scale was completed in the emergency department. A note appears under R40.2 (Coma) indicating that the appropriate seventh character is to be added to each code from subcategory R40.21-, R40.22-, R40.23- to specify where the coma scale was completed. There is also a note that a code from each subcategory is required to complete the coma scale. The code for motor response is R40.2312, for opening of eyes is R40.2112, and for verbal response is R40.2212.

The documentation indicates that there was cerebral edema with the intracranial injury. Therefore, the intracranial injury codes to S06.1X7A. The sixth character of the code indicates the level of loss of consciousness with 7 defined as loss of consciousness of any duration with death due to brain injury prior to regaining consciousness. The hypotension, hypoxemia, and apnea are all symptoms of the severe intracranial injury and are not coded separately. Code G93.89, Brain death, is not assigned because the S06.1X7A code indicates the death.

The external cause of injury code is V20.0XXA. Documentation indicates that the patient was the driver of a motorcycle and hit an elk while driving in the mountains. Since the documentation indicates that this accident did not occurred on the highway it is classified as a nontraffic accident. The place of occurrence code is Y92.828. A note under category Y92 states that place of occurrence codes should be used in conjunction with an activity code and should be recorded only at the initial encounter for treatment. An activity code (category Y93) was not coded as there is no applicable activity code for driving a motorcycle. Additionally, a status code (category Y99) was not coded due to the fact that this information was not documented.

Procedures: The root operation for a ventilator is Performance, which is a root operation in the Extracorporeal Assistance and Performance section. *Performance* is defined as completely taking over a physiological function by extracorporeal means. The code for the ventilator is 5A1955Z. The fifth character of the code specifies the duration that the patient was on the ventilator and, in this case, 5 indicates the patient was on the ventilator for greater than 96 consecutive hours. *Coding Clinic* Q4 2014 directs the coder to code the insertion of the endotracheal tube when a patient is intubated and begun on mechanical ventilation. The root operation is Insertion with the body part Trachea. Since no scope is indicated, the approach is Via Natural or Artificial Opening and the Device left in place is an Endotracheal Airway, which codes to 0BH17EZ.

The patient's intracranial pressures were monitored, which codes to 4A103BD. Additionally, measurement of the patient's brain waves was performed, which codes to 4A00X4Z.

| **3.30.** | D35.01 | Neoplasm Table, Adrenal, cortex, right side, benign |
|---|---|---|
| | E24.8 | Cushing's, syndrome or disease, specified NEC |
| | I10 | Hypertension, hypertensive (accelerated) (benign) (essential) (idiopathic) (malignant) (systemic) |
| | 0GB30ZZ | Excision, Gland, Adrenal, Right (0GB3) |
| | | Adrenalectomy, *see* Excision, Endocrine System (0GB) |

**Rationale:**
Diagnoses: The tumor of the adrenal gland was benign and codes to D35.01. The fifth character of the code specifies the right adrenal gland. The Neoplasm Table provides code D35.0- for benign tumor of cortex of adrenal gland. When verifying the code in the Tabular you will note that D35.01 is the correct code for the right side. The Cushing's syndrome codes to E24.8. The physician should be queried regarding whether or not the Cushing's is related to the ACTH, which would result in this code being E24.3.The patient also has hypertension which was treated with medication during the stay and is coded as a secondary diagnosis (I10). Note: The patient is also on other medications. The physician could be queried as to the underlying conditions if they are pertinent to this encounter.

Procedure: The code for resection of the tumor of the right adrenal gland is 0GB30ZZ with the fourth character specifying that the tumor was removed from the right adrenal gland. Excision is the appropriate root operation because only the tumor was removed and not the entire adrenal gland.

**3.31.**

| | |
|---|---|
| I25.10 | Arteriosclerosis, arteriosclerotic, coronary (artery) |
| I49.5 | Syndrome, sick, sinus |
| I11.0 | Hypertension, heart (disease), with heart failure (congestive) |
| I50.9 | Failure, heart, congestive |
| 027034Z | Dilation, Artery, Coronary, One Site (0270) |
| 02703ZZ | Dilation, Artery, Coronary, One Site (0270) |
| | Angioplasty, *see* Dilation, Heart and Great Vessels (027) |
| | Percutaneous transluminal coronary angioplasty (PTCA), *see* Dilation, Heart and Great Vessels (027) |
| 0JH606Z | Insertion of device in, Subcutaneous Tissue and Fascia, Chest (0JH6) |
| | Pacemaker, Dual Chamber, Chest (0JH6) |
| 02H63JZ | Insertion of device in, Atrium, Right (02H6) |
| 02HK3JZ | Insertion of device in, Ventricle, Right (02HK) |

**Rationale**:

Diagnoses: In accordance with UHDDS definition for principal diagnosis, the reason (after study) the patient is admitted to the hospital is to undergo the PTCA for the CAD; therefore, I25.10 is the principal diagnosis. The sick sinus syndrome was also treated and codes to I49.5. Additionally, the hypertensive heart disease with CHF was also monitored and treated during the hospital stay with hypertensive heart disease being coded to I11.0. A note under this subcategory instructs the coder to use an additional code to identify the type of heart failure. Following this instructional note, an additional code of I50.9 is coded to identify the heart failure as congestive heart failure.

Procedures: Two codes are needed for the angioplasty due to the fact that only an angioplasty was performed on the left anterior descending artery and both an angioplasty and insertion of drug-eluting stent were performed on the right coronary artery. The device character value is different for each of the arteries. The code for angioplasty of the left anterior descending artery is 02703ZZ with the device character indicating that no device was left in this artery. The code for the angioplasty and insertion of a drug-eluting stent of the right coronary artery is 027034Z with the device character indicating that a drug-eluting stent was left in this artery.

Three codes are needed for the dual chambered pacemaker insertion. The first of the three codes is for the insertion of the pacemaker generator into the subcutaneous pocket in the chest wall with the code 0JH606Z. The body part character (fourth character) specifies that the generator was placed in the subcutaneous tissue and fascia of the chest and the device character (sixth character) specifies that this is a dual chamber pacemaker. The second code is for the percutaneous insertion of the electrode into the right atrium with the code 02H63JZ. The body part character specifies the right atrium and the device character (sixth character) indicates that a pacemaker cardiac lead was the device left at the operative site. The third code is for the percutaneous insertion of the electrode into the right ventricle with the code 02HK3JZ. The body part character specifies the right ventricle and the device character indicates that the device remaining at the operative site is a pacemaker cardiac lead.

**3.32.**

| | |
|---|---|
| O03.38 | Abortion (complete) (spontaneous), incomplete (spontaneous), complicated (by) (following), infection, urinary tract |
| B96.20 | Infection, infected, infective (opportunistic), Escherichia (E.) coli NEC, as cause of disease classified elsewhere |
| Z3A.12 | Pregnancy, weeks of gestation, 12 weeks |
| 10D17ZZ | Extraction, Products of Conception, Retained (10D1) |

**Rationale:**

Diagnoses: The patient developed a urinary tract infection following the incomplete spontaneous abortion; therefore, the code O03.38 for complicated spontaneous abortion is coded. B96.2 is coded as a secondary diagnosis to show that E. coli was the organism causing the UTI. In the Tabular at the beginning of Chapter 15, the following note appears: "Use additional code from category Z3A, Weeks of gestation, to identify specific week of pregnancy."

Procedure: The code for the D&C is 10D17ZZ. Coding Guideline C2 states "Procedures performed following a delivery or abortion for curettage of the endometrium or evacuation of retained products of conception are all coded in the Obstetrics section, to the root operation Extraction and the body part Products of Conception, Retained." The approach to perform the D&C was Via a Natural Opening (7).

**3.33.**

| | |
|---|---|
| N92.0 | Menorrhagia (primary) |
| 0UDB7ZZ | Extraction, Endometrium (0UDB) |
| | Curettage, *see* Extraction |
| 0UDB8ZX | Extraction, Endometrium (0UDB) |

**Rationale:**

Diagnosis: Menorrhagia with no further specificity codes to N92.0

Procedures: Two procedures were performed, dilatation and curettage and endometrial biopsy. The D&C codes to 0UDB7ZZ with the root operation being Extraction. The approach for the D&C was Via the Natural Opening. The endometrial biopsy codes to 0UDB8ZX. The approach for the endometrial biopsy was Via Natural Opening Endoscopic because a hysteroscope was inserted before the biopsy was taken. The qualifier is X to identify that the procedure performed was a biopsy. The correct root operation for the endometrial biopsy is Extraction, not Excision. *Extraction* is defined as pulling or stripping out or off all or a portion of a body part by the use of force. Additionally, in this training manual under the definition of Excision there is a coding note stating that bone marrow and endometrial biopsies are not coded to Excision. They are coded to Extraction, with the qualifier Diagnostic.

**3.34.**

| | |
|---|---|
| S83.212A | Tear, torn (traumatic) meniscus (knee) (current injury), medial, bucket-handle |
| W03.XXXA | Tackle in sports |
| 0SBD4ZZ | Excision, Joint, Knee, Left (0SBD) |
| | Meniscectomy, *see* Excision, Lower Joints (0SB) |

Diagnoses: The code for the bucket-handle tear of the medial meniscus is S83.212A. A note under category S83 indicates that codes from this category require a seventh character extension. The seventh character A for initial encounter is appropriate. Coding Guideline I.C.19.a. states that extension A, initial encounter, is used while the patient is receiving active treatment for the condition. Examples of active treatment are: surgical treatment, emergency department encounter, and evaluation and treatment by a new physician. An additional guideline states the need to code an external cause code, with the appropriate seventh character, for each encounter for which the injury or condition is being treated. No place of occurrence, activity, or external cause status codes are assigned because this is not the initial encounter for treatment.

Procedure: The root operation is Excision since only a portion (anterior) of the medial meniscus was removed. The approach is Percutaneous Endoscopic because the procedure was done arthroscopically.

**3.35.**    I25.5          Cardiomyopathy, ischemic

         I25.2          History, personal, myocardial infarction (old)

         Z98.61       Status, angioplasty, coronary artery

         0JH808Z    Insertion of device in, Subcutaneous Tissue and Fascia, Abdomen (0JH8)

                              Defibrillator Generator, Abdomen (0JH8)

         02HK3KZ   Insertion of device in, Ventricle, Right (02HK)

         02H63KZ   Insertion of device in, Atrium, Right (02H6)

**Rationale:**

Diagnoses: The reason for the insertion of the cardiovert-defibrillator was the ischemic cardiomyopathy, which codes to I25.5. The patient also has a history of previous MI (I25.2) and PTCA (Z98.61).

Procedure: Three distinct procedures were performed during this operative episode. ICD-10-PCS Root Operation Coding Guideline B3.2a states to code multiple procedures during the same operative episode if the same root operation is performed on different body parts as defined by distinct values of the body part character. The first procedure performed was the insertion of the defibrillator generator into the subcutaneous tissue in the abdominal area, which codes to 0JH808Z. The additional procedures performed were the insertion of defibrillator leads into both the right ventricle and atrium. The code for the right ventricle is 02HK3KZ and the right atrium is 02H63KZ.

**3.36.**    L97.214    Ulcer, lower limb, calf, right, with bone necrosis

         A41.51      Sepsis, Escherichia coli (E. coli)

         R65.20      Sepsis, severe

         J96.00       Failure, respiration, respiratory, acute

         0Y6H0Z1   Detachment, Leg, Lower, Right (0Y6H0Z)

                            Amputation *see* Detachment

**Rationale:**

Diagnoses: The chronic skin ulcer of the right calf with bone necrosis codes to L97.214. The patient also had E. coli sepsis (A41.51) with acute respiratory failure. ICD-10-CM Coding Guideline I.C.1.d.1.a states that if a patient has sepsis and associated acute organ dysfunction or multiple organ dysfunction, follow the instructions for coding severe sepsis. ICD-10-CM Coding Guideline I.C.1.d.1.b states the coding of severe sepsis requires a minimum of two codes: first a code for the underlying systemic infection, followed by a code from subcategory R65.2, Severe sepsis. Additional code(s) for the associated organ dysfunction are also required. Following the guidelines, R65.20 (Severe sepsis) and J96.00 (Acute respiratory failure) are also coded.

Procedures: The code for the below-the-knee amputation is 0Y6H0Z1 with the seventh character (qualifier) being 1 for a High amputation of the lower leg. The definition of *High amputation of the lower leg* is amputation at the proximal portion of the shaft of the tibia and fibula. The operative report specifies that the amputation occurs directly below the tibial tubercle. The tibial tubercle, also known as the tibial tuberosity, is a large oblong elevation on the proximal, anterior aspect of the tibia, just below where the anterior surfaces of the lateral and medial tibial condyles end. Detachment is the correct root operation for all amputation procedures. *Detachment* is defined as cutting off all or a portion of the upper or lower extremities. Per ICD-10-PCS Coding Guideline B6.1b temporary postop wound drains are considered integral to the performance of a procedure and are not coded as devices.

**3.37.**    K57.20      Diverticulitis, intestine, large, with abscess, perforation or peritonitis
         K50.112     Enteritis, regional, large intestine, with, intestinal obstruction
                       Crohn's disease *see* Enteritis, regional
         0DTN0ZZ    Resection, Colon, Sigmoid (0DTN)
                       Colectomy *see* Resection, Gastrointestinal System (0DT)
         0DTF0ZZ    Resection, Intestine, Large, Right (0DTF)
                       Hemicolectomy *see* Resection, Gastrointestinal System (0DT)
         0D1M0Z4    Bypass, Colon, Descending (0D1M)
                       Colostomy *see* Bypass, Gastrointestinal System (0D1)

**Rationale:**

Diagnoses: K57.20 is the correct code for diverticulitis of the sigmoid colon (large intestine) with perforation and K50.112 for Crohn's disease with perforation of the right colon and proximal transverse colon.

Procedures: During this procedure, a laparotomy is performed followed by a sigmoid colectomy, extended hemicolectomy, and colostomy. The laparotomy is considered the approach to reach the operative site and is therefore not coded separately. Coding Guideline B3.1b states that procedural steps necessary to reach the operative site and close the operative site are not coded separately. The code for the sigmoid colectomy is 0DTN0ZZ. The root operation Resection is used for the sigmoid colectomy since the entire sigmoid colon was removed. The next procedure performed was an extended hemicolectomy. During this procedure the entire right colon and part of the transverse colon are removed. The correct body part character is the right large intestine (F) instead of the ascending colon (K) as the right colon anatomical boundaries span from the cecum to the proximal transverse colon. The root operation for removal of the entire right colon is Resection, resulting in code 0DTF0ZZ. The final procedure performed is a colostomy which codes to 0D1M0Z4. The ICD-10-PCS Coding Guideline for Bypass Procedures states that bypass procedures are coded by identifying the body part bypassed from and the body part bypassed to. The fourth character body part specifies the body part passed from, and the qualifier specifies the body part bypassed to. For this colostomy, the body part bypassed from is the Descending Colon (M) and the body part bypassed to is the Abdominal Wall (4).

**3.38.**    M17.11      Osteoarthritis, primary, knee
         0SRC0J9    Replacement, Joint, Knee, Right (0SRC)
                       Arthroplasty *see* Replacement, Lower Joints (0SR)

**Rationale:**

Diagnosis: The code for primary osteoarthritis of the right knee is M17.11.

Procedure: During a total arthroplasty of the knee the patient's natural knee components are removed and replaced with a prosthetic device. The replacement code includes the taking out of the patient's own body part and therefore is not coded separately. ICD-10-PCS Coding Guideline B3.1.b states components of a procedure specified in the root operation definition and explanation are not coded separately

**3.39.**    M51.36      Degeneration, degenerative, intervertebral disc, Lumbar region
                       Disease, disc, degenerative *see* Degeneration, Intervertebral disc
         0SG10AJ    Fusion, Lumbar Vertebral, 2 or more (0SG1)
         0QB30ZZ    Excision, Bone, Pelvic, Left (0QB3) Iliac Crest *use* Bone, Pelvic, Left

**Rationale:**

Diagnoses: The code for degenerative disc disease of the lumbar region is M51.36.

Procedures: Spinal fusions are classified by the anatomic portion (column) fused and technique (approach) used. For the anterior column, the body (corpus) of adjacent vertebrae are fused (interbody fusion). The anterior column can be fused using an anterior, lateral or posterior technique. The technique for this procedure was posterior: 0SG10AJ. The laminectomy was not coded separately, as the excision of the lamina is a component of the fusion. Prior to the fusion, the surgeon removes the lamina bones covering the back of the spinal canal to see the nerve roots. During an interbody fusion, once the cages are in place, the surgeon will fix the bones in place using pedicle screws, which hold the vertebrae together and prevents them from moving. The combination of the graft material with pedicle screws holds the spine steady as the interbody fusion heals. The insertion of pedicle screws is coded separately. Per ICD-10-PCS Guideline 3.10c the use of autologous bone graft material for the fusion is not coded separately. The third procedure code is 0QB30ZZ for excising bone from the left iliac crest for the graft material. Guideline B3.9 states "If an autograft is obtained from a different body part in order to complete the objective of the procedure, a separate procedure is coded." The Alphabetic Index can be utilized to find the correct body part value: Iliac crest – see Bone, Pelvic, Left.

# Procedures in the Medical and Surgical-related Sections

## Coding Procedures in the Obstetrics Section – Section 1

**3.41.**    10A07Z6        Root Operation: Abortion
Abortion, Vacuum (10A07Z6)

**3.42.**    10E0XZZ        Root Operation: Delivery
Delivery, Manually assisted (10E0XZZ)

**3.43.**    10903ZA        Root Operation: Drainage
Drainage, Products of Conception, Fetal Cerebrospinal Fluid (1090)

**Rationale:**

The correct body part for a fetal spinal tap is Products of Conception, which is the body part for all the Obstetrics codes.

## Coding Procedures in the Placement Section – Section 2

**3.44.**    2Y41X5Z        Root Operation: Packing
Packing, Nasal (2Y41X5Z)

**3.45.**    2W3FX1Z        Root Operation: Immobilization
Immobilization, Hand, Left (2W3FX)

**3.46.**    2W1RX7Z        Root Operation: Compression
Compression, Leg, Lower, Left (2W1RX)

**Rationale:**

The correct body part is the Lower Leg, Left and not the Lower Extremity, Left. In this case, the compression device was only placed on the lower portion of the left leg and not the entire left leg (lower extremity).

**3.47.** 2W24X4Z Root Operation: Dressing
Dressing, Chest Wall (2W24X4Z)

**3.48.** 2W6LX0Z Root Operation: Traction
Traction, Extremity, Lower, Right (2W6LX)

## Coding Procedures in the Administration Section – Section 3

**3.49.** 30243G1 Root Operation: Transfusion
Transfusion, Vein, Central, Bone Marrow (3024)
Bone Marrow Transplant, *see* Transfusion

**3.50.** 30243N0 Root Operation: Transfusion
Transfusion, Vein, Central, Blood, Red Cells (3024)

**Rationale:**
In the Alphabetic Index the main term Administration has a cross reference note "Blood products see Transfusion." Autotransfusion is a process in which a person receives his or her own blood for a transfusion. Blood can be predonated before a surgery or can be collected during and after the surgery using a device commonly known as a *cell saver*. The intraoperative cell saver machine suctions, washes, and filters blood so it can be given back into the patient's body. The cell saver is used in operations in which there is expected to be a large volume blood loss.

**3.51.** 3E1M39Z Root Operation: Irrigation
Irrigation, Peritoneal Cavity, Dialysate (3E1M39Z)
Dialysis, Peritoneal (3E1M39Z)

**3.52.** 3E1U38Z Root Operation: Irrigation
Irrigation, Joint, Irrigating Substance (3E1U38Z)

**3.53.** 3E0S33Z Root Operation: Introduction
Introduction of substance in or on, Epidural Space, Anti-inflammatory (3E0S33Z)
Injection, *see* Introduction of substance in or on

## Coding Procedures in the Measurement and Monitoring Section – Section 4

**3.54.** 4A023N7 Measurement, Cardiac, Sampling and Pressure, Left Heart (4A02)
Catheterization, Heart *see* Measurement, Cardiac (4A02)

**Rationale:**
During a left heart catheterization, a catheter enters through either the femoral or brachial artery (note it is usually the femoral artery). A small incision is made, again usually in the groin area, and the catheter is percutaneously threaded into the left ventricle under fluoroscopy. During the procedure, the catheter tip is moved into various positions while the physician watches its progress on the imaging screen. Measurements of pressures within the left heart chamber are carried out during this procedure. In addition, the physician might also collect blood samples from the heart. Additional codes would be required if other image procedures were performed during the left heart catheterization such as left ventriculogram or coronary arteriography

**3.55.**   4A12X45   Root Operation: Monitoring
Monitoring, Cardiac, Electrical Activity, Ambulatory (4A12X45)
Holter Monitoring (4A12X45)

**3.56.**   4A1H7CZ   Root Operation: Monitoring
Monitoring, Products of Conception, Cardiac, Rate (4A1H)

## Coding Procedures in the Extracorporeal Assistance and Performance Section – Section 5

**3.57.**   5A02210   Root Operation: Assistance
Assistance, Cardiac, Continuous, Balloon Pump (5A02210)
IABP (Intra-aortic balloon pump), *see* Assistance, Cardiac (5A02)

**3.58.**   5A1D00Z   Root Operation: Performance
Performance, Urinary, Single, Filtration (5A1D00Z)
Hemodialysis (5A1D00Z)
Dialysis, Hemodialysis (5A1D00Z)

**3.59.**   5A1221Z   Root Operation: Performance
Performance, Cardiac, Continuous, Output (5A1221Z)
Bypass, Cardiopulmonary (5A1221Z)

**Rationale:**
Cardiopulmonary bypass is a technique that mechanically circulates and oxygenates blood from the body while bypassing the heart and lungs. This technique uses a heart-lung machine to continuously maintain perfusion to other body organs and tissues during surgery. In selecting the duration character for this procedure, the selections are Single, Intermittent, or Continuous, with Continuous (2) being the correct selection. Staying in the row in the Table under Duration, and Continuous, the selections for the function character are Output and Pacing. Output is the correct selection because during this technique, the machine continuously takes over the output of the heart and lungs.

**3.60.**   I25.10   Arteriosclerosis, arteriosclerotic (diffuse) (obliterans) (of) (senile) (with calcification), coronary (artery), native vessel
I21.09   Infarct, infarction, myocardium, ST elevation, anterior (anteroapical) (anterolateral) (anteroseptal) (Q wave) (wall)
E11.9   Diabetes, diabetic (mellitus) (sugar), type 2
E78.0   Hypercholesterolemia (essential) (familial) (hereditary) (primary) (pure)
Z92.21   History, personal (of), chemotherapy for neoplastic condition
Z85.038   History, personal (of), malignant neoplasm, colon NEC
Z79.4   Long-term (current) drug therapy (use of), insulin
Z90.49   Absence (of) (organ or part) (complete or partial), intestine (acquired), large
021209W   Bypass, Artery, Coronary, Three Sites (0212)
02100Z9   Bypass, Artery, Coronary, One Site (0210)
5A1221Z   Performance, Cardiac, Continuous, Output (5A1221Z)
Bypass, Cardiopulmonary (5A1221Z)
06BQ4ZZ   Excision, Vein, Greater Saphenous, Left (06BQ)

**Rationale:**
Diagnoses: The reason the patient was transferred to this hospital was to have the CABG procedure for the four-vessel CAD; therefore, I25.10 is the principal diagnosis. A secondary code for the myocardial infarction, I21.09, is required since the myocardial infarction is still less than 4 weeks old. In the Tabular under category I21, there is a note that states "myocardial infarction specified as acute or with a stated duration of 4 weeks (28 days) or less from onset." Patient also has type 2 diabetes mellitus (E11.9) and hypercholesterolemia (E78.0). In the Tabular, under category E11, the following note appears: "Use additional code to identify any insulin use (Z79.4)." Patient also has a history of colon cancer (Z85.038) and chemotherapy (Z92.21). An additional code for absence of the sigmoid colon can also be coded as Z90.49.

Procedures: Coding Guideline B3.6c states that if multiple coronary artery sites are bypassed, a separate procedure is coded for each coronary artery site that uses a different device and/or qualifier. In this case both aortocoronary artery bypass and internal mammary coronary artery bypass were done. Applying the guideline, these bypasses are coded separately. 021209W is the code for bypassing three coronary sites via aortocoronary artery bypass and 02100Z9 for the internal mammary bypass. The patient was placed on cardiopulmonary bypass, code 5A1221Z. Per Coding Guideline B3.9 an additional code, 06BQ4ZZ, is needed for the harvesting of the saphenous vein graft material. Coding Guideline B3.9 states that if an autograft is obtained from a different body part, a separate procedure is coded. The cardioplegia and hypothermia are inherent in cardiopulmonary bypass procedures and are not coded separately. Additionally, the pacing wires and mediastinal tubes are considered to be integral to the performance of the procedure and are not coded as devices. Coding Guideline B6.1b states that materials such as sutures, ligatures, radiological markers, and temporary postoperative wound drains are considered integral to the performance of a procedure and are not coded as devices.

**3.61.**    5A2204Z      Root Operation: Restoration
Restoration, Cardiac, Single, Rhythm (5A2204Z)
Cardioversion (5A2204Z)

## Coding Procedures in the Extracorporeal Therapies Section – Section 6

**3.62.**    6A4Z0ZZ      Root Operation: Hypothermia
Hypothermia, Whole Body (6A4Z)

**3.63.**    6A800ZZ      Root Operation: Ultraviolet Light Therapy
Ultraviolet Light Therapy, Skin (6A80)

## Coding Procedures in the Osteopathic Section – Section 7

**3.64.**    7W04X4Z      Root Operation: Osteopathic Treatment
Osteopathic Treatment, Sacrum (7W04X)

## Coding Procedures in the Other Procedures Section – Section 8

**3.65.**    8E0W8CZ      Root Operation: Other Procedures
Robotic-Assisted Procedure, Trunk Region (8E0W)

**Rationale:**
For this question, only the robotic assistance portion of the procedure was coded to illustrate coding root operations in the Other Procedures section. To completely code this procedure, two codes are required—one for the transurethral prostatectomy (primary procedure) and one for the robotic assistance.

**3.66.**     8E0YXY8     Root Operation: Other Procedures
Suture Removal, Extremity, Lower (8E0YXY8)

## Coding Procedures in the Chiropractic Section – Section 9

**3.67.**     9WB3XJZ     Root Operation: Manipulation
Manipulation, Chiropractic, *see* Chiropractic Manipulation
Chiropractic Manipulation, Lumbar (9WB3X)

# Procedures in the Ancillary Sections

## Coding Procedures in the Imaging Section – Section B

**3.68.**     BG34Y0Z     Root Operation: Magnetic Resonance Imaging (MRI)
Magnetic Resonance Imaging (MRI), Gland, Thyroid (BG34)

**3.69.**     BW03ZZZ     Root Operation: Plain Radiography
Plain Radiography, Chest (BW03ZZZ)
X-ray, *see* Plain Radiography
Radiography, *see* Plain Radiography
Imaging, diagnostic, *see* Plain Radiography

**3.70.**     I25.110     Arteriosclerosis, arteriosclerotic (diffuse) (obliterans) (of) (senile) (with calcification), coronary (artery), native vessel, with, angina pectoris, unstable

            I10     Hypertension, hypertensive (accelerated) (benign) (essential) (idiopathic) (malignant) (systemic)

            Z82.49     History, family, disease or disorder (of), cardiovascular NEC
            Z72.0     Tobacco, use
Use, tobacco

            4A023N7     Measurement, Cardiac, Sampling and Pressure, Left Heart (4A02)
Catheterization, Heart *see* Measurement, Cardiac (4A02)

            B2151ZZ     Fluoroscopy, Heart, Left (B215)
Ventriculogram, cardiac, Left Ventricle *see* Fluoroscopy, Heart, Left (B215)

            B2111ZZ     Fluoroscopy, Artery, Coronary, Multiple (B211)
Angiography, *see* Fluoroscopy, Heart (B21)

**Rationale:**

Diagnoses: ICD-10-CM provides a combination code for the arteriosclerosis and unstable angina, I25.110. Secondary diagnosis codes for the hypertension (I10), family history of heart disease (Z82.49), and tobacco use (Z72.0) are also assigned.

Procedures: A cardiac catheterization involves the use of catheters, x-ray imaging (fluoroscopy) and contrast dye. A catheter is inserted, usually in the groin area, and threaded into the heart using an x-ray machine that produces real time pictures (fluoroscopy). During the procedure the catheter tip is moved into various positions in the patient's vessels and chambers while the physician watches its progress on the imaging screen. Measurements of pressures within the left heart chamber are carried out during this procedure. In addition to measuring pressures and blood in the heart chamber, a physician usually also collects blood samples from the heart during a heart catheterization. The root operation for the left heart catheterization is measurement with the code being 4A023N7. The sixth character (N) is for sampling and pressure. The seventh character 7 indicates the heart chamber which was catheterized, left heart. In addition to the cardiac catheterization, a left ventriculogram (B2151ZZ) and coronary angiography (B2111ZZ) were performed. Once the catheter reaches the coronary arteries, dye is injected into them. This dye shows up on the x-ray screen and allows the physician to see if there is any blockage. The physician will repeat the injection of the dye several times, looking at the arteries from various angles. Once the physician completes examining the coronary arteries, the catheter is redirected to the left ventricle, dye is injected, and x-rays are taken.

## *Coding Procedures in the Nuclear Medicine Section – Section C*

**3.71.**    C23GKZZ     Root Operation: Positron Emission Tomographic (PET) Imaging
Positron Emission Tomographic (PET) Imaging, Myocardium (C23G)
PET Scan, *see* Positron Emission Tomographic (PET) Imaging

**3.72.**    C7221ZZ     Root Operation: Tomographic (Tomo) Nuclear Medicine Imaging
Tomographic (Tomo) Nuclear Medicine Imaging, Spleen (C722)

## *Coding Procedures in the Radiation Therapy Section – Section D*

**3.73.**    DV1097Z     Root Operation: Brachytherapy
Brachytherapy, Prostate (DV10)

**3.74.**    DDY07ZZ     Root Operation: Contact Radiation
Contact Radiation, Esophagus (DDY07ZZ)

## *Coding Procedures in the Physical Rehabilitation and Diagnostic Audiology Section – Section F*

**3.75.**    F08L5BZ     Root Operation: Activities of Daily Living Treatment
Activities of Daily Living Treatment (F08)

**3.76.**    F13Z31Z     Root Operation: Hearing Assessment
Hearing Assessment (F13Z)
Assessment, Hearing, *see* Hearing Assessment, Diagnostic Audiology (F13)
Audiometry, *see* Hearing Assessment, Diagnostic Audiology (F13)

## Coding Procedures in the Mental Health Section – Section G

**3.77.**    GZB3ZZZ    Root Operation: Electroconvulsive Therapy
Electroconvulsive Therapy, Bilateral-Multiple
Seizures (GZB3ZZZ)

**3.78.**    GZ11ZZZ    Root Operation: Psychological Tests
Psychological Tests, Personality and Behavioral (GZ11ZZZ)
Testing, Mental health, *see* Psychological Tests

## Coding Procedures in the Substance Abuse Treatment Section – Section H

**3.79.**    HZ2ZZZZ    Root Operation: Detoxification Services
Detoxification Services, for substance abuse (HZ2ZZZZ)

**3.80.**    HZ53ZZZ    Root Operation: Psychotherapy
Psychotherapy, Individual, for substance abuse, 12-step (HZ53ZZZ)

# Appendix A

## Medical and Surgical Body Parts

| Section 0 - Medical and Surgical - Character 4 - Body Part | |
|---|---|
| **1st** Toe, Left<br>**1st** Toe, Right | **Includes:**<br>Hallux |
| **Abdomen** Muscle, Left<br>**Abdomen** Muscle, Right | **Includes:**<br>External oblique muscle<br>Internal oblique muscle<br>Pyramidalis muscle<br>Rectus abdominis muscle<br>Transversus abdominis muscle |
| **Abdominal** Aorta | **Includes:**<br>Inferior phrenic artery<br>Lumbar artery<br>Median sacral artery<br>Middle suprarenal artery<br>Ovarian artery<br>Testicular artery |
| **Abdominal** Sympathetic Nerve | **Includes:**<br>Abdominal aortic plexus<br>Auerbach's (myenteric) plexus<br>Celiac (solar) plexus<br>Celiac ganglion<br>Gastric plexus<br>Hepatic plexus<br>Inferior hypogastric plexus<br>Inferior mesenteric ganglion<br>Inferior mesenteric plexus<br>Meissner's (submucous) plexus<br>Myenteric (Auerbach's) plexus<br>Pancreatic plexus<br>Pelvic splanchnic nerve<br>Renal plexus<br>Solar (celiac) plexus<br>Splenic plexus<br>Submucous (Meissner's) plexus<br>Superior hypogastric plexus<br>Superior mesenteric ganglion<br>Superior mesenteric plexus<br>Suprarenal plexus |
| **Abducens** Nerve | **Includes:**<br>Sixth cranial nerve |
| **Accessory** Nerve | **Includes:**<br>Eleventh cranial nerve |
| **Acoustic** Nerve | **Includes:**<br>Cochlear nerve<br>Eighth cranial nerve<br>Scarpa's (vestibular) ganglion<br>Spiral ganglion<br>Vestibular (Scarpa's) ganglion<br>Vestibular nerve<br>Vestibulocochlear nerve |

| Section 0 - Medical and Surgical - Character 4 - Body Part ||
|---|---|
| **Adenoids** | **Includes:**<br>Pharyngeal tonsil |
| **Adrenal** Gland<br>**Adrenal** Gland, Left<br>**Adrenal** Gland, Right<br>**Adrenal** Glands, Bilateral | **Includes:**<br>Suprarenal gland |
| **Ampulla** of Vater | **Includes:**<br>Duodenal ampulla<br>Hepatopancreatic ampulla |
| **Anal** Sphincter | **Includes:**<br>External anal sphincter<br>Internal anal sphincter |
| **Ankle** Bursa and Ligament, Left<br>**Ankle** Bursa and Ligament, Right | **Includes:**<br>Calcaneofibular ligament<br>Deltoid ligament<br>Ligament of the lateral malleolus<br>Talofibular ligament |
| **Ankle** Joint, Left<br>**Ankle** Joint, Right | **Includes:**<br>Inferior tibiofibular joint<br>Talocrural joint |
| **Anterior** Chamber, Left<br>**Anterior** Chamber, Right | **Includes:**<br>Aqueous humour |
| **Anterior** Tibial Artery, Left<br>**Anterior** Tibial Artery, Right | **Includes:**<br>Anterior lateral malleolar artery<br>Anterior medial malleolar artery<br>Anterior tibial recurrent artery<br>Dorsalis pedis artery<br>Posterior tibial recurrent artery |
| **Anus** | **Includes:**<br>Anal orifice |
| **Aortic** Valve | **Includes:**<br>Aortic annulus |
| **Appendix** | **Includes:**<br>Vermiform appendix |
| **Ascending** Colon | **Includes:**<br>Hepatic flexure |
| **Atrial** Septum | **Includes:**<br>Interatrial septum |
| **Atrium,** Left | **Includes:**<br>Atrium pulmonale<br>Left auricular appendix |
| **Atrium,** Right | **Includes:**<br>Atrium dextrum cordis<br>Right auricular appendix<br>Sinus venosus |
| **Auditory** Ossicle, Left<br>**Auditory** Ossicle, Right | **Includes:**<br>Incus<br>Malleus<br>Ossicular chain<br>Stapes |

| Section 0 - Medical and Surgical - Character 4 - Body Part | |
|---|---|
| **Axillary** Artery, Left<br>**Axillary** Artery, Right | **Includes:**<br>Anterior circumflex humeral artery<br>Lateral thoracic artery<br>Posterior circumflex humeral artery<br>Subscapular artery<br>Superior thoracic artery<br>Thoracoacromial artery |
| **Azygos** Vein | **Includes:**<br>Right ascending lumbar vein<br>Right subcostal vein |
| **Basal** Ganglia | **Includes:**<br>Basal nuclei<br>Claustrum<br>Corpus striatum<br>Globus pallidus<br>Substantia nigra<br>Subthalamic nucleus |
| **Basilic** Vein, Left<br>**Basilic** Vein, Right | **Includes:**<br>Median antebrachial vein<br>Median cubital vein |
| **Bladder** | **Includes:**<br>Trigone of bladder |
| **Brachial** Artery, Left<br>**Brachial** Artery, Right | **Includes:**<br>Inferior ulnar collateral artery<br>Profunda brachii<br>Superior ulnar collateral artery |
| **Brachial** Plexus | **Includes:**<br>Axillary nerve<br>Dorsal scapular nerve<br>First intercostal nerve<br>Long thoracic nerve<br>Musculocutaneous nerve<br>Subclavius nerve<br>Suprascapular nerve |
| **Brachial** Vein, Left<br>**Brachial** Vein, Right | **Includes:**<br>Radial vein<br>Ulnar vein |
| **Brain** | **Includes:**<br>Cerebrum<br>Corpus callosum<br>Encephalon |
| **Breast,** Bilateral<br>**Breast,** Left<br>**Breast,** Right | **Includes:**<br>Mammary duct<br>Mammary gland |
| **Buccal** Mucosa | **Includes:**<br>Buccal gland<br>Molar gland<br>Palatine gland |
| **Carotid** Bodies, Bilateral<br>**Carotid** Body, Left<br>**Carotid** Body, Right | **Includes:**<br>Carotid glomus |

| Section 0 - Medical and Surgical - Character 4 - Body Part | |
|---|---|
| **Carpal** Joint, Left<br>**Carpal** Joint, Right | Includes:<br>Intercarpal joint<br>Midcarpal joint |
| **Carpal,** Left<br>**Carpal,** Right | Includes:<br>Capitate bone<br>Hamate bone<br>Lunate bone<br>Pisiform bone<br>Scaphoid bone<br>Trapezium bone<br>Trapezoid bone<br>Triquetral bone |
| **Celiac** Artery | Includes:<br>Celiac trunk |
| **Cephalic** Vein, Left<br>**Cephalic** Vein, Right | Includes:<br>Accessory cephalic vein |
| **Cerebellum** | Includes:<br>Culmen |
| **Cerebral** Hemisphere | Includes:<br>Frontal lobe<br>Occipital lobe<br>Parietal lobe<br>Temporal lobe |
| **Cerebral** Meninges | Includes:<br>Arachnoid mater<br>Leptomeninges<br>Pia mater |
| **Cerebral** Ventricle | Includes:<br>Aqueduct of Sylvius<br>Cerebral aqueduct (Sylvius)<br>Choroid plexus<br>Ependyma<br>Foramen of Monro (intraventricular)<br>Fourth ventricle<br>Interventricular foramen (Monro)<br>Left lateral ventricle<br>Right lateral ventricle<br>Third ventricle |
| **Cervical** Nerve | Includes:<br>Greater occipital nerve<br>Spinal nerve, cervical<br>Suboccipital nerve<br>Third occipital nerve |
| **Cervical** Plexus | Includes:<br>Ansa cervicalis<br>Cutaneous (transverse) cervical nerve<br>Great auricular nerve<br>Lesser occipital nerve<br>Supraclavicular nerve<br>Transverse (cutaneous) cervical nerve |

| Section 0 - Medical and Surgical - Character 4 - Body Part ||
|---|---|
| **Cervical** Vertebra | **Includes:**<br>Spinous process<br>Vertebral arch<br>Vertebral foramen<br>Vertebral lamina<br>Vertebral pedicle |
| **Cervical** Vertebral Joint | **Includes:**<br>Atlantoaxial joint<br>Cervical facet joint |
| **Cervical** Vertebral Joints, 2 or more | **Includes:**<br>Cervical facet joint |
| **Cervicothoracic** Vertebral Joint | **Includes:**<br>Cervicothoracic facet joint |
| **Cisterna** Chyli | **Includes:**<br>Intestinal lymphatic trunk<br>Lumbar lymphatic trunk |
| **Coccygeal** Glomus | **Includes:**<br>Coccygeal body |
| **Colic** Vein | **Includes:**<br>Ileocolic vein<br>Left colic vein<br>Middle colic vein<br>Right colic vein |
| **Conduction** Mechanism | **Includes:**<br>Atrioventricular node<br>Bundle of His<br>Bundle of Kent<br>Sinoatrial node |
| **Conjunctiva,** Left<br>**Conjunctiva,** Right | **Includes:**<br>Plica semilunaris |
| **Dura** Mater | **Includes:**<br>Cranial dura mater<br>Dentate ligament<br>Diaphragma sellae<br>Falx cerebri<br>Spinal dura mater<br>Tentorium cerebelli |
| **Elbow** Bursa and Ligament, Left<br>**Elbow** Bursa and Ligament, Right | **Includes:**<br>Annular ligament<br>Olecranon bursa<br>Radial collateral ligament<br>Ulnar collateral ligament |
| **Elbow** Joint, Left<br>**Elbow** Joint, Right | **Includes:**<br>Distal humerus, involving joint<br>Humeroradial joint<br>Humeroulnar joint<br>Proximal radioulnar joint |
| **Epidural** Space | **Includes:**<br>Cranial epidural space<br>Extradural space<br>Spinal epidural space |

| Section 0 - Medical and Surgical - Character 4 - Body Part | |
|---|---|
| **Epiglottis** | **Includes:**<br>Glossoepiglottic fold |
| **Esophagogastric** Junction | **Includes:**<br>Cardia<br>Cardioesophageal junction<br>Gastroesophageal (GE) junction |
| **Esophagus,** Lower | **Includes:**<br>Abdominal esophagus |
| **Esophagus,** Middle | **Includes:**<br>Thoracic esophagus |
| **Esophagus,** Upper | **Includes:**<br>Cervical esophagus |
| **Ethmoid** Bone, Left<br>**Ethmoid** Bone, Right | **Includes:**<br>Cribriform plate |
| **Ethmoid** Sinus, Left<br>**Ethmoid** Sinus, Right | **Includes:**<br>Ethmoidal air cell |
| **Eustachian** Tube, Left<br>**Eustachian** Tube, Right | **Includes:**<br>Auditory tube<br>Pharyngotympanic tube |
| **External** Auditory Canal, Left<br>**External** Auditory Canal, Right | **Includes:**<br>External auditory meatus |
| **External** Carotid Artery, Left<br>**External** Carotid Artery, Right | **Includes:**<br>Ascending pharyngeal artery<br>Internal maxillary artery<br>Lingual artery<br>Maxillary artery<br>Occipital artery<br>Posterior auricular artery<br>Superior thyroid artery |
| **External** Ear, Bilateral<br>**External** Ear, Left<br>**External** Ear, Right | **Includes:**<br>Antihelix<br>Antitragus<br>Auricle<br>Earlobe<br>Helix<br>Pinna<br>Tragus |
| **External** Iliac Artery, Left<br>**External** Iliac Artery, Right | **Includes:**<br>Deep circumflex iliac artery<br>Inferior epigastric artery |
| **External** Jugular Vein, Left<br>**External** Jugular Vein, Right | **Includes:**<br>Posterior auricular vein |
| **Extraocular** Muscle, Left<br>**Extraocular** Muscle, Right | **Includes:**<br>Inferior oblique muscle<br>Inferior rectus muscle<br>Lateral rectus muscle<br>Medial rectus muscle<br>Superior oblique muscle<br>Superior rectus muscle |

| Section 0 - Medical and Surgical - Character 4 - Body Part | |
|---|---|
| **Eye,** Left<br>**Eye,** Right | **Includes:**<br>Ciliary body<br>Posterior chamber |
| **Face** Artery | **Includes:**<br>Angular artery<br>Ascending palatine artery<br>External maxillary artery<br>Facial artery<br>Inferior labial artery<br>Submental artery<br>Superior labial artery |
| **Face** Vein, Left<br>**Face** Vein, Right | **Includes:**<br>Angular vein<br>Anterior facial vein<br>Common facial vein<br>Deep facial vein<br>Frontal vein<br>Posterior facial (retromandibular) vein<br>Supraorbital vein |
| **Facial** Muscle | **Includes:**<br>Buccinator muscle<br>Corrugator supercilii muscle<br>Depressor anguli oris muscle<br>Depressor labii inferioris muscle<br>Depressor septi nasi muscle<br>Depressor supercilii muscle<br>Levator anguli oris muscle<br>Levator labii superioris alaeque nasi<br>Levator labii superioris alaeque nasi<br>Levator labii superioris alaeque nasi<br>Levator labii superioris muscle<br>Mentalis muscle<br>Nasalis muscle<br>Occipitofrontalis muscle<br>Orbicularis oris muscle<br>Procerus muscle<br>Risorius muscle<br>Zygomaticus muscle |
| **Facial** Nerve | **Includes:**<br>Chorda tympani<br>Geniculate ganglion<br>Greater superficial petrosal nerve<br>Nerve to the stapedius<br>Parotid plexus<br>Posterior auricular nerve<br>Seventh cranial nerve<br>Submandibular ganglion |
| **Fallopian** Tube, Left<br>**Fallopian** Tube, Right | **Includes:**<br>Oviduct<br>Salpinx<br>Uterine tube |

| Section 0 - Medical and Surgical - Character 4 - Body Part | |
| --- | --- |
| **Femoral** Artery, Left<br>**Femoral** Artery, Right | **Includes:**<br>Circumflex iliac artery<br>Deep femoral artery<br>Descending genicular artery<br>External pudendal artery<br>Superficial epigastric artery |
| **Femoral** Nerve | **Includes:**<br>Anterior crural nerve<br>Saphenous nerve |
| **Femoral** Shaft, Left<br>**Femoral** Shaft, Right | **Includes:**<br>Body of femur |
| **Femoral** Vein, Left<br>**Femoral** Vein, Right | **Includes:**<br>Deep femoral (profunda femoris) vein<br>Popliteal vein<br>Profunda femoris (deep femoral) vein |
| **Fibula,** Left<br>**Fibula,** Right | **Includes:**<br>Body of fibula<br>Head of fibula<br>Lateral malleolus |
| **Finger** Nail | **Includes:**<br>Nail bed<br>Nail plate |
| **Finger** Phalangeal Joint, Left<br>**Finger** Phalangeal Joint, Right | **Includes:**<br>Interphalangeal (IP) joint |
| **Foot** Artery, Left<br>**Foot** Artery, Right | **Includes:**<br>Arcuate artery<br>Dorsal metatarsal artery<br>Lateral plantar artery<br>Lateral tarsal artery<br>Medial plantar artery |
| **Foot** Bursa and Ligament, Left<br>**Foot** Bursa and Ligament, Right | **Includes:**<br>Calcaneocuboid ligament<br>Cuneonavicular ligament<br>Intercuneiform ligament<br>Interphalangeal ligament<br>Metatarsal ligament<br>Metatarsophalangeal ligament<br>Subtalar ligament<br>Talocalcaneal ligament<br>Talocalcaneonavicular ligament<br>Tarsometatarsal ligament |
| **Foot** Muscle, Left<br>**Foot** Muscle, Right | **Includes:**<br>Abductor hallucis muscle<br>Adductor hallucis muscle<br>Extensor digitorum brevis muscle<br>Extensor hallucis brevis muscle<br>Flexor digitorum brevis muscle<br>Flexor hallucis brevis muscle<br>Quadratus plantae muscle |

| Section 0 - Medical and Surgical - Character 4 - Body Part | |
|---|---|
| **Foot** Vein, Left<br>**Foot** Vein, Right | **Includes:**<br>Common digital vein<br>Dorsal metatarsal vein<br>Dorsal venous arch<br>Plantar digital vein<br>Plantar metatarsal vein<br>Plantar venous arch |
| **Frontal** Bone, Left<br>**Frontal** Bone, Right | **Includes:**<br>Zygomatic process of frontal bone |
| **Gastric** Artery | **Includes:**<br>Left gastric artery<br>Right gastric artery |
| **Glenoid** Cavity, Left<br>**Glenoid** Cavity, Right | **Includes:**<br>Glenoid fossa (of scapula) |
| **Glomus** Jugulare | **Includes:**<br>Jugular body |
| **Glossopharyngeal** Nerve | **Includes:**<br>Carotid sinus nerve<br>Ninth cranial nerve<br>Tympanic nerve |
| **Greater** Omentum | **Includes:**<br>Gastrocolic ligament<br>Gastrocolic omentum<br>Gastrophrenic ligament<br>Gastrosplenic ligament |
| **Greater** Saphenous Vein, Left<br>**Greater** Saphenous Vein, Right | **Includes:**<br>External pudendal vein<br>Great saphenous vein<br>Superficial circumflex iliac vein<br>Superficial epigastric vein |
| **Hand** Artery, Left<br>**Hand** Artery, Right | **Includes:**<br>Deep palmar arch<br>Princeps pollicis artery<br>Radialis indicis<br>Superficial palmar arch |
| **Hand** Bursa and Ligament, Left<br>**Hand** Bursa and Ligament, Right | **Includes:**<br>Carpometacarpal ligament<br>Intercarpal ligament<br>Interphalangeal ligament<br>Lunotriquetral ligament<br>Metacarpal ligament<br>Metacarpophalangeal ligament<br>Pisohamate ligament<br>Pisometacarpal ligament<br>Scapholunate ligament<br>Scaphotrapezium ligament |
| **Hand** Muscle, Left<br>**Hand** Muscle, Right | **Includes:**<br>Hypothenar muscle<br>Palmar interosseous muscle<br>Thenar muscle |

| Section 0 - Medical and Surgical - Character 4 - Body Part | |
|---|---|
| **Hand** Vein, Left<br>**Hand** Vein, Right | **Includes:**<br>Dorsal metacarpal vein<br>Palmar (volar) digital vein<br>Palmar (volar) metacarpal vein<br>Superficial palmar venous arch<br>Volar (palmar) digital vein<br>Volar (palmar) metacarpal vein |
| **Head** and Neck Bursa and Ligament | **Includes:**<br>Alar ligament of axis<br>Cervical interspinous ligament<br>Cervical intertransverse ligament<br>Cervical ligamentum flavum<br>Lateral temporomandibular ligament<br>Sphenomandibular ligament<br>Stylomandibular ligament<br>Transverse ligament of atlas |
| **Head** and Neck Sympathetic Nerve | **Includes:**<br>Cavernous plexus<br>Cervical ganglion<br>Ciliary ganglion<br>Internal carotid plexus<br>Otic ganglion<br>Pterygopalatine (sphenopalatine) ganglion<br>Sphenopalatine (pterygopalatine) ganglion<br>Stellate ganglion<br>Submandibular ganglion<br>Submaxillary ganglion |
| **Head** Muscle | **Includes:**<br>Auricularis muscle<br>Masseter muscle<br>Pterygoid muscle<br>Splenius capitis muscle<br>Temporalis muscle<br>Temporoparietalis muscle |
| **Heart,** Left | **Includes:**<br>Left coronary sulcus<br>Obtuse margin |
| **Heart,** Right | **Includes:**<br>Right coronary sulcus |
| **Hemiazygos** Vein | **Includes:**<br>Left ascending lumbar vein<br>Left subcostal vein |
| **Hepatic** Artery | **Includes:**<br>Common hepatic artery<br>Gastroduodenal artery<br>Hepatic artery proper |
| **Hip** Bursa and Ligament, Left<br>**Hip** Bursa and Ligament, Right | **Includes:**<br>Iliofemoral ligament<br>Ischiofemoral ligament<br>Pubofemoral ligament<br>Transverse acetabular ligament<br>Trochanteric bursa |

| Section 0 - Medical and Surgical - Character 4 - Body Part ||
|---|---|
| **Hip** Joint, Left<br>**Hip** Joint, Right | **Includes:**<br>Acetabulofemoral joint |
| **Hip** Muscle, Left<br>**Hip** Muscle, Right | **Includes:**<br>Gemellus muscle<br>Gluteus maximus muscle<br>Gluteus medius muscle<br>Gluteus minimus muscle<br>Iliacus muscle<br>Obturator muscle<br>Piriformis muscle<br>Psoas muscle<br>Quadratus femoris muscle<br>Tensor fasciae latae muscle |
| **Humeral** Head, Left<br>**Humeral** Head, Right | **Includes:**<br>Greater tuberosity<br>Lesser tuberosity<br>Neck of humerus (anatomical)(surgical) |
| **Humeral** Shaft, Left<br>**Humeral** Shaft, Right | **Includes:**<br>Distal humerus<br>Humerus, distal<br>Lateral epicondyle of humerus<br>Medial epicondyle of humerus |
| **Hypogastric** Vein, Left<br>**Hypogastric** Vein, Right | **Includes:**<br>Gluteal vein<br>Internal iliac vein<br>Internal pudendal vein<br>Lateral sacral vein<br>Middle hemorrhoidal vein<br>Obturator vein<br>Uterine vein<br>Vaginal vein<br>Vesical vein |
| **Hypoglossal** Nerve | **Includes:**<br>Twelfth cranial nerve |
| **Hypothalamus** | **Includes:**<br>Mammillary body |
| **Inferior** Mesenteric Artery | **Includes:**<br>Sigmoid artery<br>Superior rectal artery |
| **Inferior** Mesenteric Vein | **Includes:**<br>Sigmoid vein<br>Superior rectal vein |
| **Inferior** Vena Cava | **Includes:**<br>Postcava<br>Right inferior phrenic vein<br>Right ovarian vein<br>Right second lumbar vein<br>Right suprarenal vein<br>Right testicular vein |
| **Inguinal** Region, Bilateral<br>**Inguinal** Region, Left<br>**Inguinal** Region, Right | **Includes:**<br>Inguinal canal<br>Inguinal triangle |

| Section 0 - Medical and Surgical - Character 4 - Body Part ||
|---|---|
| **Inner** Ear, Left<br>**Inner** Ear, Right | **Includes:**<br>Bony labyrinth<br>Bony vestibule<br>Cochlea<br>Round window<br>Semicircular canal |
| **Innominate** Artery | **Includes:**<br>Brachiocephalic artery<br>Brachiocephalic trunk |
| **Innominate** Vein, Left<br>**Innominate** Vein, Right | **Includes:**<br>Brachiocephalic vein<br>Inferior thyroid vein |
| **Internal** Carotid Artery, Left<br>**Internal** Carotid Artery, Right | **Includes:**<br>Caroticotympanic artery<br>Carotid sinus<br>Ophthalmic artery |
| **Internal** Iliac Artery, Left<br>**Internal** Iliac Artery, Right | **Includes:**<br>Deferential artery<br>Hypogastric artery<br>Iliolumbar artery<br>Inferior gluteal artery<br>Inferior vesical artery<br>Internal pudendal artery<br>Lateral sacral artery<br>Middle rectal artery<br>Obturator artery<br>Superior gluteal artery<br>Umbilical artery<br>Uterine artery<br>Vaginal artery |
| **Internal** Mammary Artery, Left<br>**Internal** Mammary Artery, Right | **Includes:**<br>Anterior intercostal artery<br>Internal thoracic artery<br>Musculophrenic artery<br>Pericardiophrenic artery<br>Superior epigastric artery |
| **Intracranial** Artery | **Includes:**<br>Anterior cerebral artery<br>Anterior choroidal artery<br>Anterior communicating artery<br>Basilar artery<br>Circle of Willis<br>Middle cerebral artery<br>Posterior cerebral artery<br>Posterior communicating artery<br>Posterior inferior cerebellar artery (PICA) |

| Section 0 - Medical and Surgical - Character 4 - Body Part | |
|---|---|
| **Intracranial** Vein | **Includes:**<br>Anterior cerebral vein<br>Basal (internal) cerebral vein<br>Dural venous sinus<br>Great cerebral vein<br>Inferior cerebellar vein<br>Inferior cerebral vein<br>Internal (basal) cerebral vein<br>Middle cerebral vein<br>Ophthalmic vein<br>Superior cerebellar vein<br>Superior cerebral vein |
| **Jejunum** | **Includes:**<br>Duodenojejunal flexure |
| **Kidney** | **Includes:**<br>Renal calyx<br>Renal capsule<br>Renal cortex<br>Renal segment |
| **Kidney** Pelvis, Left<br>**Kidney** Pelvis, Right | **Includes:**<br>Ureteropelvic junction (UPJ) |
| **Kidney,** Left<br>**Kidney,** Right<br>**Kidneys,** Bilateral | **Includes:**<br>Renal calyx<br>Renal capsule<br>Renal cortex<br>Renal segment |
| **Knee** Bursa and Ligament, Left<br>**Knee** Bursa and Ligament, Right | **Includes:**<br>Anterior cruciate ligament (ACL)<br>Lateral collateral ligament (LCL)<br>Ligament of head of fibula<br>Medial collateral ligament (MCL)<br>Patellar ligament<br>Popliteal ligament<br>Posterior cruciate ligament (PCL)<br>Prepatellar bursa |
| **Knee** Joint, Femoral Surface, Left<br>**Knee** Joint, Femoral Surface, Right | **Includes:**<br>Femoropatellar joint<br>Patellofemoral joint |
| **Knee** Joint, Left<br>**Knee** Joint, Right | **Includes:**<br>Femoropatellar joint<br>Femorotibial joint<br>Lateral meniscus<br>Medial meniscus<br>Patellofemoral joint<br>Tibiofemoral joint |
| **Knee** Joint, Tibial Surface, Left<br>**Knee** Joint, Tibial Surface, Right | **Includes:**<br>Femorotibial joint<br>Tibiofemoral joint |
| **Knee** Tendon, Left<br>**Knee** Tendon, Right | **Includes:**<br>Patellar tendon |

| Section 0 - Medical and Surgical - Character 4 - Body Part ||
|---|---|
| **Lacrimal** Duct, Left<br>**Lacrimal** Duct, Right | **Includes:**<br>Lacrimal canaliculus<br>Lacrimal punctum<br>Lacrimal sac<br>Nasolacrimal duct |
| **Larynx** | **Includes:**<br>Aryepiglottic fold<br>Arytenoid cartilage<br>Corniculate cartilage<br>Crlcoid cartilage<br>Cuneiform cartilage<br>False vocal cord<br>Glottis<br>Rima glottidis<br>Thyroid cartilage<br>Ventricular fold |
| **Lens,** Left<br>**Lens,** Right | **Includes:**<br>Zonule of Zinn |
| **Lesser** Omentum | **Includes:**<br>Gastrohepatic omentum<br>Hepatogastric ligament |
| **Lesser** Saphenous Vein, Left<br>**Lesser** Saphenous Vein, Right | **Includes:**<br>Small saphenous vein |
| **Liver** | **Includes:**<br>Quadrate lobe |
| **Lower** Arm and Wrist Muscle, Left<br>**Lower** Arm and Wrist Muscle, Right | **Includes:**<br>Anatomical snuffbox<br>Brachioradialis muscle<br>Extensor carpi radialis muscle<br>Extensor carpi ulnaris muscle<br>Flexor carpi radialis muscle<br>Flexor carpi ulnaris muscle<br>Flexor pollicis longus muscle<br>Palmaris longus muscle<br>Pronator quadratus muscle<br>Pronator teres muscle |
| **Lower** Eyelid, Left<br>**Lower** Eyelid, Right | **Includes:**<br>Inferior tarsal plate<br>Medial canthus |
| **Lower** Femur, Left<br>**Lower** Femur, Right | **Includes:**<br>Lateral condyle of femur<br>Lateral epicondyle of femur<br>Medial condyle of femur<br>Medial epicondyle of femur |

## Section 0 - Medical and Surgical - Character 4 - Body Part

| | |
|---|---|
| **Lower** Leg Muscle, Left<br>**Lower** Leg Muscle, Right | **Includes:**<br>Extensor digitorum longus muscle<br>Extensor hallucis longus muscle<br>Fibularis brevis muscle<br>Fibularis longus muscle<br>Flexor digitorum longus muscle<br>Flexor hallucis longus muscle<br>Gastrocnemius muscle<br>Peroneus brevis muscle<br>Peroneus longus muscle<br>Popliteus muscle<br>Soleus muscle<br>Tibialis anterior muscle<br>Tibialis posterior muscle |
| **Lower** Leg Tendon, Left<br>**Lower** Leg Tendon, Right | **Includes:**<br>Achilles tendon |
| **Lower** Lip | **Includes:**<br>Frenulum labii inferioris<br>Labial gland<br>Vermilion border |
| **Lumbar** Nerve | **Includes:**<br>Lumbosacral trunk<br>Spinal nerve, lumbar<br>Superior clunic (cluneal) nerve |
| **Lumbar** Plexus | **Includes:**<br>Accessory obturator nerve<br>Genitofemoral nerve<br>Iliohypogastric nerve<br>Ilioinguinal nerve<br>Lateral femoral cutaneous nerve<br>Obturator nerve<br>Superior gluteal nerve |
| **Lumbar** Spinal Cord | **Includes:**<br>Cauda equina<br>Conus medullaris |
| **Lumbar** Sympathetic Nerve | **Includes:**<br>Lumbar ganglion<br>Lumbar splanchnic nerve |
| **Lumbar** Vertebra | **Includes:**<br>Spinous process<br>Vertebral arch<br>Vertebral foramen<br>Vertebral lamina<br>Vertebral pedicle |
| **Lumbar** Vertebral Joint | **Includes:**<br>Lumbar facet joint |
| **Lumbosacral** Joint | **Includes:**<br>Lumbosacral facet joint |

| Section 0 - Medical and Surgical - Character 4 - Body Part ||
|---|---|
| **Lymphatic,** Aortic | **Includes:**<br>Celiac lymph node<br>Gastric lymph node<br>Hepatic lymph node<br>Lumbar lymph node<br>Pancreaticosplenic lymph node<br>Paraaortic lymph node<br>Retroperitoneal lymph node |
| **Lymphatic,** Head | **Includes:**<br>Buccinator lymph node<br>Infraauricular lymph node<br>Infraparotid lymph node<br>Parotid lymph node<br>Preauricular lymph node<br>Submandibular lymph node<br>Submaxillary lymph node<br>Submental lymph node<br>Subparotid lymph node<br>Suprahyoid lymph node |
| **Lymphatic,** Left Axillary | **Includes:**<br>Anterior (pectoral) lymph node<br>Apical (subclavicular) lymph node<br>Brachial (lateral) lymph node<br>Central axillary lymph node<br>Lateral (brachial) lymph node<br>Pectoral (anterior) lymph node<br>Posterior (subscapular) lymph node<br>Subclavicular (apical) lymph node<br>Subscapular (posterior) lymph node |
| **Lymphatic,** Left Lower Extremity | **Includes:**<br>Femoral lymph node<br>Popliteal lymph node |
| **Lymphatic,** Left Neck | **Includes:**<br>Cervical lymph node<br>Jugular lymph node<br>Mastoid (postauricular) lymph node<br>Occipital lymph node<br>Postauricular (mastoid) lymph node<br>Retropharyngeal lymph node<br>Supraclavicular (Virchow's) lymph node<br>Virchow's (supraclavicular) lymph node |
| **Lymphatic,** Left Upper Extremity | **Includes:**<br>Cubital lymph node<br>Deltopectoral (infraclavicular) lymph node<br>Epitrochlear lymph node<br>Infraclavicular (deltopectoral) lymph node<br>Supratrochlear lymph node |
| **Lymphatic,** Mesenteric | **Includes:**<br>Inferior mesenteric lymph node<br>Pararectal lymph node<br>Superior mesenteric lymph node |

| Section 0 - Medical and Surgical - Character 4 - Body Part | |
|---|---|
| **Lymphatic,** Pelvis | **Includes:**<br>Common iliac (subaortic) lymph node<br>Gluteal lymph node<br>Iliac lymph node<br>Inferior epigastric lymph node<br>Obturator lymph node<br>Sacral lymph node<br>Subaortic (common iliac) lymph node<br>Suprainguinal lymph node |
| **Lymphatic,** Right Axillary | **Includes:**<br>Anterior (pectoral) lymph node<br>Apical (subclavicular) lymph node<br>Brachial (lateral) lymph node<br>Central axillary lymph node<br>Lateral (brachial) lymph node<br>Pectoral (anterior) lymph node<br>Posterior (subscapular) lymph node<br>Subclavicular (apical) lymph node<br>Subscapular (posterior) lymph node |
| **Lymphatic,** Right Lower Extremity | **Includes:**<br>Femoral lymph node<br>Popliteal lymph node |
| **Lymphatic,** Right Neck | **Includes:**<br>Cervical lymph node<br>Jugular lymph node<br>Mastoid (postauricular) lymph node<br>Occipital lymph node<br>Postauricular (mastoid) lymph node<br>Retropharyngeal lymph node<br>Right jugular trunk<br>Right lymphatic duct<br>Right subclavian trunk<br>Supraclavicular (Virchow's) lymph node<br>Virchow's (supraclavicular) lymph node |
| **Lymphatic,** Right Upper Extremity | **Includes:**<br>Cubital lymph node<br>Deltopectoral (infraclavicular) lymph node<br>Epitrochlear lymph node<br>Infraclavicular (deltopectoral) lymph node<br>Supratrochlear lymph node |
| **Lymphatic,** Thorax | **Includes:**<br>Intercostal lymph node<br>Mediastinal lymph node<br>Parasternal lymph node<br>Paratracheal lymph node<br>Tracheobronchial lymph node |
| **Mandible,** Left<br>**Mandible,** Right | **Includes:**<br>Alveolar process of mandible<br>Condyloid process<br>Mandibular notch<br>Mental foramen |

| Section 0 - Medical and Surgical - Character 4 - Body Part ||
|---|---|
| **Mastoid Sinus,** Left<br>**Mastoid Sinus,** Right | **Includes:**<br>Mastoid air cells |
| **Maxilla,** Left<br>**Maxilla,** Right | **Includes:**<br>Alveolar process of maxilla |
| **Maxillary Sinus,** Left<br>**Maxillary Sinus,** Right | **Includes:**<br>Antrum of Highmore |
| **Median** Nerve | **Includes:**<br>Anterior interosseous nerve<br>Palmar cutaneous nerve |
| **Medulla** Oblongata | **Includes:**<br>Myelencephalon |
| **Mesentery** | **Includes:**<br>Mesoappendix<br>Mesocolon |
| **Metacarpocarpal** Joint, Left<br>**Metacarpocarpal** Joint, Right | **Includes:**<br>Carpometacarpal (CMC) joint |
| **Metatarsal-Phalangeal** Joint, Left<br>**Metatarsal-Phalangeal** Joint, Right | **Includes:**<br>Metatarsophalangeal (MTP) joint |
| **Metatarsal-Tarsal** Joint, Left<br>**Metatarsal-Tarsal** Joint, Right | **Includes:**<br>Tarsometatarsal joint |
| **Middle** Ear, Left<br>**Middle** Ear, Right | **Includes:**<br>Oval window<br>Tympanic cavity |
| **Minor** Salivary Gland | **Includes:**<br>Anterior lingual gland |
| **Mitral** Valve | **Includes:**<br>Bicuspid valve<br>Left atrioventricular valve<br>Mitral annulus |
| **Nasal** Bone | **Includes:**<br>Vomer of nasal septum |
| **Nasal** Septum | **Includes:**<br>Quadrangular cartilage<br>Septal cartilage<br>Vomer bone |
| **Nasal** Turbinate | **Includes:**<br>Inferior turbinate<br>Middle turbinate<br>Nasal concha<br>Superior turbinate |
| **Nasopharynx** | **Includes:**<br>Choana<br>Fossa of Rosenmuller<br>Pharyngeal recess<br>Rhinopharynx |

## Section 0 - Medical and Surgical - Character 4 - Body Part

| | |
|---|---|
| **Neck** Muscle, Left<br>**Neck** Muscle, Right | **Includes:**<br>Anterior vertebral muscle<br>Arytenoid muscle<br>Cricothyroid muscle<br>Infrahyoid muscle<br>Levator scapulae muscle<br>Platysma muscle<br>Scalene muscle<br>Splenius cervicis muscle<br>Sternocleidomastoid muscle<br>Suprahyoid muscle<br>Thyroarytenoid muscle |
| **Nipple,** Left<br>**Nipple,** Right | **Includes:**<br>Areola |
| **Nose** | **Includes:**<br>Columella<br>External naris<br>Greater alar cartilage<br>Internal naris<br>Lateral nasal cartilage<br>Lesser alar cartilage<br>Nasal cavity<br>Nostril |
| **Occipital** Bone, Left<br>**Occipital** Bone, Right | **Includes:**<br>Foramen magnum |
| **Oculomotor** Nerve | **Includes:**<br>Third cranial nerve |
| **Olfactory** Nerve | **Includes:**<br>First cranial nerve<br>Olfactory bulb |
| **Optic** Nerve | **Includes:**<br>Optic chiasma<br>Second cranial nerve |
| **Orbit,** Left<br>**Orbit,** Right | **Includes:**<br>Bony orbit<br>Orbital portion of ethmoid bone<br>Orbital portion of frontal bone<br>Orbital portion of lacrimal bone<br>Orbital portion of maxilla<br>Orbital portion of palatine bone<br>Orbital portion of sphenoid bone<br>Orbital portion of zygomatic bone |
| **Pancreatic** Duct | **Includes:**<br>Duct of Wirsung |
| **Pancreatic** Duct, Accessory | **Includes:**<br>Duct of Santorini |
| **Parotid** Duct, Left<br>**Parotid** Duct, Right | **Includes:**<br>Stensen's duct |
| **Pelvic** Bone, Left<br>**Pelvic** Bone, Right | **Includes:**<br>Iliac crest<br>Ilium<br>Ischium<br>Pubis |

| Section 0 - Medical and Surgical - Character 4 - Body Part | |
|---|---|
| **Pelvic** Cavity | **Includes:**<br>Retropubic space |
| **Penis** | **Includes:**<br>Corpus cavernosum<br>Corpus spongiosum |
| **Perineum** Muscle | **Includes:**<br>Bulbospongiosus muscle<br>Cremaster muscle<br>Deep transverse perineal muscle<br>Ischiocavernosus muscle<br>Superficial transverse perineal muscle |
| **Peritoneum** | **Includes:**<br>Epiploic foramen |
| **Peroneal** Artery, Left<br>**Peroneal** Artery, Right | **Includes:**<br>Fibular artery |
| **Peroneal** Nerve | **Includes:**<br>Common fibular nerve<br>Common peroneal nerve<br>External popliteal nerve<br>Lateral sural cutaneous nerve |
| **Pharynx** | **Includes:**<br>Hypopharynx<br>Laryngopharynx<br>Oropharynx<br>Piriform recess (sinus) |
| **Phrenic** Nerve | **Includes:**<br>Accessory phrenic nerve |
| **Pituitary** Gland | **Includes:**<br>Adenohypophysis<br>Hypophysis<br>Neurohypophysis |
| **Pons** | **Includes:**<br>Apneustic center<br>Basis pontis<br>Locus ceruleus<br>Pneumotaxic center<br>Pontine tegmentum<br>Superior olivary nucleus |
| **Popliteal** Artery, Left<br>**Popliteal** Artery, Right | **Includes:**<br>Inferior genicular artery<br>Middle genicular artery<br>Superior genicular artery<br>Sural artery |
| **Portal** Vein | **Includes:**<br>Hepatic portal vein |
| **Prepuce** | **Includes:**<br>Foreskin<br>Glans penis |
| **Pudendal** Nerve | **Includes:**<br>Posterior labial nerve<br>Posterior scrotal nerve |

| Section 0 - Medical and Surgical - Character 4 - Body Part ||
|---|---|
| **Pulmonary** Artery, Left | **Includes:**<br>Arterial canal (duct)<br>Botallo's duct<br>Pulmoaortic canal |
| **Pulmonary** Valve | **Includes:**<br>Pulmonary annulus<br>Pulmonic valve |
| **Pulmonary** Vein, Left | **Includes:**<br>Left inferior pulmonary vein<br>Left superior pulmonary vein |
| **Pulmonary** Vein, Right | **Includes:**<br>Right inferior pulmonary vein<br>Right superior pulmonary vein |
| **Radial** Artery, Left<br>**Radial** Artery, Right | **Includes:**<br>Radial recurrent artery |
| **Radial** Nerve | **Includes:**<br>Dorsal digital nerve<br>Musculospiral nerve<br>Palmar cutaneous nerve<br>Posterior interosseous nerve |
| **Radius**, Left<br>**Radius**, Right | **Includes:**<br>Ulnar notch |
| **Rectum** | **Includes:**<br>Anorectal junction |
| **Renal** Artery, Left<br>**Renal** Artery, Right | **Includes:**<br>Inferior suprarenal artery<br>Renal segmental artery |
| **Renal** Vein, Left | **Includes:**<br>Left inferior phrenic vein<br>Left ovarian vein<br>Left second lumbar vein<br>Left suprarenal vein<br>Left testicular vein |
| **Retina**, Left<br>**Retina**, Right | **Includes:**<br>Fovea<br>Macula<br>Optic disc |
| **Retroperitoneum** | **Includes:**<br>Retroperitoneal space |
| **Sacral** Nerve | **Includes:**<br>Spinal nerve, sacral |
| **Sacral** Plexus | **Includes:**<br>Inferior gluteal nerve<br>Posterior femoral cutaneous nerve<br>Pudendal nerve |
| **Sacral** Sympathetic Nerve | **Includes:**<br>Ganglion impar (ganglion of Walther)<br>Pelvic splanchnic nerve<br>Sacral ganglion<br>Sacral splanchnic nerve |

| Section 0 - Medical and Surgical - Character 4 - Body Part | |
|---|---|
| **Sacrococcygeal** Joint | **Includes:**<br>Sacrococcygeal symphysis |
| **Scapula,** Left<br>**Scapula,** Right | **Includes:**<br>Acromion (process)<br>Coracoid process |
| **Sciatic** Nerve | **Includes:**<br>Ischiatic nerve |
| **Shoulder** Bursa and Ligament, Left<br>**Shoulder** Bursa and Ligament, Right | **Includes:**<br>Acromioclavicular ligament<br>Coracoacromial ligament<br>Coracoclavicular ligament<br>Coracohumeral ligament<br>Costoclavicular ligament<br>Glenohumeral ligament<br>Glenoid ligament (labrum)<br>Interclavicular ligament<br>Sternoclavicular ligament<br>Subacromial bursa<br>Transverse humeral ligament<br>Transverse scapular ligament |
| **Shoulder** Joint, Left<br>**Shoulder** Joint, Right | **Includes:**<br>Glenohumeral joint |
| **Shoulder** Muscle, Left<br>**Shoulder** Muscle, Right | **Includes:**<br>Deltoid muscle<br>Infraspinatus muscle<br>Subscapularis muscle<br>Supraspinatus muscle<br>Teres major muscle<br>Teres minor muscle |
| **Sigmoid** Colon | **Includes:**<br>Rectosigmoid junction<br>Sigmoid flexure |
| **Skin** | **Includes:**<br>Dermis<br>Epidermis<br>Sebaceous gland<br>Sweat gland |
| **Sphenoid** Bone, Left<br>**Sphenoid** Bone, Right | **Includes:**<br>Greater wing<br>Lesser wing<br>Optic foramen<br>Pterygoid process<br>Sella turcica |
| **Spinal** Canal | **Includes:**<br>Vertebral canal |
| **Spinal** Meninges | **Includes:**<br>Arachnoid mater<br>Denticulate ligament<br>Leptomeninges<br>Pia mater |
| **Spleen** | **Includes:**<br>Accessory spleen |

| Section 0 - Medical and Surgical - Character 4 - Body Part ||
|---|---|
| **Splenic** Artery | **Includes:**<br>Left gastroepiploic artery<br>Pancreatic artery<br>Short gastric artery |
| **Splenic** Vein | **Includes:**<br>Left gastroepiploic vein<br>Pancreatic vein |
| **Sternum** | **Includes:**<br>Manubrium<br>Suprasternal notch<br>Xiphoid process |
| **Stomach,** Pylorus | **Includes:**<br>Pyloric antrum<br>Pyloric canal<br>Pyloric sphincter |
| **Subarachnoid** Space | **Includes:**<br>Cranial subarachnoid space<br>Spinal subarachnoid space |
| **Subclavian** Artery, Left<br>**Subclavian** Artery, Right | **Includes:**<br>Costocervical trunk<br>Dorsal scapular artery<br>Internal thoracic artery |
| **Subcutaneous** Tissue and Fascia, Anterior Neck | **Includes:**<br>Deep cervical fascia<br>Pretracheal fascia |
| **Subcutaneous** Tissue and Fascia, Chest | **Includes:**<br>Pectoral fascia |
| **Subcutaneous** Tissue and Fascia, Face | **Includes:**<br>Masseteric fascia<br>Orbital fascia |
| **Subcutaneous** Tissue and Fascia, Left Foot | **Includes:**<br>Plantar fascia (aponeurosis) |
| **Subcutaneous** Tissue and Fascia, Left Hand | **Includes:**<br>Palmar fascia (aponeurosis) |
| **Subcutaneous** Tissue and Fascia,<br>Left Lower Arm | **Includes:**<br>Antebrachial fascia<br>Bicipital aponeurosis |
| **Subcutaneous** Tissue and Fascia,<br>Left Upper Arm | **Includes:**<br>Axillary fascia<br>Deltoid fascia<br>Infraspinatus fascia<br>Subscapular aponeurosis<br>Supraspinatus fascia |
| **Subcutaneous** Tissue and Fascia,<br>Left Upper Leg | **Includes:**<br>Crural fascia<br>Fascia lata<br>Iliac fascia<br>Iliotibial tract (band) |
| **Subcutaneous** Tissue and Fascia,<br>Posterior Neck | **Includes:**<br>Prevertebral fascia |

| Section 0 - Medical and Surgical - Character 4 - Body Part | |
|---|---|
| **Subcutaneous** Tissue and Fascia, Right Foot | **Includes:**<br>Plantar fascia (aponeurosis) |
| **Subcutaneous** Tissue and Fascia, Right Hand | **Includes:**<br>Palmar fascia (aponeurosis) |
| **Subcutaneous** Tissue and Fascia,<br>Right Lower Arm | **Includes:**<br>Antebrachial fascia<br>Bicipital aponeurosis |
| **Subcutaneous** Tissue and Fascia,<br>Right Upper Arm | **Includes:**<br>Axillary fascia<br>Deltoid fascia<br>Infraspinatus fascia<br>Subscapular aponeurosis<br>Supraspinatus fascia |
| **Subcutaneous** Tissue and Fascia,<br>Right Upper Leg | **Includes:**<br>Crural fascia<br>Fascia lata<br>Iliac fascia<br>Iliotibial tract (band) |
| **Subcutaneous** Tissue and Fascia, Scalp | **Includes:**<br>Galea aponeurotica |
| **Subcutaneous** Tissue and Fascia, Trunk | **Includes:**<br>External oblique aponeurosis<br>Transversalis fascia |
| **Subdural** Space | **Includes:**<br>Cranial subdural space<br>Spinal subdural space |
| **Submaxillary** Gland, Left<br>**Submaxillary** Gland, Right | **Includes:**<br>Submandibular gland |
| **Superior** Mesenteric Artery | **Includes:**<br>Ileal artery<br>Ileocolic artery<br>Inferior pancreaticoduodenal artery<br>Jejunal artery |
| **Superior** Mesenteric Vein | **Includes:**<br>Right gastroepiploic vein |
| **Superior** Vena Cava | **Includes:**<br>Precava |
| **Tarsal** Joint, Left<br>**Tarsal** Joint, Right | **Includes:**<br>Calcaneocuboid joint<br>Cuboideonavicular joint<br>Cuneonavicular joint<br>Intercuneiform joint<br>Subtalar (talocalcaneal) joint<br>Talocalcaneal (subtalar) joint<br>Talocalcaneonavicular joint |
| **Tarsal,** Left<br>**Tarsal,** Right | **Includes:**<br>Calcaneus<br>Cuboid bone<br>Intermediate cuneiform bone<br>Lateral cuneiform bone<br>Medial cuneiform bone<br>Navicular bone<br>Talus bone |

| Section 0 - Medical and Surgical - Character 4 - Body Part | |
|---|---|
| **Temporal** Artery, Left<br>**Temporal** Artery, Right | **Includes:**<br>Middle temporal artery<br>Superficial temporal artery<br>Transverse facial artery |
| **Temporal** Bone, Left<br>**Temporal** Bone, Right | **Includes:**<br>Mastoid process<br>Petrous part of temoporal bone<br>Tympanic part of temoporal bone<br>Zygomatic process of temporal bone |
| **Thalamus** | **Includes:**<br>Epithalamus<br>Geniculate nucleus<br>Metathalamus<br>Pulvinar |
| **Thoracic** Aorta | **Includes:**<br>Aortic arch<br>Aortic intercostal artery<br>Ascending aorta<br>Bronchial artery<br>Esophageal artery<br>Subcostal artery |
| **Thoracic** Duct | **Includes:**<br>Left jugular trunk<br>Left subclavian trunk |
| **Thoracic** Nerve | **Includes:**<br>Intercostal nerve<br>Intercostobrachial nerve<br>Spinal nerve, thoracic<br>Subcostal nerve |
| **Thoracic** Sympathetic Nerve | **Includes:**<br>Cardiac plexus<br>Esophageal plexus<br>Greater splanchnic nerve<br>Inferior cardiac nerve<br>Least splanchnic nerve<br>Lesser splanchnic nerve<br>Middle cardiac nerve<br>Pulmonary plexus<br>Superior cardiac nerve<br>Thoracic aortic plexus<br>Thoracic ganglion |
| **Thoracic** Vertebra | **Includes:**<br>Spinous process<br>Vertebral arch<br>Vertebral foramen<br>Vertebral lamina<br>Vertebral pedicle |
| **Thoracic** Vertebral Joint | **Includes:**<br>Costotransverse joint<br>Costovertebral joint<br>Thoracic facet joint |
| **Thoracolumbar** Vertebral Joint | **Includes:**<br>Thoracolumbar facet joint |

| Section 0 - Medical and Surgical - Character 4 - Body Part | |
|---|---|
| **Thorax** Bursa and Ligament, Left<br>**Thorax** Bursa and Ligament, Right | **Includes:**<br>Costotransverse ligament<br>Costoxiphoid ligament<br>Sternocostal ligament |
| **Thorax** Muscle, Left<br>**Thorax** Muscle, Right | **Includes:**<br>Intercostal muscle<br>Levatores costarum muscle<br>Pectoralis major muscle<br>Pectoralis minor muscle<br>Serratus anterior muscle<br>Subclavius muscle<br>Subcostal muscle<br>Transverse thoracis muscle |
| **Thymus** | **Includes:**<br>Thymus gland |
| **Thyroid** Artery, Left<br>**Thyroid** Artery, Right | **Includes:**<br>Cricothyroid artery<br>Hyoid artery<br>Sternocleidomastoid artery<br>Superior laryngeal artery<br>Superior thyroid artery<br>Thyrocervical trunk |
| **Tibia,** Left<br>**Tibia,** Right | **Includes:**<br>Lateral condyle of tibia<br>Medial condyle of tibia<br>Medial malleolus |
| **Tibial** Nerve | **Includes:**<br>Lateral plantar nerve<br>Medial plantar nerve<br>Medial popliteal nerve<br>Medial sural cutaneous nerve |
| **Toe** Nail | **Includes:**<br>Nail bed<br>Nail plate |
| **Toe** Phalangeal Joint, Left<br>**Toe** Phalangeal Joint, Right | **Includes:**<br>Interphalangeal (IP) joint |
| **Tongue** | **Includes:**<br>Frenulum linguae<br>Lingual tonsil |
| **Tongue,** Palate, Pharynx Muscle | **Includes:**<br>Chondroglossus muscle<br>Genioglossus muscle<br>Hyoglossus muscle<br>Inferior longitudinal muscle<br>Levator veli palatini muscle<br>Palatoglossal muscle<br>Palatopharyngeal muscle<br>Pharyngeal constrictor muscle<br>Salpingopharyngeus muscle<br>Styloglossus muscle<br>Stylopharyngeus muscle<br>Superior longitudinal muscle<br>Tensor veli palatini muscle |
| **Tonsils** | **Includes:**<br>Palatine tonsil |

| Section 0 - Medical and Surgical - Character 4 - Body Part | |
|---|---|
| **Transverse** Colon | **Includes:**<br>Splenic flexure |
| **Tricuspid** Valve | **Includes:**<br>Right atrioventricular valve<br>Tricuspid annulus |
| **Trigeminal** Nerve | **Includes:**<br>Fifth cranial nerve<br>Gasserian ganglion<br>Mandibular nerve<br>Maxillary nerve<br>Ophthalmic nerve<br>Trifacial nerve |
| **Trochlear** Nerve | **Includes:**<br>Fourth cranial nerve |
| **Trunk** Bursa and Ligament, Left<br>**Trunk** Bursa and Ligament, Right | **Includes:**<br>Iliolumbar ligament<br>Interspinous ligament<br>Intertransverse ligament<br>Ligamentum flavum<br>Pubic ligament<br>Sacrococcygeal ligament<br>Sacroiliac ligament<br>Sacrospinous ligament<br>Sacrotuberous ligament<br>Supraspinous ligament |
| **Trunk** Muscle, Left<br>**Trunk** Muscle, Right | **Includes:**<br>Coccygeus muscle<br>Erector spinae muscle<br>Interspinalis muscle<br>Intertransversarius muscle<br>Latissimus dorsi muscle<br>Levator ani muscle<br>Quadratus lumborum muscle<br>Rhomboid major muscle<br>Rhomboid minor muscle<br>Serratus posterior muscle<br>Transversospinalis muscle<br>Trapezius muscle |
| **Tympanic** Membrane, Left<br>**Tympanic** Membrane, Right | **Includes:**<br>Pars flaccida |
| **Ulna,** Left<br>**Ulna,** Right | **Includes:**<br>Olecranon process<br>Radial notch |
| **Ulnar** Artery, Left<br>**Ulnar** Artery, Right | **Includes:**<br>Anterior ulnar recurrent artery<br>Common interosseous artery<br>Posterior ulnar recurrent artery |
| **Ulnar** Nerve | **Includes:**<br>Cubital nerve |
| **Upper** Arm Muscle, Left<br>**Upper** Arm Muscle, Right | **Includes:**<br>Biceps brachii muscle<br>Brachialis muscle<br>Coracobrachialis muscle<br>Triceps brachii muscle |

| Section 0 - Medical and Surgical - Character 4 - Body Part | |
|---|---|
| **Upper Eyelid**, Left<br>**Upper** Eyelid, Right | **Includes:**<br>Lateral canthus<br>Levator palpebrae superioris muscle<br>Orbicularis oculi muscle<br>Superior tarsal plate |
| **Upper** Femur, Left<br>**Upper** Femur, Right | **Includes:**<br>Femoral head<br>Greater trochanter<br>Lesser trochanter<br>Neck of femur |
| **Upper** Leg Muscle, Left<br>**Upper** Leg Muscle, Right | **Includes:**<br>Adductor brevis muscle<br>Adductor longus muscle<br>Adductor magnus muscle<br>Biceps femoris muscle<br>Gracilis muscle<br>Pectineus muscle<br>Quadriceps (femoris)<br>Rectus femoris muscle<br>Sartorius muscle<br>Semimembranosus muscle<br>Semitendinosus muscle<br>Vastus intermedius muscle<br>Vastus lateralis muscle<br>Vastus medialis muscle |
| **Upper** Lip | **Includes:**<br>Frenulum labii superioris<br>Labial gland<br>Vermilion border |
| **Ureter**<br>**Ureter,** Left<br>**Ureter,** Right<br>**Ureters,** Bilateral | **Includes:**<br>Ureteral orifice<br>Ureterovesical orifice |
| **Urethra** | **Includes:**<br>Bulbourethral (Cowper's) gland<br>Cowper's (bulbourethral) gland<br>External urethral sphincter<br>Internal urethral sphincter<br>Membranous urethra<br>Penile urethra<br>Prostatic urethra |
| **Uterine** Supporting Structure | **Includes:**<br>Broad ligament<br>Infundibulopelvic ligament<br>Ovarian ligament<br>Round ligament of uterus |
| **Uterus** | **Includes:**<br>Fundus uteri<br>Myometrium<br>Perimetrium<br>Uterine cornu |
| **Uvula** | **Includes:**<br>Palatine uvula |

| Section 0 - Medical and Surgical - Character 4 - Body Part | |
|---|---|
| **Vagus** Nerve | **Includes:**<br>Anterior vagal trunk<br>Pharyngeal plexus<br>Pneumogastric nerve<br>Posterior vagal trunk<br>Pulmonary plexus<br>Recurrent laryngeal nerve<br>Superior laryngeal nerve<br>Tenth cranial nerve |
| **Vas** Deferens<br>**Vas** Deferens, Bilateral<br>**Vas** Deferens, Left<br>**Vas** Deferens, Right | **Includes:**<br>Ductus deferens<br>Ejaculatory duct |
| **Ventricle**, Right | **Includes:**<br>Conus arteriosus |
| **Ventricular** Septum | **Includes:**<br>Interventricular septum |
| **Vertebral** Artery, Left<br>**Vertebral** Artery, Right | **Includes:**<br>Anterior spinal artery<br>Posterior spinal artery |
| **Vertebral** Vein, Left<br>**Vertebral** Vein, Right | **Includes:**<br>Deep cervical vein<br>Suboccipital venous plexus |
| **Vestibular** Gland | **Includes:**<br>Bartholin's (greater vestibular) gland<br>Greater vestibular (Bartholin's) gland<br>Paraurethral (Skene's) gland<br>Skene's (paraurethral) gland |
| **Vitreous,** Left<br>**Vitreous,** Right | **Includes:**<br>Vitreous body |
| **Vocal** Cord, Left<br>**Vocal** Cord, Right | **Includes:**<br>Vocal fold |
| **Vulva** | **Includes:**<br>Labia majora<br>Labia minora |
| **Wrist** Bursa and Ligament, Left<br>**Wrist** Bursa and Ligament, Right | **Includes:**<br>Palmar ulnocarpal ligament<br>Radial collateral carpal ligament<br>Radiocarpal ligament<br>Radioulnar ligament<br>Ulnar collateral carpal ligament |
| **Wrist** Joint, Left<br>**Wrist** Joint, Right | **Includes:**<br>Distal radioulnar joint<br>Radiocarpal joint |

# Appendix B

## Root Operations

Note: The Root Operation Tables listed in Appendix B contain the same information regarding Root Operations as presented in Appendix A of the 2016 ICD-10-PCS Reference Manual but are presented in a different format.

### Medical and Surgical Section Root Operation Groups

| Root Operation | Objective of Procedure | Site of Procedure | Example |
|---|---|---|---|
| **Root operations that take out some/all of a body part** | | | |
| Excision | Cutting out/off without replacement | Some of a body part | Breast lumpectomy |
| Resection | Cutting out/off without replacement | All of a body part | Total mastectomy |
| Detachment | Cutting out/off without replacement | Extremity only, any level | Amputation above elbow |
| Destruction | Eradicating without replacement | Some/all of a body part | Fulguration of endometrium |
| Extraction | Pulling out or off without replacement | Some/all of a body part | Suction D&C |
| **Root operations that take out solids/fluids/gases from a body part** | | | |
| Drainage | Taking/letting out fluids/gases | Within a body part | Incision and drainage |
| Extirpation | Taking/cutting out solid matter | Within a body part | Thrombectomy |
| Fragmentation | Breaking solid matter into pieces | Within a body part | Lithotripsy |
| **Root operations involving cutting or separation only** | | | |
| Division | Cutting into/separating a body part | Within a body part | Neurotomy |
| Release | Freeing a body part from constraint | Around a body part | Adhesiolysis |
| **Root operations that put in/put back or move some/all of a body part** | | | |
| Transplantation | Putting in a living body part from a person/animal | Some/all of a body part | Kidney transplant |
| Reattachment | Putting back a detached body part | Some/all of a body part | Reattach severed finger |
| Transfer | Moving, to function for a similar body part | Some/all of a body part | Skin transfer flap |
| Reposition | Moving, to normal or other suitable location | Some/all of a body part | Move undescended testicle |

| Root operations that alter the diameter/route of a tubular body part | | | |
|---|---|---|---|
| Restriction | Partially closing orifice/lumen | Tubular body part | Gastroesophageal fundoplication |
| Occlusion | Completely closing orifice/lumen | Tubular body part | Fallopian tube ligation |
| Dilation | Expanding orifice/lumen | Tubular body part | Percutaneous trans-luminal coronary angioplasty (PTCA) |
| Bypass | Altering route of passage | Tubular body part | Coronary artery bypass graft (CABG) |
| Root operations that always involve a device | | | |
| Insertion | Putting in non-biological device | In/on a body part | Central line insertion |
| Replacement | Putting in device that replaces a body part | Some/all of a body part | Total hip replacement |
| Supplement | Putting in device that reinforces or augments a body part | In/on a body part | Abdominal wall herni-orrhaphy using mesh |
| Change | Exchanging device w/out cutting/puncturing | In/on a body part | Drainage tube change |
| Removal | Taking out device | In/on a body part | Central line removal |
| Revision | Correcting a malfunctioning/displaced device | In/on a body part | Revision of pacemaker insertion |
| Root operations involving examination only | | | |
| Inspection | Visual/manual exploration | Some/all of a body part | Diagnostic cystoscopy |
| Map | Locating electrical impulses/functional areas | Brain/cardiac conduction mechanism | Cardiac electrophysiological study |
| Root operations that include other repairs | | | |
| Repair | Restoring body part to its normal structure | Some/all of a body part | Suture laceration |
| Control | Stopping/attempting to stop postprocedural bleed | Anatomical region | Post-prostatectomy bleeding |
| Root operations that include other objectives | | | |
| Fusion | Rendering joint immobile | Joint | Spinal fusion |
| Alteration | Modifying body part for cosmetic purposes without affecting function | Some/all of a body part | Face lift |
| Creation | Making new structure for sex change operation | Perineum | Artificial vagina/penis |

# Root Operations in the Medical and Surgical Section in Alphabetical Order

| | | |
|---|---|---|
| Alteration 0 | Definition | Modifying the anatomic structure of a body part without affecting the function of the body part |
| | Explanation | Principal purpose is to improve appearance |
| | Examples | Face lift, breast augmentation |
| Bypass 1 | Definition | Altering the route of passage of the contents of a tubular body part |
| | Explanation | Rerouting contents around an area of a body part to another distal (downstream) area in the normal route; rerouting the contents to another different but similar route and body part; or to an abnormal route and another dissimilar body part. It includes one or more concurrent anastomoses with or without the use of a device such as autografts, tissue substitutes and synthetic substitutes |
| | Examples | Coronary artery bypass graft (CABG), colostomy formation |
| Change 2 | Definition | Taking out or off a device from a body part and putting back an identical or similar device in or on the same body part without cutting or puncturing the skin or a mucous membrane |
| | Explanation | All Change procedures are coded using the approach External |
| | Examples | Urinary catheter change, gastrostomy tube change, drainage tube change |
| Control 3 | Definition | Stopping, or attempting to stop, postprocedural bleeding |
| | Explanation | The site of the bleeding is coded as an anatomical region and not to a specific body part |
| | Examples | Control of post-prostatectomy hemorrhage, control of post-tonsillectomy hemorrhage |
| Creation 4 | Definition | Making a new genital structure that does not take over the function of a body part |
| | Explanation | Used only for sex change operations |
| | Examples | Creation of vagina in a male, creation of penis in a female |
| Destruction 5 | Definition | Physical eradication of all or a portion of a body part by the direct use of energy, force or a destructive agent |
| | Explanation | None of the body part is physically taken out |
| | Examples | Fulguration of rectal polyp, cautery of skin lesion, fulguration of endometrium |
| Detachment 6 | Definition | Cutting off all or part of the upper or lower extremities |
| | Explanation | The body part value is the site of the detachment, with a qualifier if applicable to further specify the level where the extremity was detached |
| | Examples | Below knee amputation, disarticulation of shoulder, amputation above elbow |

| Dilation 7 | Definition | Expanding an orifice or the lumen of a tubular body part |
|---|---|---|
| | Explanation | The orifice can be a natural orifice or an artificially created orifice. Accomplished by stretching a tubular body part using intraluminal pressure or by cutting part of the orifice or wall of the tubular body part |
| | Examples | Percutaneous transluminal angioplasty, pyloromyotomy, percutaneous transluminal coronary angioplasty (PTCA) |
| Division 8 | Definition | Cutting into a body part without draining fluids and/or gases from the body part in order to separate or transect a body part |
| | Explanation | All or a portion of the body part is separated into two or more portions |
| | Examples | Spinal cordotomy, osteotomy, neurotomy |
| Drainage 9 | Definition | Taking or letting out fluids and/or gases from a body part |
| | Explanation | The qualifier **Diagnostic** is used to identify drainage procedures that are biopsies |
| | Examples | Thoracentesis, incision and drainage |
| Excision B | Definition | Cutting out or off, without replacement, a portion of a body part |
| | Explanation | The qualifier **Diagnostic** is used to identify excision procedures that are biopsies |
| | Examples | Partial nephrectomy, liver biopsy, breast lumpectomy |
| Extirpation C | Definition | Taking or cutting out solid matter from a body part |
| | Explanation | The solid matter may be an abnormal byproduct of a biological function or a foreign body; it may be embedded in a body part, or in the lumen of a tubular body part. The solid matter may or may not have been previously broken into pieces. |
| | Examples | Thrombectomy, choledocholithotomy, excision foreign body |
| Extraction D | Definition | Pulling or stripping out or off all or a portion of a body part by the use of force |
| | Explanation | The qualifier **Diagnostic** is used to identify extraction procedures that are biopsies |
| | Examples | Dilation and curettage, vein stripping, suction D&C |
| Fragmentation F | Definition | Breaking solid matter in a body part into pieces |
| | Explanation | The solid matter may be an abnormal byproduct of a biological function or a foreign body. Physical force (e.g., manual, ultrasonic) applied directly or indirectly through intervening body parts is used to break the solid matter into pieces. The pieces of solid matter are not taken out, but are eliminated or absorbed through normal biological functions |
| | Examples | Extracorporeal shockwave lithotripsy, transurethral lithotripsy |

| Fusion G | Definition | Joining together portions of an articular body part rendering the articular body part immobile |
|---|---|---|
| | Explanation | The body part is joined together by fixation device, bone graft, or other means |
| | Examples | Spinal fusion, ankle arthrodesis |
| Insertion H | Definition | Putting in a non-biological device that monitors, assists, performs or prevents a physiological function but does not physically take the place of a body part |
| | Explanation | N/A |
| | Examples | Insertion of radioactive implant, insertion of central venous catheter |
| Inspection J | Definition | Visually and/or manually exploring a body part |
| | Explanation | Visual exploration may be performed with or without optical instrumentation. Manual exploration may be performed directly or through intervening body layers |
| | Examples | Diagnostic arthroscopy, exploratory laparotomy, diagnostic cystoscopy |
| Map K | Definition | Locating the route of passage of electrical impulses and/or locating functional areas in a body part |
| | Explanation | Applicable only to the cardiac conduction mechanism and the central nervous system |
| | Examples | Cardiac mapping, cortical mapping, cardiac electrophysiological study |
| Occlusion L | Definition | Completely closing an orifice or the lumen of a tubular body part |
| | Explanation | The orifice can be a natural orifice or an artificially created orifice |
| | Examples | Fallopian tube ligation, ligation of inferior vena cava |
| Reattachment M | Definition | Putting back in or on all or a portion of a separated body part to its normal location or other suitable location |
| | Explanation | Vascular circulation and nervous pathways may or may not be reestablished |
| | Examples | Reattachment of hand, reattachment of avulsed kidney, reattachment of finger |
| Release N | Definition | Freeing a body part from an abnormal physical constraint by cutting or by use of force |
| | Explanation | Some of the restraining tissue may be taken out but none of the body part is taken out |
| | Examples | Adhesiolysis, carpal tunnel release |

| Removal<br>P | Definition | Taking out or off a device from a body part |
|---|---|---|
| | Explanation | If the device is taken out and a similar device is put in without cutting or puncturing the skin or mucous membrane, the procedure is coded to the root operation Change. Otherwise, the procedure for taking out the device is coded to the root operation Removal and the procedure for putting in the new device is coded to the root operation performed. |
| | Examples | Drainage tube removal, cardiac pacemaker removal, central line removal |
| Repair<br>Q | Definition | Restoring, to the extent possible, a body part to its normal anatomic structure and function |
| | Explanation | Used only when the method to accomplish the repair is not one of the other root operations |
| | Examples | Herniorrhaphy, suture of laceration, colostomy takedown |
| Replacement<br>R | Definition | Putting in or on biological or synthetic material that physically takes the place and/or function of all or a portion of a body part |
| | Explanation | The biological material is non-living, or the biological material is living and from the same individual. The body part may have been previously taken out, previously replaced, or may be taken out concomitantly with the Replacement procedure. **If the body part has been previously replaced, a separate Removal procedure is coded for taking out the device used in the previous replacement.** |
| | Examples | Total hip replacement, bone graft, free skin graft |
| Reposition<br>S | Definition | Moving to its normal location, or other suitable location, all or a portion of a body part |
| | Explanation | The body part is moved to a new location from an abnormal location, or from a normal location where it is not functioning correctly. The body part may or may not be cut out or off to be moved to the new location. |
| | Examples | Reposition of undescended testicle, fracture reduction |
| Resection<br>T | Definition | Cutting out or off, without replacement, all of a body part |
| | Explanation | N/A |
| | Examples | Total nephrectomy, total lobectomy of lung, total mastectomy |
| Restriction<br>V | Definition | Partially closing an orifice or the lumen of a tubular body part |
| | Explanation | The orifice can be a natural orifice or an artificially created orifice |
| | Examples | Esophagogastric fundoplication, cervical cerclage |

| | | |
|---|---|---|
| Revision W | Definition | Correcting, to the extent possible, a portion of a malfunctioning device or the position of a displaced device |
| | Explanation | Revision can include correcting a malfunctioning or displaced device by taking out or putting in components of the device such as a screw or pin |
| | Examples | Adjustment of pacemaker lead, adjustment of hip prosthesis, revision of pacemaker insertion |
| Supplement U | Definition | Putting in or on biologic or synthetic material that physically reinforces and/or augments the function of a portion of a body part |
| | Explanation | The biological material is non-living, or the biological material is living and from the same individual. The body part may have been previously replaced. If the body part has been previously replaced, the Supplement procedure is performed to physically reinforce and/or augment the function of the replaced body part. |
| | Examples | Herniorrhaphy using mesh, free nerve graft, mitral valve ring annuloplasty, put a new acetabular liner in a previous hip replacement, abdominal wall herniorrhaphy using mesh |
| Transfer X | Definition | Moving, without taking out, all or a portion of a body part to another location to take over the function of all or a portion of a body part |
| | Explanation | The body part transferred remains connected to its vascular and nervous supply |
| | Examples | Tendon transfer, skin pedicle flap transfer, skin transfer flap |
| Transplantation Y | Definition | Putting in or on all or a portion of a living body part taken from another individual or animal to physically take the place and/or function of all or a portion of a similar body part |
| | Explanation | The native body part may or may not be taken out, and the transplanted body part may take over all or a portion of its function |
| | Examples | Kidney transplant, heart transplant |

# Appendix C

## Approaches

Note: The Approach Table listed here contains the same information regarding approaches as presented in Appendix A of the 2016 ICD-10-PCS Reference Manual but is presented in a different format.

### ICD-10-PCS Approaches

| Value | Approach | Definition | Examples |
|---|---|---|---|
| 0 | Open | Cutting through the skin or mucous membrane and any other body layers necessary to expose the site of the procedure | Open CABG<br>Open endarterectomy<br>Open resection cecum<br>Abdominal hysterectomy |
| 3 | Percutaneous | Entry, by puncture or minor incision, of instrumentation through the skin or mucous membrane and any other body layers necessary to reach the site of the procedure | Percutaneous needle core biopsy of kidney<br>Liposuction<br>Percutaneous drainage of ascites<br>Needle biopsy of liver |
| 4 | Percutaneous Endoscopic | Entry, by puncture or minor incision, of instrumentation through the skin or mucous membrane and any other body layers necessary to reach and visualize the site of the procedure | Laparoscopic cholecystectomy<br>Laparoscopy with destruction of endometriosis<br>Endoscopic drainage of sinus<br>Arthroscopy |
| 7 | Via Natural or Artificial Opening | Entry of instrumentation through a natural or artificial external opening to reach the site of the procedure | Foley catheter placement<br>Transvaginal intraluminal cervical cerclage<br>Digital rectal exam<br>Endotracheal intubation |
| 8 | Via Natural or Artificial Opening Endoscopic | Entry of instrumentation through a natural or artificial external opening to reach and visualize the site of the procedure | Transurethral cystoscopy with removal of bladder stone<br>Endoscopic ERCP<br>Hysteroscopy<br>EGD<br>Colonoscopy |
| F | Via Natural or Artificial Opening with Percutaneous Endoscopic Assistance | Entry of instrumentation through a natural or artificial external opening and entry, by puncture or minor incision, of instrumentation through the skin or mucous membrane and any other body layers necessary to aid in the performance of the procedure | Laparoscopic-assisted vaginal hysterectomy |
| X | External | Procedures performed directly on the skin or mucous membrane and procedures performed indirectly by the application of external force through the skin or mucous membrane | Resection of tonsils<br>Closed reduction of fracture<br>Excision of skin lesion<br>Cautery nosebleed |

# Appendix D

## ICD-10-PCS Device and Substance Classification

Note: The information in this appendix contains the same information regarding device and substance classification as presented in Appendix B of the 2016 ICD-10-PCS Reference Manual.

This appendix discusses the distinguishing features of device, substance and equipment as classified in ICD-10-PCS, to provide further guidance for correct identification and coding. It includes discussion of the PCS definitions and classification of device, substance and equipment, and is accompanied by specific coding instruction and examples.

### PCS Device Classification

In most PCS codes, the sixth character of the code is used to classify device. The sixth character device value defines the material or appliance used to accomplish the objective of the procedure that remains in or on the procedure site at the end of the procedure. If the device is the means by which the procedural objective is accomplished, then a specific device value is coded in the sixth character. If no device is used to accomplish the objective of the procedure, the device value No Device is coded in the sixth character.

For example, an aortocoronary bypass that uses saphenous vein graft to accomplish the bypass is coded to the device value Autologous Venous Tissue in the sixth character of the PCS code. A coronary bypass that uses the patient's internal mammary artery directly to accomplish the bypass uses the device value No Device in the sixth character of the PCS code.

### Device and Procedural Objective

Whether the material used in a procedure should be coded using a specific PCS device value can be determined primarily by asking this question:

> Is this material central to achieving the objective of the procedure, or does it only support the performance of the procedure?

For example, radiological markers are put in the procedure site to guide the performance of a primary procedure such as excision of a tumor, whereas radioactive brachytherapy seeds are put in the procedure site as an end in themselves, to treat a malignant tumor. In the first example, a radiological marker placed during the primary procedure to assist in performing the procedure is not classified as a device in PCS and so is not separately coded. In the second example, where insertion of brachytherapy seeds is the objective of the procedure, the brachytherapy seeds are recorded in the PCS code with the device value Radioactive Element in the root operation Insertion.

The same device coded as a specific device value for one procedure may not be coded at all for another procedure where it is not central to the procedural objective. For example, a procedure performed specifically to place a drain in a body part for diagnostic or therapeutic purposes is coded to the root operation Drainage with the specific device value Drainage Device in the sixth character of the code. However, a wound drain placed at an incision site at the conclusion of the procedure to promote healing is not central to the procedural objective and therefore not coded separately as a device in PCS. For this reason, materials such as wound dressings and operative site drains that support the performance of the procedure are not coded separately.

Sutures and suture alternatives (e.g., fibrin glue, dermabond, specialized vessel closures) are not coded as devices in PCS, because in most cases using material to bring the edges of a procedure site together is not central to the procedural objective, but is used to support the performance of the procedure (to close the site). For procedures where the sole objective is to close a wound created by trauma or other incident, the procedure is coded to the root operation Repair with the device value No Device in the sixth character of the PCS code.

## Device and Location

Whether material or an appliance is coded as a device cannot be determined by the size, shape, or complexity of the object or material being used. A device may be too small to be seen with the naked eye (microcoils used to occlude a vessel) or two feet long (external fixator for a long bone). A device may be of a predetermined shape (prosthetic heart valve) or no particular shape (morsellized bone graft). A device may be a highly complex machine (cardiac synchronization pacemaker/defibrillator) or a simple piece of hardware (internal fixation bone screw).

However, material that is classified as a PCS device is distinguished from material classified as a PCS substance by the fact that it has a specific location. A device is intended to maintain a fixed location at the procedure site where it was put, whereas a substance is intended to disperse or be absorbed in the body. Indeed, a device that does not stay where it was put may need to be "revised" in a subsequent procedure, to move the device back to its intended location.

## Device and Removability

Material that is classified as a PCS device is also distinguishable by the fact that it is removable. Although it may not be *practical* to remove some types of devices once they become established at the site, it is *physically possible* to remove a device for some time after the procedure. A skin graft, once it "takes," may be nearly indistinguishable from the surrounding skin and no longer clearly identifiable as a device. Nevertheless, procedures that involve material coded as a device can for the most part be "reversed" by removing the device from the procedure site.

## Device Distribution in PCS

The general distribution and use of the sixth character when specified as a device is summarized in the following table. The sections and root operations that specify device in the sixth character are listed along with examples of sixth character values and corresponding procedure examples.

| PCS Section | Root Operation | Device Value Example | Procedure Example |
|---|---|---|---|
| Medical and Surgical | Alteration | Autologous Tissue Substitute | Nasal tip elevation using fat autograft |
| Medical and Surgical | Bypass | Synthetic Substitute | Femoral-popliteal bypass using synthetic graft |
| Medical and Surgical | Change | Drainage Device | Foley catheter exchange |
| Medical and Surgical | Creation | Nonautologous Tissue Substitute | Sex change operation using tissue bank graft material |
| Medical and Surgical | Dilation | Intraluminal Device | Percutaneous coronary angioplasty using stent |
| Medical and Surgical | Drainage | Drainage Device | Drainage of pleural effusion using chest tube |
| Medical and Surgical | Fusion | Interbody Fusion Device | Spinal interbody fusion |
| Medical and Surgical | Insertion | Infusion Pump | Insertion of infusion pump for pain control |
| Medical and Surgical | Occlusion | Extraluminal Device | Fallopian tube ligation using clips |
| Medical and Surgical | Removal | Spacer | Removal of joint spacer |
| Medical and Surgical | Replacement | Autologous Tissue Substitute | Skin graft using patient's own skin |
| Medical and Surgical | Reposition | Internal Fixation Device | Fracture reduction with plate and screw fixation |
| Medical and Surgical | Restriction | Extraluminal Device | Laparoscopic gastric banding, adjustable band |
| Medical and Surgical | Revision | Neurostimulator Lead | Reposition of spinal neurostimulator lead |
| Medical and Surgical | Supplement | Zooplastic Tissue | Pulmonary artery patch graft using bovine pericardium |
| Obstetrics | Insertion, Removal | Monitoring Electrode | Insertion of fetal monitoring electrode |
| Placement | Change | Cast | Forearm cast change |
| Placement | Compression | Pressure Dressing | Application of pressure dressing to lower leg |
| Placement | Dressing | Bandage | Application of bandage to chest wall |
| Placement | Immobilization | Splint | Splint placement to wrist |
| Placement | Packing | Packing Material | Nasal packing |
| Placement | Removal | Brace | Removal of back brace |
| Placement | Traction | Traction Apparatus | Skin traction of lower leg using traction device |

## PCS Substance Classification

The sixth character, substance value, defines the blood component or other liquid put in or on the body to accomplish the objective of the procedure. The sixth character is defined as *substance* in the Administration section. Administration is the only section where a substance is classified as a separate code, and not included as information in a more definitive procedure.

## Substance and Procedural Objective

Many different substances are typically put in or on the body in the course of an inpatient hospital stay, both during surgical procedures and at the bedside. Only those which meet UHDDS and facility coding guidelines are coded separately. Most material classified as a substance in the Administration section is in liquid form and intended to be immediately absorbed by the body or, in the case of blood and blood products, disseminated in the circulatory system. An exception is the substance value Adhesion Barrier. It is a non-liquid substance classified in the Administration section, and coded separately for tracking purposes.

## Substance and Removability

Most substances cannot be removed once they are administered, because the whole point of administering them is for them to be dispersed and/or absorbed by the body. Imaging contrast is sometimes extracted from the bloodstream at the conclusion of a procedure to minimize the possibility of adverse effects.

## Substance Distribution in Administration Section

The general distribution and use of the sixth character specified as a substance in the Administration section is summarized in the following table. All root operations that specify substance in the sixth character are listed along with examples of sixth character values and corresponding procedure examples.

### Substance value example

- Introduction: Nutritional substance
- Irrigation: Irrigating Substance
- Transfusion: Frozen Plasma

### Procedure example

- Introduction: Infusion of total parenteral nutrition
- Irrigation: Irrigation of eye
- Transfusion: Transfusion of frozen plasma

## Classification of Substances in Ancillary Sections

Three Ancillary sections record their own specific substance values as part of the PCS code, where a substance is used to support the objective of the procedure. They are the Imaging, Nuclear Medicine, and Radiation Oncology sections, and they specify Contrast, Radionuclide, and Radioisotope, respectively. However, these substance values are unambiguously included as part of a more definitive procedure code, to be recorded when the substance is used to support the objective of the procedure. Substances in these three Ancillary sections are therefore not likely to be confused with separately coded substances in the Administration section.

## Substance Distribution in Ancillary Sections

The three Ancillary sections that specify a type of substance used in the procedure are summarized in the following table. The sections and the type of substance classified are listed along with the PCS character where this information is recorded. Also included are examples of the values used and corresponding procedure examples.

### Imaging

- Substance classified: Contrast (fifth character)
- Substance value example: Low Osmolar Contrast
- Procedure example: Left heart ventriculography using low osmolar contrast

### Nuclear Medicine

- Substance classified: Radionuclide (fifth character)
- Substance value example: Fluorine 18
- Procedure example: PET scan of brain using Fluorine 18

### Radiation Therapy

- Substance classified: Isotope (sixth character)
- Substance value example: Iodine 125
- Procedure example: HDR brachytherapy of thyroid using Iodine 125

## Equipment and PCS Coding

For the most part, equipment used to assist in the performance of the procedure is not coded in PCS. The *only* exception to this rule occurs in the Rehabilitation and Diagnostic Audiology section, where the sixth character is specified as *equipment*. The sixth character values in the Rehabilitation and Diagnostic Audiology section are used to capture information about the machine, physical aid, or other equipment used to assist in performing the procedure.

## Equipment and Procedural Objective

For all other sections in PCS, equipment is distinguished from a codeable device by the fact that equipment is a method used to support the performance of a procedure. For example, the machine used to maintain cardiovascular circulation during an open heart bypass procedure is equipment that performs the circulatory functions for the heart so that the heart bypass can be performed. This support procedure is coded to the root operation Performance in the Extracorporeal Assistance and Performance section, and the type of equipment used is not captured in the code. The primary procedure is coded to the root operation Bypass in the Medical and Surgical section, and any graft material used is coded to the appropriate sixth character device value.

## Equipment and Location

Equipment is also distinguished from a device in PCS by the fact that equipment resides primarily outside the body during the procedure. Cardiopulmonary circulatory support is coded to the Extracorporeal Assistance and Performance section and the type of equipment used is not recorded in the PCS code. With cardiovascular support equipment, the machinery resides primarily outside the body. The outtake and return cannulae are the only portions of the machine directly connected to the patient.

Hemodialysis is also coded to the Extracorporeal Assistance and Performance section and the equipment used is not recorded in the PCS code. As with cardiovascular support equipment, the hemodialysis machine resides primarily outside the body. The blood lines connected to the patient's dialysis fistula are the only portion of the machine directly connected to the patient. Insertion of the lines into the fistula are not coded as a separate device insertion procedure, because establishing vascular access is the interface between the patient and the equipment used to perform the procedure, rather than an end in itself.

On the other hand, insertion of a vascular catheter to give a patient a blood transfusion is the central objective of the procedure. The vascular catheter in such cases is classified as a device.

## Equipment and Removability

Equipment used solely to support the performance of a procedure and therefore not coded in PCS can be further distinguished by the fact that the equipment is used only for the duration of the procedure. Once the procedure is completed, any portions of the equipment attached to the patient are disconnected. For example, a patient no longer requiring mechanical ventilation is "extubated," or disconnected from the equipment that provides ventilation support.

## Summary

Three distinguishing features have been identified to enable correct identification and coding of device, substance, and equipment: procedural objective, location, and removability. The procedural objective alone is sufficient in most cases to determine whether material or an appliance used in a procedure should be coded in PCS. Once it is determined that the information should be coded in PCS, location and removability are useful in determining whether the item is classified as a device or substance. The following table summarizes the distinguishing features of device, substance and equipment in relation to each other, along with examples.

### Device

- Procedural objective: Material or appliance put in or on the body is central to accomplishing the procedural objective
- Location: Resides at the site of the procedure, not intended to change location
- Removability: In most cases, capable of being removed from the procedure site
- Procedure example: Neurostimulator lead insertion

### Substance

- Procedural objective: Administration of the substance is the procedural objective
- Location: A liquid or blood product has no fixed position, but is intended to be absorbed or dispersed
- Removability: A liquid or blood product may not be removable, once dispersed or absorbed
- Procedure example: Antibiotic injection

### Equipment

- Procedural objective: Machinery or other aid used to perform a procedure
- Location: Resides primarily outside the body, though interfaces with the body via tube or other means
- Removability: Temporary, used for the duration of the procedure only
- Procedure example: Mechanical ventilation

# AHIMA ICD-10 Products
## Available at www.ahimastore.org

## Books from AHIMA Press
- *ICD-10-CM Code Book, 2016* (AC221015)
- *ICD-10-PCS Code Book, 2016* (AC222015)
- *Implementing ICD-10-CM/PCS for Hospitals* (AC201009)
- *Pocket Guide of ICD-10-CM and ICD-10-PCS* (AC203010)
- *ICD-10-CM and ICD-10-PCS Preview*, Second Edition (AC206009)
- *ICD-10-CM and ICD-10-PCS Preview Exercises*, Second Edition (AC216011)
- *ICD-10-CM Coder Training Manual 2016* (AC206816)
- *ICD-10-PCS Coder Training Manual 2016* (AC207816)
- *Transitioning to ICD-10-CM/PCS: The Essential Guide to General Equivalence Mappings (GEMs)* (AC202810)
- *Root Operations: Key to Procedure Coding in ICD-10-PCS* (AC211010)
- *ICD-10-PCS: An Applied Approach,* 2015 Edition (AC201114)
- *Basic ICD-10-CM/PCS Coding Exercises,* Fifth Edition (AC210514)
- *Diagnostic Coding for Physician Services: ICD-10-CM* 2014 Edition (AC201213)
- *Basic ICD-10-CM/PCS Coding*, 2016 (AC200515; **available early 2016**)
- *Clinical Coding Workout with Answers,* 2016 Edition (AC201516)

## AHIMA Online Education
AHIMA offers a complete program of online ICD-10 training for organizational and non-coding staff, acute-care coders, and specialty coding settings
- ICD-10-CM Overview: Deciphering the Code
- ICD-10-PCS Overview: Deciphering the Code
- ICD-10-CM Chapter Courses (22 hours)
- ICD-10-PCS Root Operations Courses (17 hours)
- ICD-10 A&P Focus Coding Assessments and Courses by System
- ICD-10-CM, ICD-10-PCS and ICD-10-CM/PCS Post Training E-Assessments

## AHIMA Meetings, Audio Seminars, and Webinars
- Brushing Up on ICD-10: A Refresher Workshop (multiple dates and locations)
- Advanced ICD-10-PCS Skills Workshop (multiple dates and locations)
- ICD-10 Academy: Building Expertise in Coding (multiple dates and locations)
- AHIMA Academy for ICD-10-CM/PCS: Building Expert Trainers in Diagnosis and Procedure Coding (multiple dates and locations)
- Annual Clinical Coding Meeting
- AHIMA Annual Convention and Exhibit

AHIMA is constantly developing products and resources to meet the needs of HIM professionals. Check ahima.org for updates and announcements of new products.